Color and Fluorescein Angiographic Atlas of Retinal Vascular Disorders

Color and Fluorescein Angiographic Atlas of Retinal Vascular Disorders

DAVID H. ORTH, M.D.

Director, Retinal Vascular Service
  Ingalls Memorial Hospital

Co-director, Fluorescein Angiography Laboratory
  Michael Reese Hospital & Medical Center

Assistant Clinical Professor
  Abraham Lincoln School of Medicine
  University of Illinois
    Eye and Ear Infirmary
  Chicago, Illinois

WILLIAMS & WILKINS
Baltimore/London

Editor: Barbara Tansill
Associate Editor: Carol-Lynn Brown
Copy Editor: Deborah K. Tourtlotte
Design: Joanne Janowiak
Illustration Planning: Wayne Hubbel
Production: Raymond E. Reter

Made in the United States of America

Library of Congress Cataloging in Publication Data

Orth, David H.
    Color and fluorescein angiographic atlas of retinal vascular disorders.

    Bibliography: p.
    Includes index.
    1. Retina—Blood vessels—Diseases—Diagnosis—Atlases. 2. Retina—Blood ves-
sels—Radiography—Atlases. 3. Fluorescence angiography—Atlases. I. Title.
[DNLM: 1. Retinal diseases—Diagnosis—Atlases. 2. Fluorescein angiography—
Atlases. WW 17 077c]
RE661.V3077   1983   617.7′3   82-17504
ISBN 0-683-06641-2

Composed and printed at the
Waverly Press, Inc.
Mt. Royal and Guilford Aves.
Baltimore, MD 21202, U.S.A.

Dedicated to my wife and children

Barbara, Joel, and Dina

For their understanding and unselfishness in providing me the time to complete this work.

Foreword

In this volume, Dr. Orth has prepared a highly useful and well organized presentation on disorders of the retinal vasculature. The text accompanying the fundus photographs and fluorescein angiograms is presented in a lucid manner. An interesting aspect of the atlas is the author's comments. Dr. Orth presents many of his own opinions on some of the disorders. These comments are up-to-date and authoritative, based on the author's extensive personal experience.

The fundus photographs and fluorescein angiograms are of outstanding quality and are well selected. The author has used several drawings and schematic diagrams prepared by Amalie Dunker, one of the leading ophthalmic illustrators in this country. These augment the text and clarify, in many instances, the basic processes involved.

This volume will prove valuable for the ophthalmologist during residency or fellowship training and to the practicing ophthalmologist who deals with retinal vascular disorders in his daily practice. It will also prove to be a useful resource to the internist who deals with diabetes and other systemic vascular diseases. The sections on arterial and venous insufficiency and cystoid macular edema are especially noteworthy and provide material not readily available in other publications.

Arnall Patz, M.D.

Preface

This atlas is designed for the clinician, resident, and fellow. Color photographs with accompanying fluorescein angiograms in a systematic fashion are presented to help in (1) recognizing different retinal vascular disorders seen in everyday practice and (2) correlating the clinical funduscopic picture with the fluorescein angiograms. Each chapter is arranged in terms of a modified differential diagnosis.

While organizing the format of the atlas, it became obvious that certain interesting features existed regarding some of the different entities. Therefore, the concept of an "author's note" is included to present some interesting anecdotal material to supplement the color photographs and angiograms. The remarks are by no means intended either to be dogmatic or to be the last word regarding diagnosis and management. As with many atlases, its limitations and usefulness are frequently dictated by the passage of time as ideas and approaches to different diseases change. Every attempt has been made to gather useful information from published material and from personal interchange between retinal specialists around the world.

I am grateful to Manuel Stillerman, M.D., for providing me with my initial exposure to ophthalmology. I am especially indebted to Arnall Patz, M.D., who nurtured my interest in macular and retinal vascular diseases. And besides being my teacher, Dr. Patz has been a close personal friend and has advised me and guided me through my initial years of practice.

A commitment to clinical research originated during my fellowship in the Retinal Vascular Center at the Wilmer Ophthalmological Institute. I am grateful to both Stuart L. Fine, M.D., and Daniel Finkelstein, M.D., for introducing me to prospective clinical trials. Many of the comments in this atlas reflect the philosophy of the Branch Vein Occlusion Study, the Macular Photocoagulation Study, and the Early Treatment Diabetic Retinopathy Study.

I am especially thankful to Morton F. Goldberg, M.D., for providing me the opportunity to continue my interest in clinical trials at the University of Illinois and for providing his expertise and time in discussing and seeing many of the patients presented in this publication.

No atlas of this type could be compiled without the support of the general ophthalmic community. I am indebted to all those ophthalmologists in the metropolitan Chicago area and Indiana who have unselfishly referred patients for consultation. I am particularly indebted to the clinicians, residents, and fellows associated with the Retinal Vascular Service at Ingalls Memorial Hospital, Michael Reese Hospital and Medical Center, and the University of Illinois Eye and Ear Infirmary.

A most important part of the atlas is the accompanying artistic schematics to help readers better understand the different disease entities. This work could not have been completed without the assistance of Ms. Amalie Dunker of the Johns Hopkins University and Hospital. I am indebted to Ms. Dunker for her outstanding contribution to this atlas and the superb quality of her work. I have worked with Ms. Dunker on other projects, and, as always, she has devoted endless hours and bountiful energy to this project and has provided a most integral part of the text.

As with any atlas, the core of the text is the photographs. Certainly, without the professional expertise of David Baczewski, Chief Ophthalmic Photographer at the Retinal Vascular Service at Ingalls Memorial Hospital, this project would never have come to realization. A special thanks to Douglas Bryant, Thomas Quirk, and Andrew Wheeler for also taking excellent photographs and for helping to organize the atlas.

I am most thankful and appreciative for the dedicated help and assistance provided by Teri Fitzgerald. Ms. Fitzgerald spent endless hours typing and retyping the material for publication as well as doing much of the proofreading and editing.

Acknowledgments

This work could not have been completed without the dedicated assistance of

Amalie P. Dunker
Medical Illustrator
Johns Hopkins Medical Institution
Baltimore, Maryland

David J. Baczewski
Chief Ophthalmic Photographer
Retinal Vascular Department
Ingalls Memorial Hospital
Harvey, Illinois

Contents

Introduction to Nomenclature and Principles of Fluorescein Angiography

In the past few decades, our technological advances have not only improved our methods for diagnosis and treatment of lesions of the posterior pole, but have also served to highlight some general confusion with regard to the anatomic terminology in this important region of the eye. Until there is a consensus on the terminology of this region, it seems useful to employ a simple equation in which the terms used are specified as either anatomic or clinical (*Figure 1*).

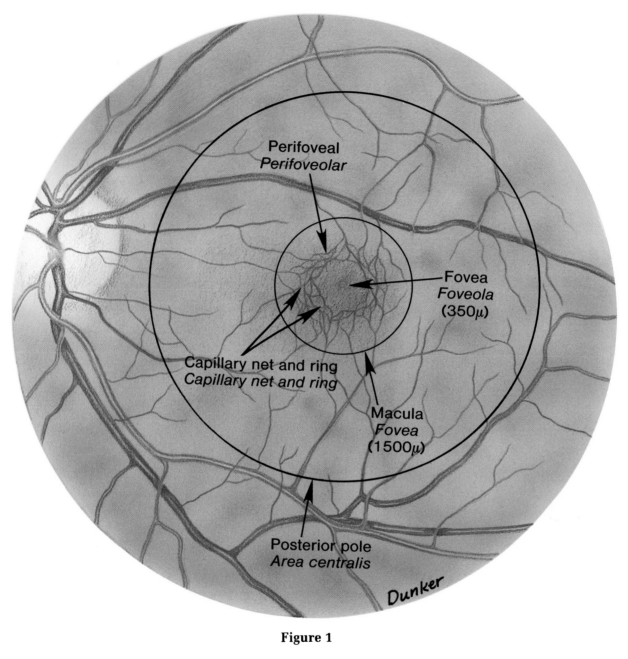

Figure 1

ANATOMIC		CLINICAL
area centralis	⟷	posterior pole
fovea (centralis)	⟷	macula
foveola	⟷	fovea
perifoveolar	⟷	perifoveal
capillary net and ring	⟷	capillary net and ring

The sensory retina is supplied by two separate vascular systems. The inner portion of the sensory retina extending from the internal limiting membrane including the inner portion of the inner nuclear layer is supplied by the retinal vascular circulation. The remainder of the sensory retina is supplied by the choroidal circulation (*Figure 2*).

The larger retinal arteries and veins and precapillary arterioles are located under the internal limiting membrane in the nerve fiber layer. The retinal capillaries and postcapillary venules are located in the deeper aspect of the inner half of the retina, i.e. the inner aspect of the inner nuclear layer.

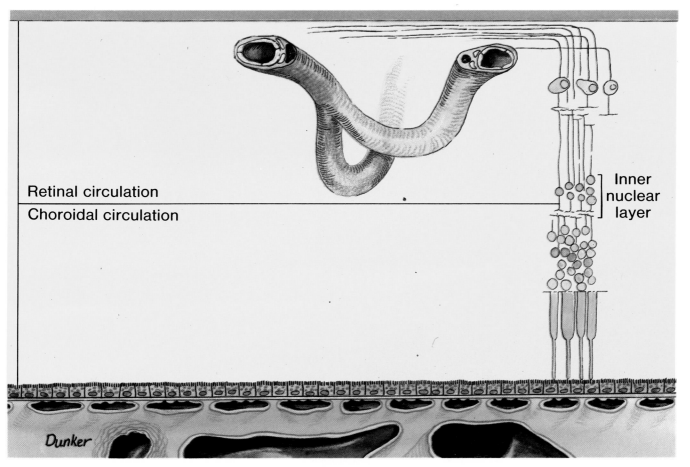

Retinal circulation
Choroidal circulation

Inner nuclear layer

Dunker

Figure 2

In understanding disorders of the retinal vasculature, it is worthwhile understanding certain normal characteristics of the retinal vasculature (*Figure 3*).

1. In the vicinity of an arterio-venous crossing, there is a common adventitial sheath.

2. There is a normal occurring capillary free zone along the retinal arteries.

3. The retinal or foveal avascular zone is bounded by a single thickness of capillaries called the perifoveal capillary net whose innermost capillary border along its free margin might usefully be termed the perifoveal capillary ring.

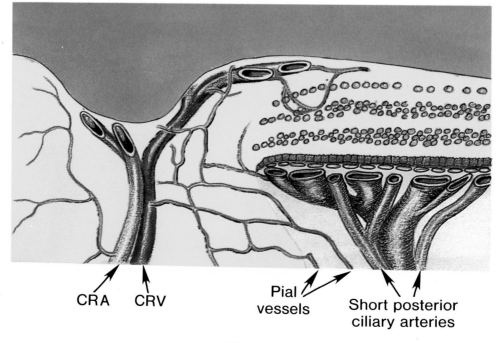

CRA   CRV   Pial vessels   Short posterior ciliary arteries

Figure 3

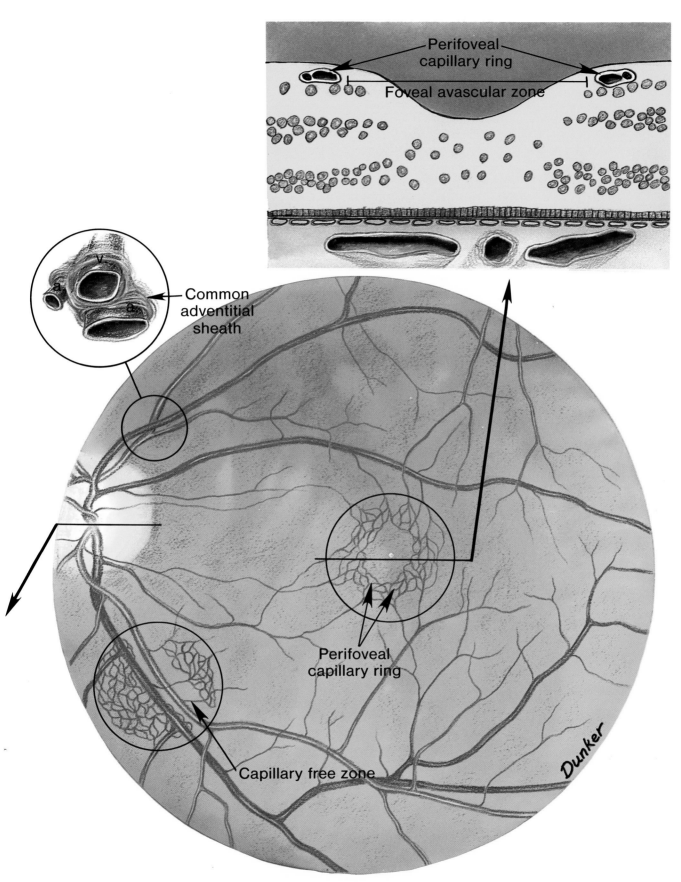

Perifoveal
capillary ring

Foveal avascular zone

Common
adventitial
sheath

Perifoveal
capillary ring

Capillary free zone

Dunker

Figure 3—*Continued*

Normal Fluorescein Angiogram

The excitation peak of the fluorescein molecule is 490 nm or 4900 Å. This is in the blue part of the spectrum and represents the wavelength for maximum absorption of light energy by fluorescein. The fluorescein molecules are stimulated by this wavelength and are excited to a higher energy level where a longer wavelength of light with a peak of 530 nm or 5300 Å is emitted. This fluorescent peak is in the green portion of the spectrum.

During fluorescein angiography, a flash of white light from the retinal camera passes through the blue excitation filter; it strikes and excites the fluorescein molecules so that a yellow-green light emerges from the patient's eye along with the blue light. The yellow-green barrier filter blocks the reflected blue light and transmits only the yellow-green wavelengths onto the film within the camera body.

There are two normal occurring barriers to the passage of fluorescein molecules. These two regions are frequently referred to as the blood-retinal barriers. They are the zonula occludens between adjacent retinal pigment epithelial cells and the tight junctions of the retinal capillary endothelial cells (*Figures 4 and 5*).

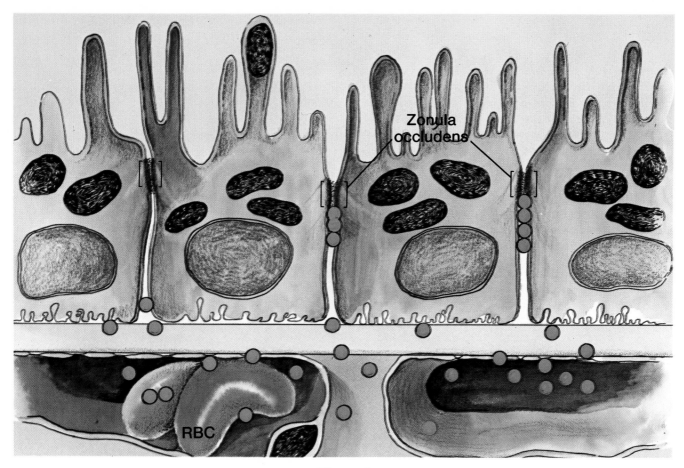

Figure 4

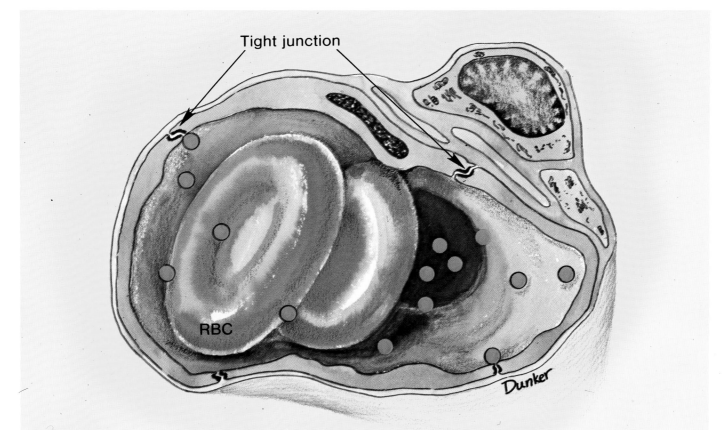

Figure 5

In the normal fluorescein angiogram, the initial signs of fluorescence begin to appear in the choroid approximately 10 to 12 seconds after injection of the fluorescein dye. The early phase is referred to as the "choroidal flush." This choroidal fluorescence is seen because unbound fluorescein molecules pass freely through the fenestra of the choriocapillaris and fill the extracellular choroidal space. A second or two after the fluorescein is seen in the choroid, fluorescence appears in the central retinal artery and the larger precapillary arteriole branches (*Figure 6*). Fluorescein then passes into the retinal capillaries, the postcapillary venules, and the major retinal veins and central retinal vein (*Figure 7*). The early phase of the retinal venous fluorescein pattern is frequently referred to as *laminar flow*. This characteristic picture occurs because the vascular flow is faster in the center of the larger retinal veins than on the sides. The fluorescence along the walls of the veins becomes thicker, and eventually there is complete fluorescence within the lumen of the vein (*Figure 8*).

Fluorescence of the disc originates from the posterior ciliary vascular system and from the capillaries of the central retinal artery on the surface of the disc.

The macular region of a normal fluorescein angiogram characteristically has a darker appearance than the surrounding region. Xanthophyll in the sensory retina partially blocks the transmission of blue light needed to excite the fluorescein molecules in the choroid. In addition, the increased density of the pigment granules in the retinal pigment epithelium underlying the macula also blocks some of the background choroidal fluorescence (*Figure 9*).

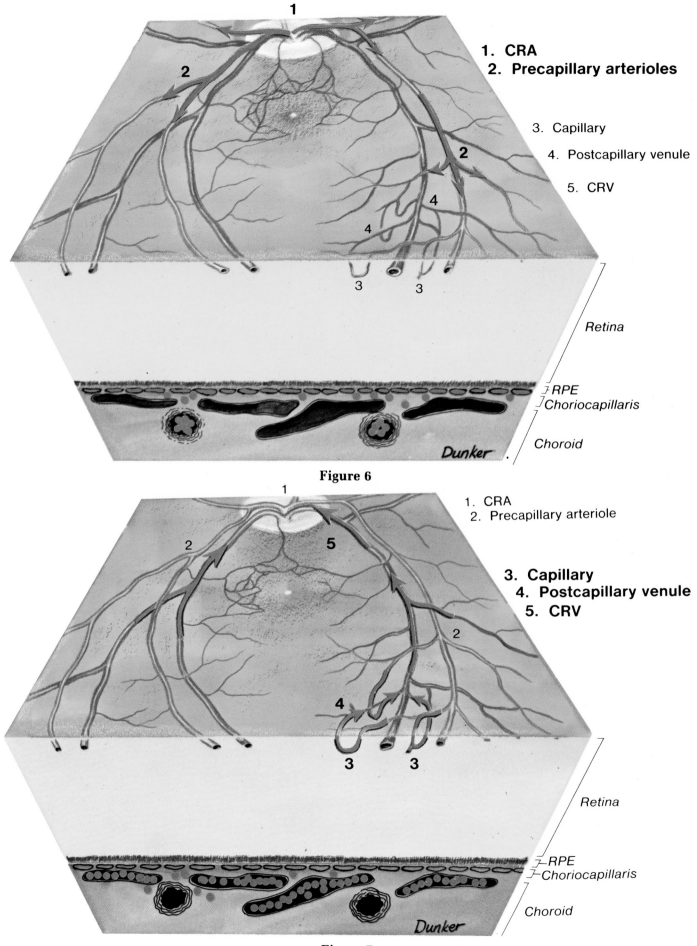

1. CRA
  2. Precapillary arterioles

3. Capillary

4. Postcapillary venule

5. CRV

Retina

RPE
Choriocapillaris

Choroid

Dunker

Figure 6

1. CRA
  2. Precapillary arteriole

3. Capillary
  4. Postcapillary venule
  5. CRV

Retina

RPE
Choriocapillaris

Choroid

Dunker

Figure 7

NOMENCLATURE AND PRINCIPLES OF FLUORESCEIN ANGIOGRAPHY

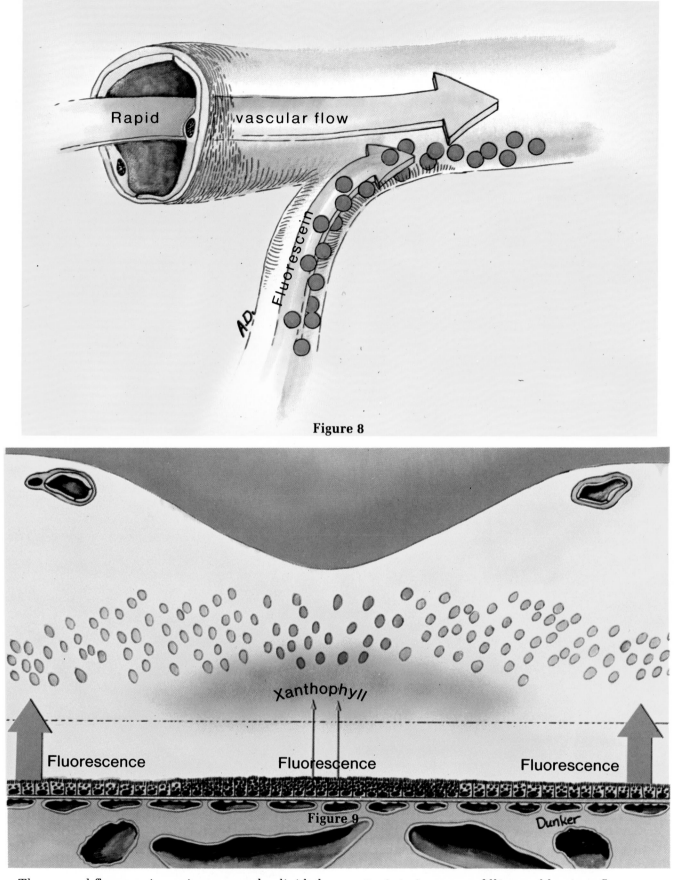

Figure 8

Figure 9

Xanthophyll

Fluorescence   Fluorescence   Fluorescence

Dunker

The normal fluorescein angiogram can be divided into the following phases:
1. Early choroidal filling and choroidal flush
2. Retinal artery filling and increased choroidal filling
3. Arterio-venous filling and laminar flow
4. Full arterio-venous filling
5. Retinal venous phase
6. Late arterio-venous recirculation phase with decreased retinal and choroidal fluorescence

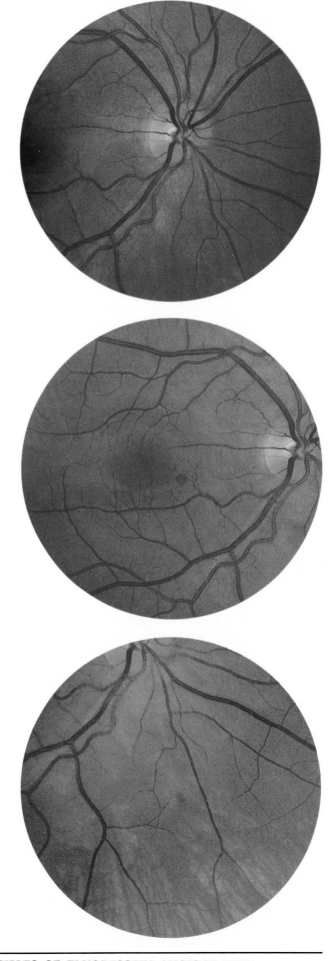

The normal disc with the retinal arteries and veins in their normal caliber ratio.

The posterior pole and macular region. A normal macular ring reflex is present.

The normal caliber ratio between arteries and veins inferior to the optic nerve and outside the temporal arcades.

AUTHOR'S NOTE

A small round artifact can be seen on the color photographs. It is located inferior nasal to the fovea. Artifacts can be distinguished from pathology by the fact that they appear the same configuration on different areas of the fundus.

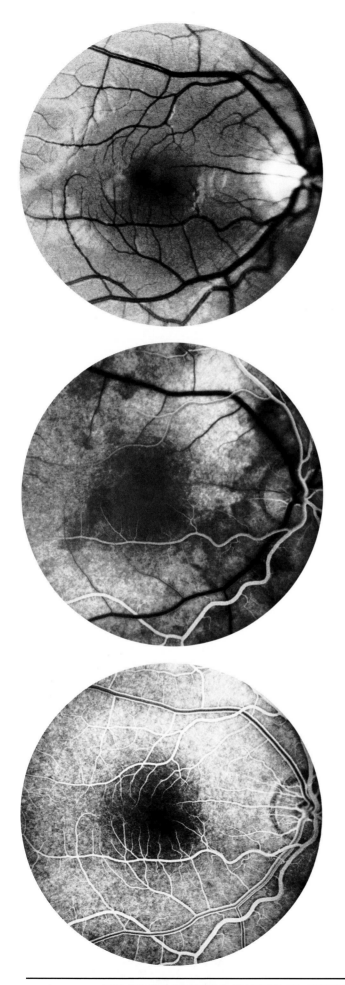

The red-free photograph shows a view of the optic nerve, the retinal vasculature, and the posterior pole. The nerve fiber layer can be seen.

The choroidal filling phase and the retinal arterial phase are seen. There is patchy filling of the choriocapillaris. There is no fluorescein dye in the retinal veins.

The choroid shows increased filling. In the early retinal arterial phase, the retinal arteries are completely fluorescent and the retinal veins show laminar flow.

The mid-arterio-venous phase shows further filling of the retinal veins with almost complete disappearance of laminar flow. There is greater fluorescence within the retinal arteries as compared with the retinal veins.

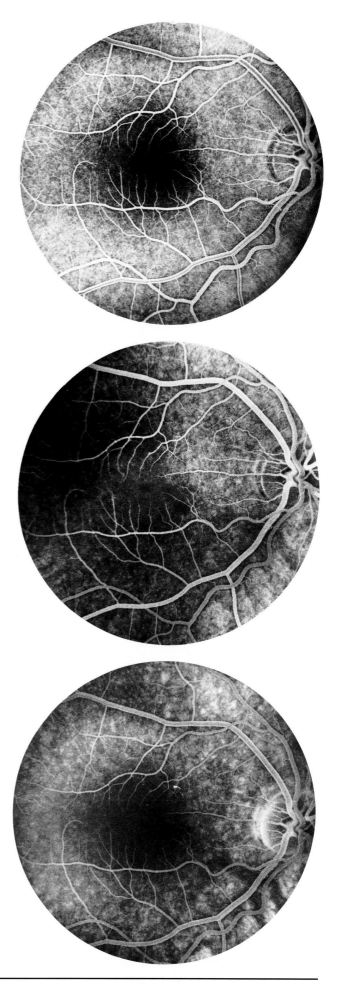

The venous phase of the angiogram begins to show some slight fading of the choroidal fluorescence. The retinal veins are more hyperfluorescent than the retinal arteries.

Late phase of the angiogram shows diminished choroidal fluorescence. There is equal fluorescence in both retinal arteries and veins, but it is less intense than in the earlier phases of the angiogram.

Normal (dark fundus) (with cilioretinal artery)

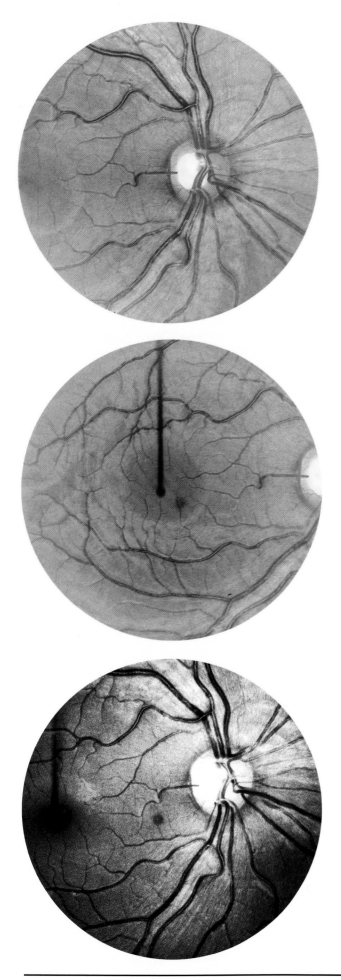

The optic nerve and retinal vasculature appear normal. There is a cilioretinal artery emanating from the temporal aspect of the optic cup at the 9 o'clock position.

The cilioretinal vessel can be seen extending toward the macula. The normal macular ring reflex is clearly visible. A fixation pointer is present.

The red-free photograph shows the cilioretinal vessel. The normal retinal sheen from the internal limiting membrane and the nerve fiber layer can be seen. The fixation pointer is also present, with the tip of the pointer in the center of the macula. The small grayish dot just temporal to the optic nerve is an artifact.

During the choroidal phase of the angiogram there is filling of the cilioretinal artery and its branches.

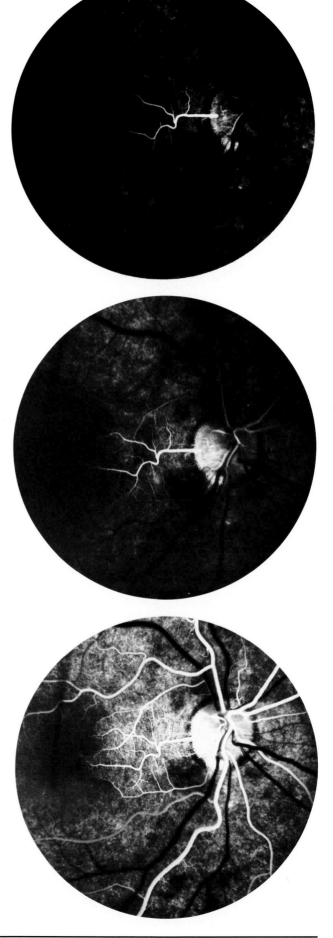

Several seconds later more of the branches from the cilioretinal artery fill with fluorescein as there is beginning flow of the fluorescein dye into the central retinal artery and its main branches.

The central retinal artery and the larger precapillary arteriolar branches are filled with fluorescein. Fluorescein also is present in the retinal capillaries. There appears to be a normal segmental filling of the capillaries on the surface of the optic nerve.

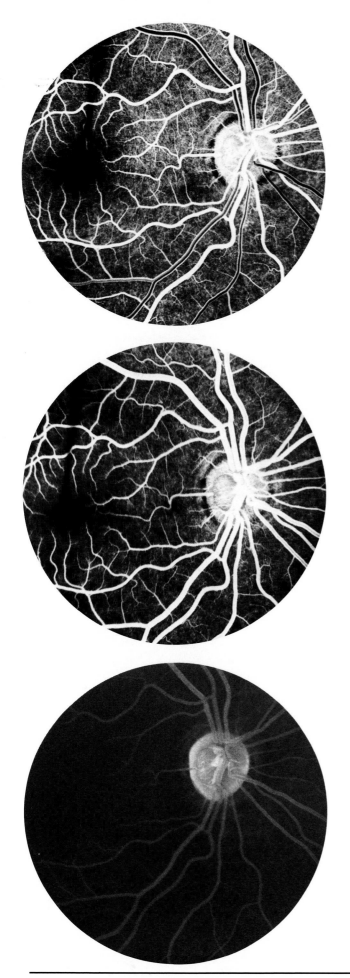

The normal filling of the postcapillary venules and the laminar flow of the major retinal veins can be seen. The perifoveal capillary net and ring are well delineated by being filled with the fluorescein dye.

The full arterio-venous phase of the angiogram is seen with equal fluorescence of the retinal arteries and veins. The fixation pointer appears as a black line extending into the center of the fovea.

The late retinal venous phase with recirculation and decreased retinal vascular and choroidal fluorescence.

Variant of Normal (small retinal avascular zone)

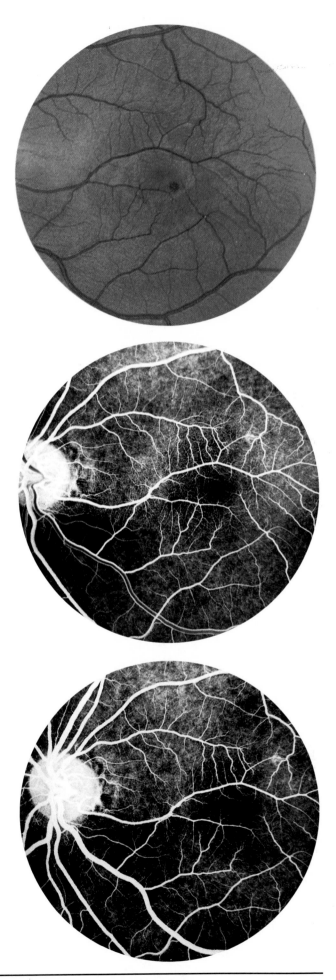

Normal macular region with normal retinal vasculature.

Laminar phase shows a smaller than normal retinal avascular zone.

Later phase of the angiogram shows a small retinal avascular zone. There is no significant pathology.

AUTHOR'S NOTE

Several terms have been used to describe the avascular region surrounded by the perifoveal capillary net seen on fluorescein angiography. Retinal avascular zone, capillary free zone, and foveal-retinal capillary free zone are all synonymous.

Bibliography

Amalric P, Bonin P: L'Angiographie fluoresceinique. *Bull Soc Ophthalmol Fr* (Numero special):219–318, 1969.

Archer D, Krill AE, Newell FW: Fluorescein studies of normal choroidal circulation. *Am J Ophthalmol* 69:543, 1970.

Bird AC, Weale RA: On the retinal vasculature of the human fovea. *Exp Eye Res* 19:409–417, 1974.

Friedenwald JS: Retinal vascular dynamics. *Am J Ophthalmol* 17:387–395, 1934.

Gass JDM, Sever RJ, Sparks D, Goren J: A combined technique of fluorescein funduscopy and angiography of the eye. *Arch Ophthalmol* 78:455–461, 1967.

Haining WM, Lancaster RC: Advanced technique for fluorescein angiography. *Arch Ophthalmol* 79:10–15, 1968.

Justice J Jr: Basic interpretations of fluorescein angiography. *Int Ophthalmol Clin* 16:41, 1976.

Justice J Jr: Fluorescein angiography. *Int Ophthalmol Clin* 16:33, 1976.

Novotny HR, Alvis DL: A method of photographing fluorescence in circulating blood in the human retina. *Circulation* 24:82–86, 1961.

Oosterhuis JA, Boen-Tan TN: Choroidal fluorescence in the normal human eye. *Ophthalmologica* 162:246, 1971.

Orth DH, Fine BS, Fagman W: Clarification of foveomacular nomenclature and grid for quantitation of macular disorders. *Trans Am Acad Ophthalmol Otolaryngol* 83:506–514, 1977.

Yannuzzi LA, Fisher YL, Levy JH: A classification of abnormal fundus fluorescence. *Ann Ophthalmol* 3:711, 1971.

CHAPTER 1

Arterial Insufficiency or Occlusion

Differential Diagnosis

A. EMBOLISM
B. RETINAL ARTERIOSCLEROSIS
C. HYPERTENSIVE RETINOPATHY
D. DIABETES MELLITUS
E. GIANT CELL ARTERITIS
F. CAROTID ARTERY DISEASE
G. COLLAGEN VASCULAR DISEASE

H. PHOTOCOAGULATION
I. TRAUMA
J. INFLAMMATORY
   (TOXOPLASMOSIS, ETC.)
K. PULSELESS DISEASE
L. OTHER

Embolism

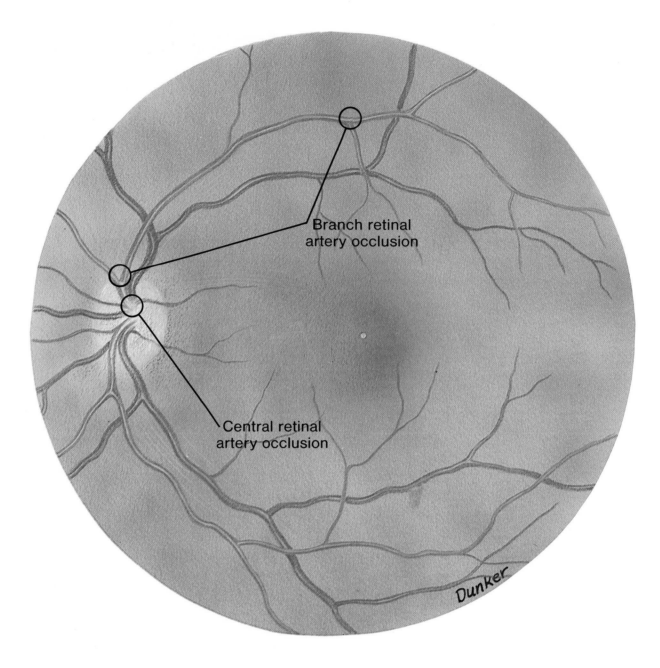

Branch retinal artery occlusion

Central retinal artery occlusion

Dunker

Embolism can be manifested as a central retinal artery occlusion or branch retinal artery occlusion (*figure*). Retinal arterial emboli can be divided into endogenous and exogenous causes:

EXOGENOUS	
silicone	oil
air	cornstarch
mercury	glassbeads
	talc

ENDOGENOUS	
cholesterol	bacteria
calcium	tumor
platelets	amniotic fluid
fibrin	parasites
lipids	fungi

The most common endogenous causes are cholesterol, fibrin, and platelet emboli. Cholesterol crystal emboli are more frequently seen in patients with arteriosclerosis of the carotid arteries. Clinically, cholesterol emboli appear as highly refractile, glistening deposits within the dimensions of the blood vessel. Frequently, the embolus appears larger than the width of the blood vessel due to the reflection from its surface. Occasionally the emboli can be dislodged through a smaller bifurcation or may even be caused to disappear by tapping on the globe or using more aggressive manipulation such as paracentesis. Showers of cholesterol emboli can be seen after carotid angiography or arterial bypass surgery. Hollenhorst plaques or cholesterol plaques frequently lodge in arterial bifurcations (A).

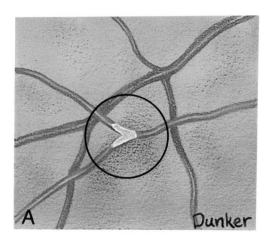

Calcific emboli are small, irregular, and appear as white or yellow deposits within the retinal arterial tree. They are less refractile than cholesterol emboli and usually do not obstruct the flow of blood in the vessel (B).

Platelet emboli are dull, white material often elongated to a certain degree within a retinal branch artery. There may be multiple platelet emboli within the same arterial branch. These emboli can move quickly to smaller branches of the central retinal artery with improvement of visual symptoms (C).

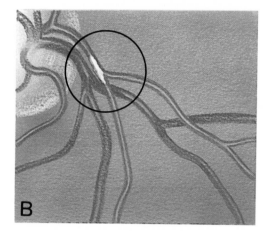

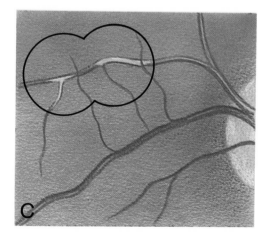

Acute Central Retinal Artery Occlusion

  I. Disc margins blurred.
 II. Sensory retina pale (thickened secondary to is-
     chemic retinal whitening).
III. Vessels are narrowed, irregular, and appear
     slightly blurred in the thickened retina.
 IV. "Cherry-red spot."

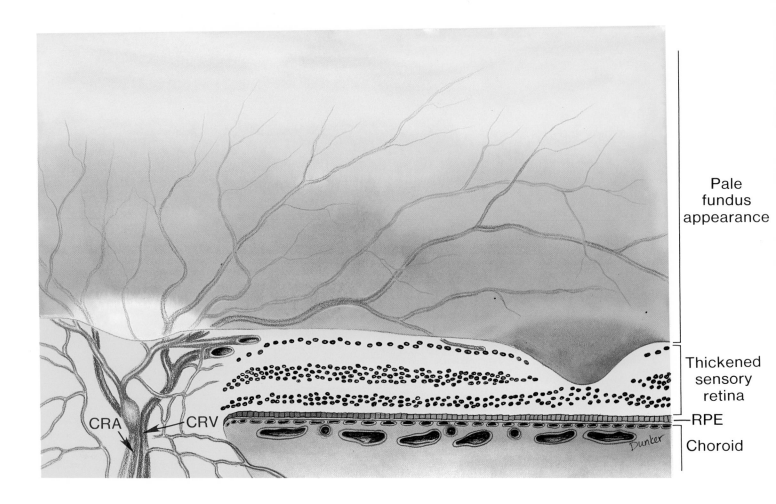

Old Central Retinal Artery Occlusion

I. The disc is pale.
II. The sensory retina is thin.
III. The retinal vessels are narrowed. A faint "cherry-red spot" may be present.

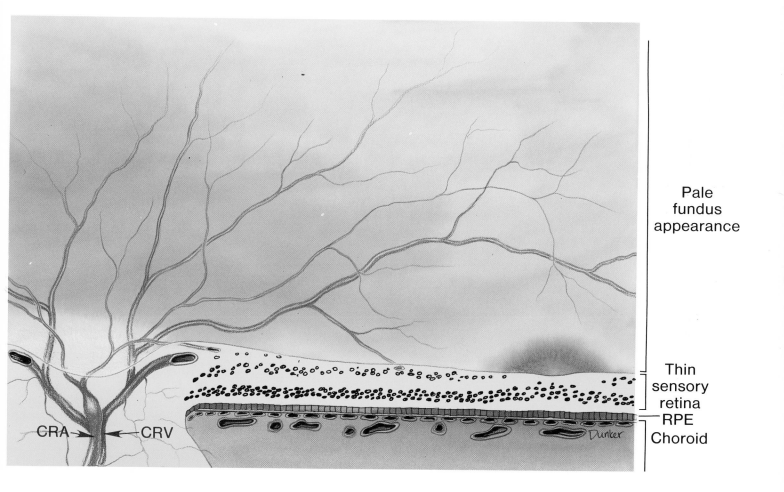

Pale fundus appearance

Thin sensory retina

RPE
Choroid

CRA ← → CRV

Central Retinal Artery Occlusion with Preservation of Papillomacular Bundle

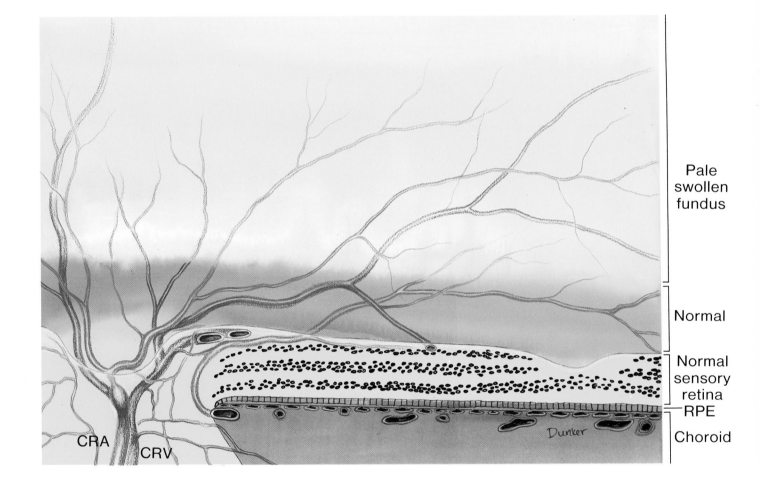

Cilioretinal Artery Occlusion

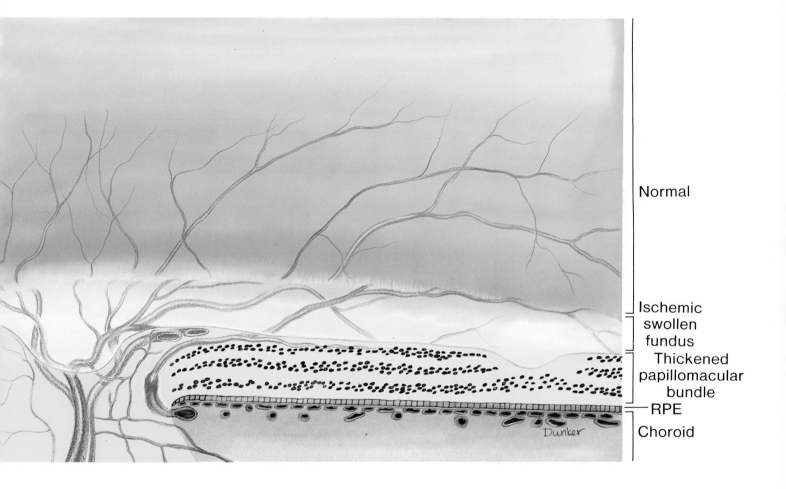

Normal

Ischemic swollen fundus

Thickened papillomacular bundle

RPE

Choroid

Dunker

Acute Central Retinal Artery Occlusion

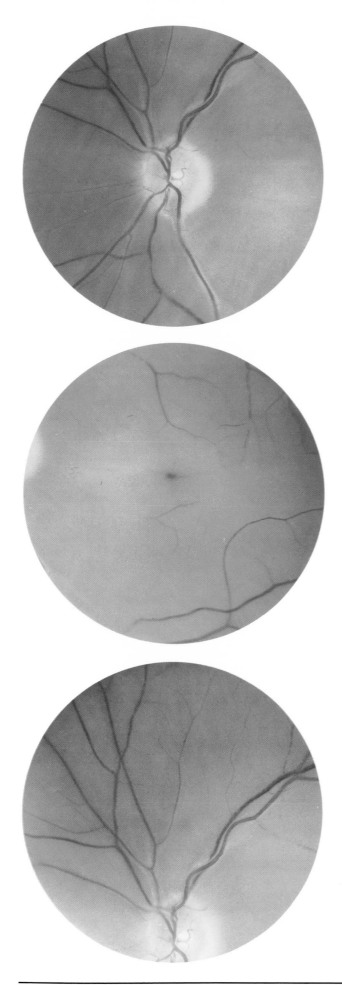

The disc margins are slightly blurred. There is a mild, pale edema of the nerve. The retinal arteries appear narrowed and irregular in caliber. There is irregularity in the blood flow within the retinal veins.

The posterior pole shows opacification or ischemic retinal whitening. A "cherry-red spot" can be seen in the foveal region.

The peripheral branches of both the arteries and veins show segmentation of blood flow ("box-carring").

AUTHOR'S NOTE
The opacification or ischemic retinal whitening of the sensory retina is also referred to as cloudy swelling of the retina.

Thirty seconds after injection of fluorescein dye, there is hyperfluorescence of some of the capillaries on the surface of the nerve. However, the central retinal artery shows very little fluorescein. There is blockage of the choroidal fluorescence due to the edematous sensory retina.

One minute after injection of the dye, the fluorescein dye fills the branches of the central retinal artery in an irregular fashion.

As the more peripheral branches of the arterial tree fill with the fluorescein dye there is the beginning of laminar flow in the retinal veins.

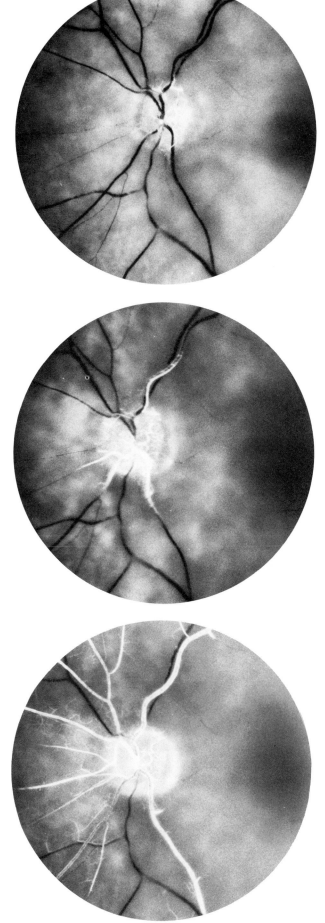

Reader's Notes

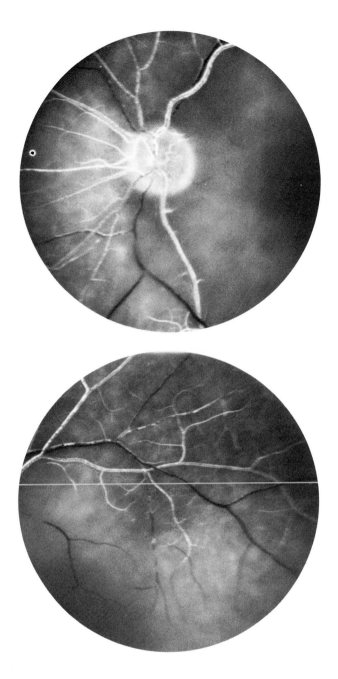

Five minutes after injection, there is irregularity in the flow of the fluorescein molecules in the central retinal artery and its branches. The retinal veins also show an irregularity in the flow of the fluorescein dye.

Ten minutes after fluorescein injection there are branches of both the arterial and venous side of the circulation which do not fill with the fluorescein dye or show an irregular filling pattern.

Central Retinal Artery Occlusion (chronic)

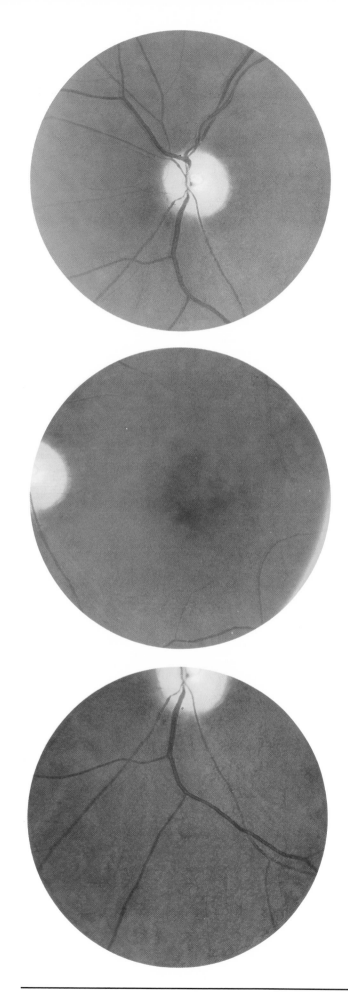

There is optic atrophy. The retinal arteries are very narrow with caliber irregularities.

The sensory retina in the posterior pole has lost its normal sheen. There is a loss of the macular ring reflex and foveal reflex.

All the branches of the central retinal artery are narrowed and show caliber irregularities.

Dilated capillaries are present on the surface of the nerve. The arterial phase of the angiogram shows a patchy choroidal filling with irregularities in the caliber of the retinal arteries.

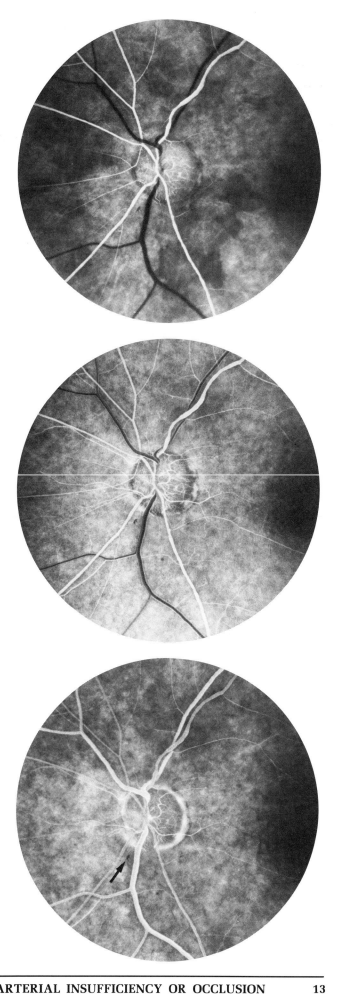

Laminar phase of the angiogram demonstrates a "smoked glass" appearance to the choroidal fluorescence due to a lack of capillary filling of the sensory retina and loss of the sensory retinal sheen.

The optic nerve appears hypofluorescent, compatible with optic atrophy. A small punctate hemorrhage inferior to the optic nerve (*arrow*) blocks the background fluorescence.

Central Retinal Artery Occlusion (incomplete)

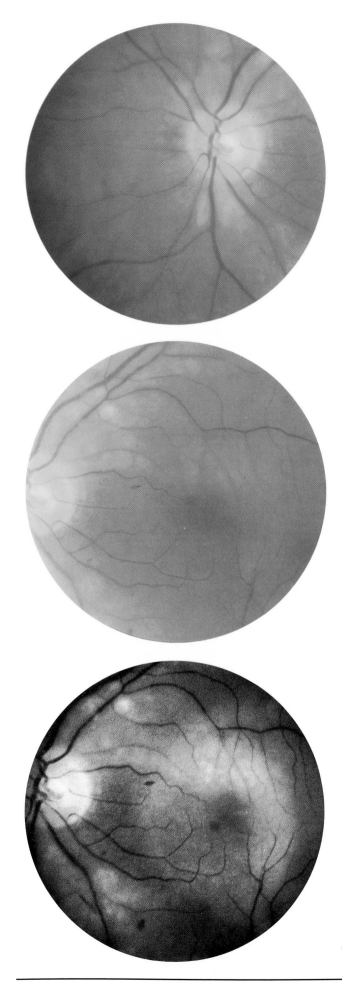

The retinal arteries are markedly narrowed and show caliber irregularities.

Retinal opacification or ischemic retinal whitening is seen primarily superior to the fovea. An area of soft exudate and a few intraretinal hemorrhages can be seen.

Red-free photograph shows retinal opacification appearing as a grayish area. The intraretinal hemorrhages appear as small black areas. An area of soft exudate is seen along the superior temporal arcade.

During the choroidal phase of the angiogram, there is preferential filling of the vessels supplying the papillomacular bundle. The remainder of the branches of the central retinal artery show no evidence of fluorescein dye.

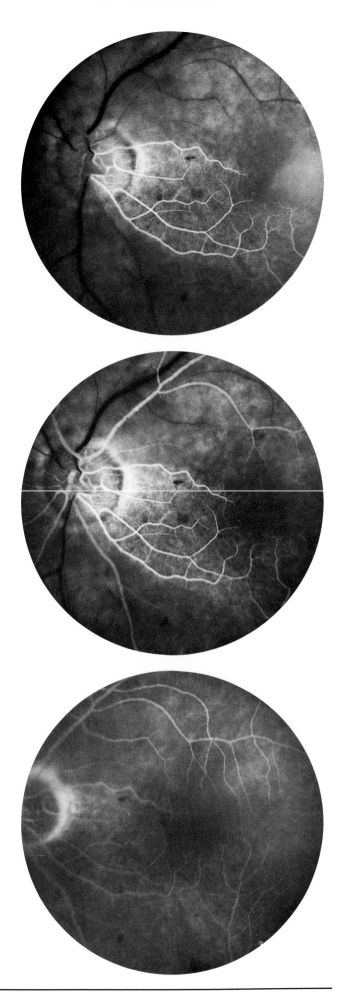

The arterial phase of the angiogram shows irregularities in the walls of the retinal arteries. There is some dilatation of the capillary bed in the papillomacular bundle. The intraretinal hemorrhages block the background choroidal fluorescence.

Late phase reveals some very subtle leakage of fluorescein dye in the papillomacular bundle. Subtle irregularities in the caliber of the retinal arteries are present.

AUTHOR'S NOTE

In cases of arterial occlusion, the timer on many of the fluorescein cameras is frequently valuable in demonstrating a prolongation in the filling of the retinal arteries. (Normally the retinal arteries fill 10 to 12 seconds after injection of the fluorescein dye.)

Central Retinal Artery Occlusion (secondary to trauma)

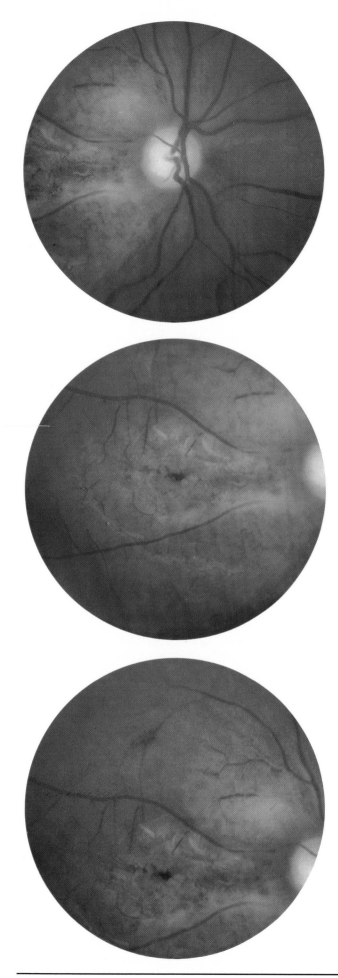

There is marked attenuation of the branches of the central retinal artery.

Ischemic retinal whitening can be seen involving the macula and most of the inferior posterior pole.

Specks of intraretinal hemorrhage are present. There is discontinuity of the smaller branched arteries.

During the arterial phase of the angiogram, there is definite delay in filling of the smaller branches of the central retinal artery. Increased blockage of the background choroidal fluorescence can be seen temporal to the optic nerve due to ischemic swelling of the sensory retina.

There is increased dilatation of the capillaries on the temporal aspect of the optic nerve. During the laminar phase of venous flow there is still evidence of delayed filling of the smaller branches of the central retinal artery.

There is slight leakage from the dilated capillaries on the temporal aspect of the nerve. The branches of the central retinal artery extending through the papillomacular bundle are definitely attenuated. The veins are filled with fluorescein, while many of the smaller arterial branches are still void of the dye.

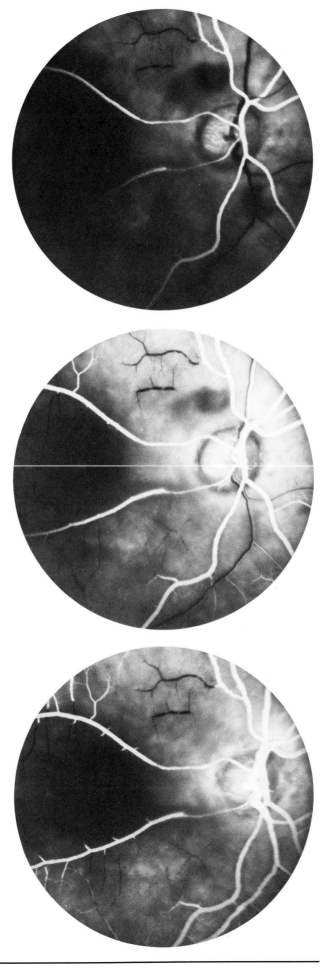

Central Retinal Artery Occlusion with Sparing of the Papillomacular Bundle

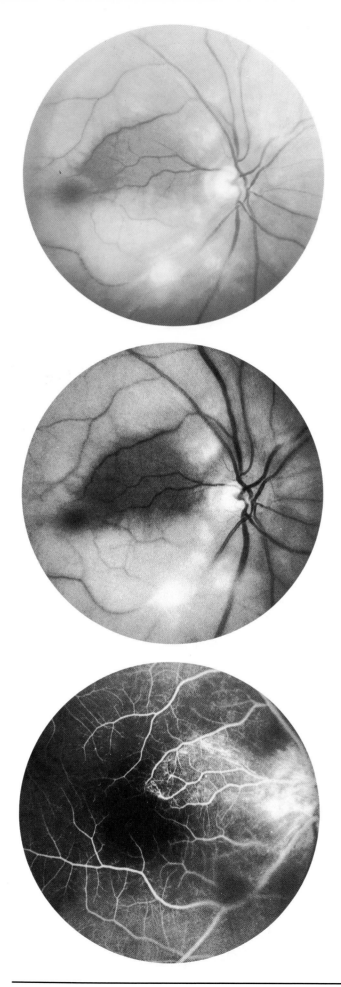

Color photograph shows ischemic retinal whitening with a "cherry-red spot." There is a triangular area of normal sensory retina in the superior aspect of the papillomacular bundle. Several confluent areas of soft exudate are present. The retinal arteries are irregular in their caliber and narrowed.

The red-free photograph shows ischemic retinal whitening which appears as opacification except for the triangular area in the papillomacular bundle. The soft exudates appear as increased opacification as compared to the other areas of ischemic retinal whitening.

The mid-arterio-venous phase of the angiogram shows filling of the retinal arteries and branches. There is dilatation of the capillary bed in the papillomacular bundle, corresponding to the normal looking retina on the color photograph. There also is dilatation of the capillaries on the surface of the optic nerve.

In the late arterio-venous phase there is further leakage of fluorescein from the dilated capillaries on the surface of the optic nerve and in the superior aspect of the papillomacular bundle. Along the inferior temporal vessels, there is an area of capillary dropout or nonperfusion, corresponding to the soft exudate (cotton-wool spot) seen on the color photograph.

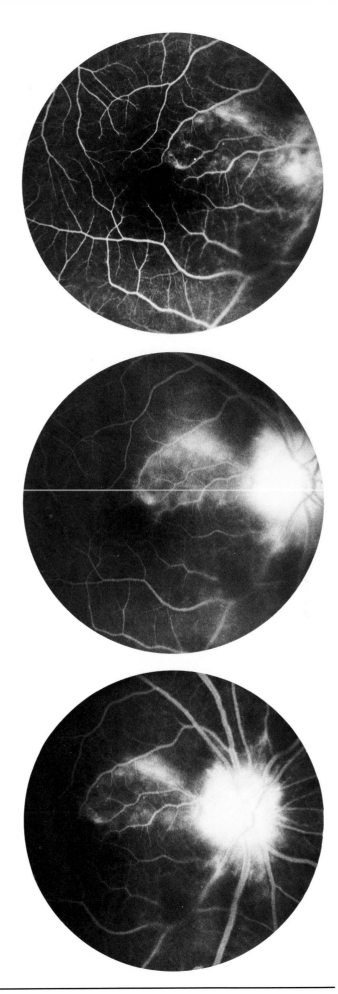

There is accumulation of fluorescein within the sensory retina secondary to leakage from the dilated capillaries.

There is evidence of leakage both in the papillomacular bundle and from the dilated capillaries on the surface of the optic nerve.

AUTHOR'S NOTE

Leakage of fluorescein from the capillaries both on the surface of the nerve and in the papillomacular bundle indicates a breakdown in the blood-retinal barrier due to loss of integrity between endothelial junctions.

Cilioretinal Artery Occlusion

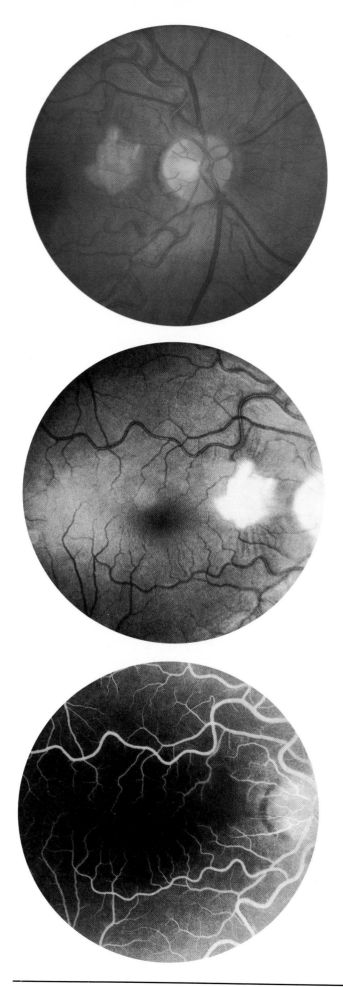

An area of ischemic retinal whitening or a large soft exudate can be seen in the papillomacular bundle.

Red-free photograph clearly shows the opaque retina. There are some striae of the sensory retina above and below the area of soft exudate.

There is an area of capillary dropout or nonperfusion in the papillomacular bundle corresponding to the ischemic retinal whitening seen on the color and red-free photographs.

Later in the angiogram there is some filling of the cilioretinal vessel (*arrow*) leading to the area of non-perfusion.

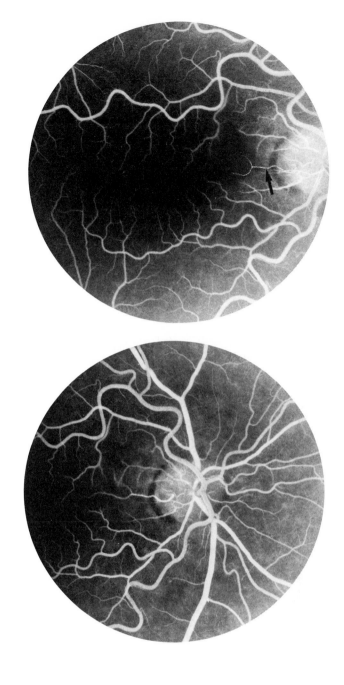

Three weeks later there is filling of the cilioretinal vessel with no evidence of nonperfusion. The vessel shows some very slight irregularity in its caliber.

AUTHOR'S NOTE

This patient had a mitral valve replacement with ocular symptoms developing shortly after surgery. Three weeks after the initial presentation with the cilioretinal occlusion, there was improvement in both the scotoma and fundus picture with absence of the ischemic retinal whitening. Vision during the acute symptoms was 20/20, and there was a paracentral scotoma.

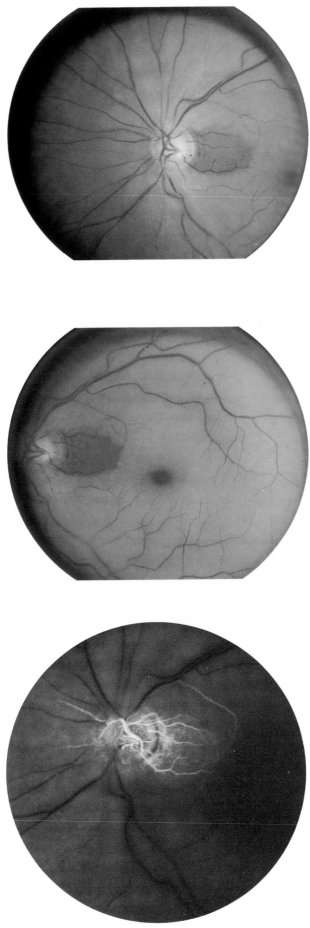

Central Retinal Artery Occlusion (sparing of the papillomacular bundle)

The branches of the central retinal artery are markedly attenuated. The ischemic retinal whitening is more apparent temporal to the optic nerve, with the nasal retina appearing essentially normal.

Sparing of the papillomacular bundle is obvious. There is extensive ischemic retinal whitening throughout the posterior pole with a "cherry-red spot" in the vicinity of the fovea.

Initially after injection of fluorescein, there is filling of the vessels in the papillomacular bundle. The remainder of the branches of the central retinal artery show no fluorescein dye.

Later in the transit time, there is irregular filling of the branches of the central retinal artery. There is slight blockage of the background choroidal fluorescence along the inferior temporal arcade due to edema of the sensory retina.

The filling of the more peripheral branches of the central retinal artery is irregular due to attenuation of the arteries. There is marked delay in filling of the retinal veins.

Branches of the retinal arteries and veins show marked delay in filling in the mid-periphery (arrows).

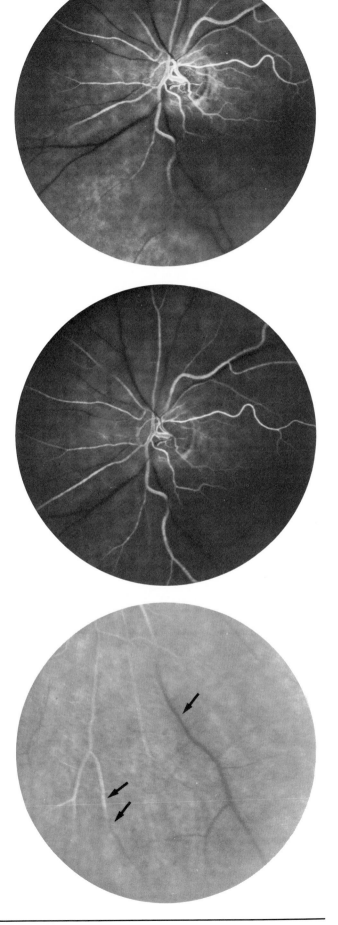

Branch Retinal Artery Occlusion (single embolus)

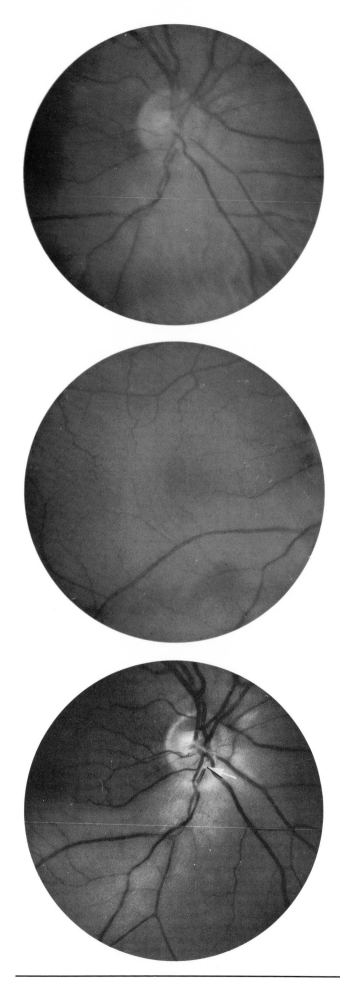

A yellow glistening embolus can be seen within the inferior temporal retinal artery as it branches from the central retinal artery.

Ischemic retinal whitening extending along the inferior arcades up to the horizontal raphe can be seen.

The red-free photograph clearly shows the embolus (*arrow*) and the inferior opaque sensory retina. The inferior temporal artery shows caliber irregularities.

The inferior retinal vasculature, including the arteries and veins, shows no filling with the fluorescein dye. The superior retinal arteries and veins show normal filling with fluorescein.

There is irregular filling of the inferior temporal artery. There is marked delay in filling of the inferior temporal retinal vein. There is staining of the walls of the inferior nasal artery secondary to a breakdown in the blood-retinal barrier.

The late fluorescein angiogram shows some irregular hyperfluorescence within the lumen of the inferior temporal artery. The remainder of the retinal vasculature shows fading of the fluorescence.

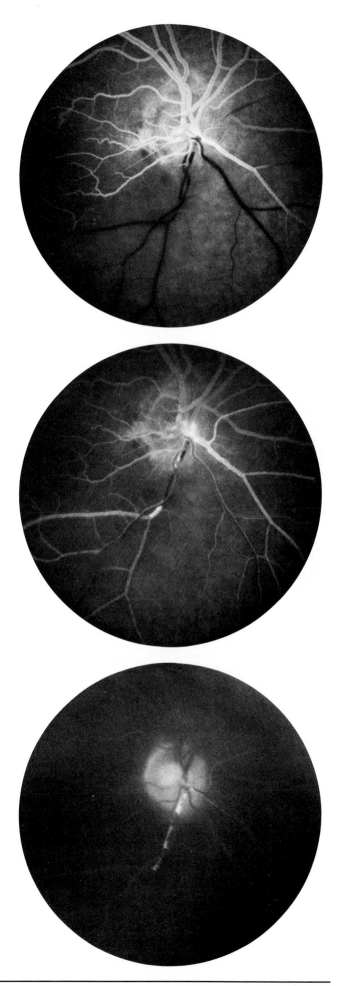

Branch Retinal Artery Occlusion (secondary to embolization)

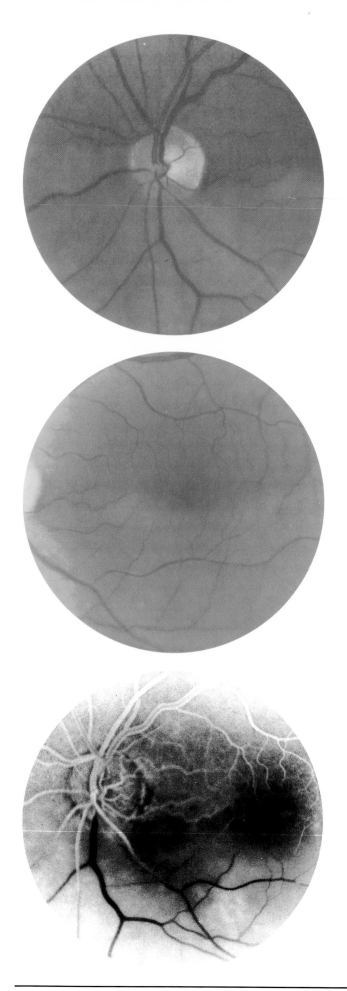

An embolus can be seen at the branching of the central retinal artery. The inferior branches are more attenuated than the normal caliber superior branch arteries.

Ischemic retinal whitening can be seen extending along the inferior temporal arcades. This swelling extends approximately to the horizontal raphe with the superior sensory retina being normal.

During the laminar phase of the angiogram, there is delay of filling of the inferior branch retinal arteries. There is increased blocked choroidal fluorescence along the inferior temporal arcade.

The superior temporal vein fills in normal fashion, while the inferior temporal vein is void of the fluorescein dye. There is slight staining of the embolus.

Irregular filling of the first branching of the inferior temporal artery is obvious.

Very late in the angiogram the inferior retinal veins finally begin to show some laminar flow. Staining of the embolus at the bifurcation of the central retinal artery can be seen.

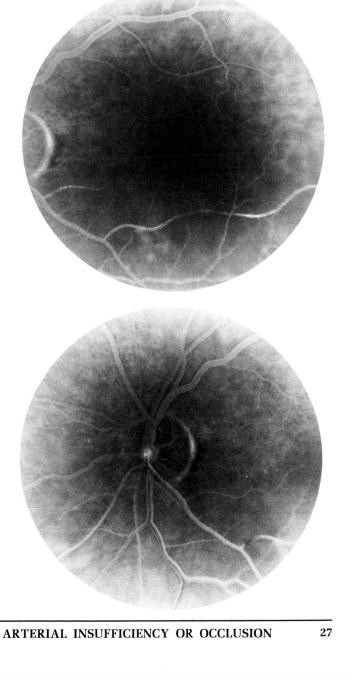

Branch Retinal Artery Occlusion (multiple emboli)

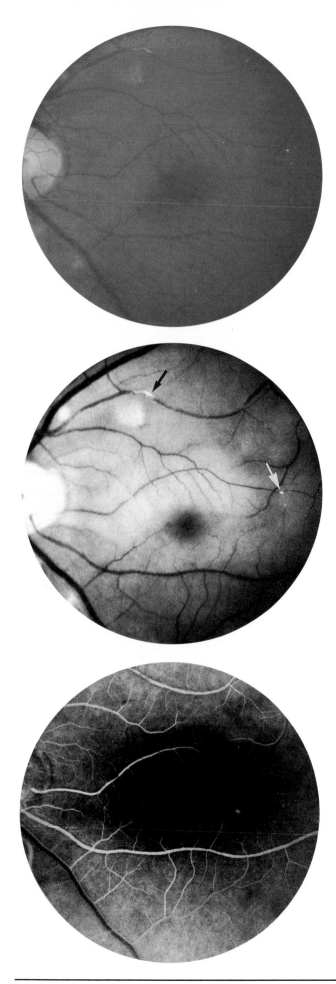

Multiple emboli can be seen temporal to the macula. There is also embolization of the superior temporal artery. There are several areas of soft exudate.

The red-free photograph demonstrates opaque retina appearing white and being primarily above the horizontal raphe. The multiple emboli can be seen (*arrow*).

During the laminar phase of the angiogram there is incomplete filling of several small retinal arterial branches. There is increased blockage of the background choroidal fluorescence by the ischemic retinal whitening.

There is some irregularity in the superior temporal artery. Terminal branches temporal to the macula (*arrows*) still have no fluorescein dye.

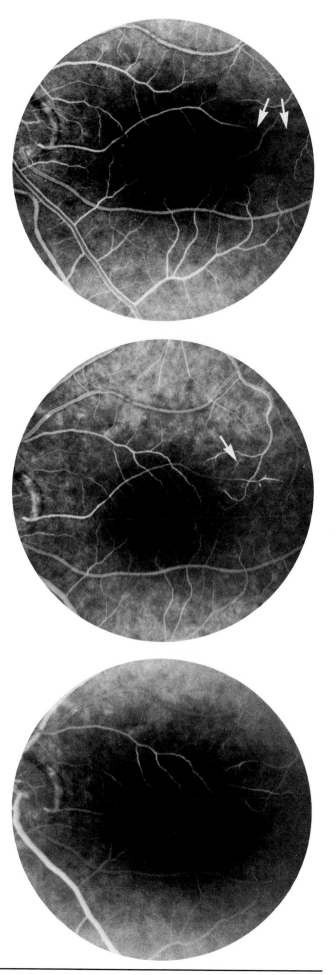

The arterio-venous phase of the angiogram shows some hyperfluorescence of the walls of several of the retinal arteries secondary to a breakdown in the blood-retinal barrier. There is some dilatation of the capillaries temporal to the macula (*arrow*).

Late angiogram shows irregularity in the fading of the fluorescent pattern in several of the retinal arterial branches.

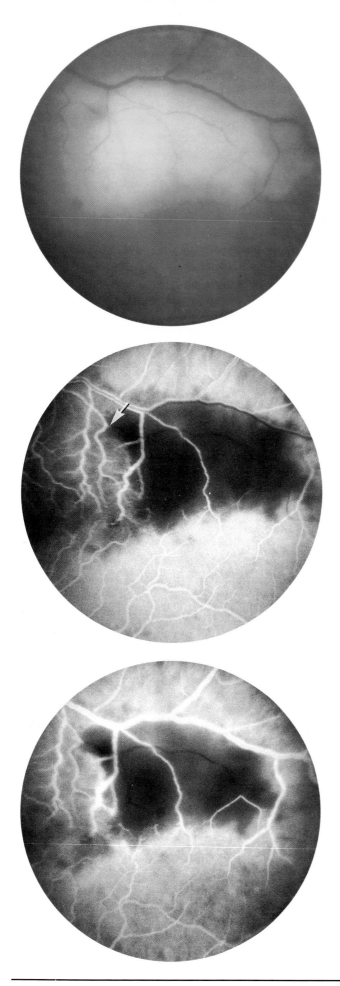

Small Branch Retinal Artery Occlusion (secondary to toxoplasmosis chorioretinitis)

A wedge-like area of ischemic retinal whitening can be seen. The view is somewhat obscured due to intraocular inflammation from ocular toxoplasmosis.

The normal choroidal filling cannot be seen due to the wedge-like blockage by the ischemic retinal whitening from a small branch artery occlusion (*arrow*). The laminar phase filling is obvious.

Late in the angiogram there is still significant blockage of the background fluorescence with delay of filling of the artery supplying this portion of the retina. The retinal branch veins show staining of the venous walls, indicating a breakdown in the blood-retinal barrier from inflammation.

AUTHOR'S NOTE:

This is a 22-year-old white female who has had repeated attacks of chorioretinitis from toxoplasmosis. The intraocular inflammation was brought under control with conventional treatment for ocular toxoplasmosis. However, an absolute scotoma remained, corresponding to the wedge-like area of occlusion.

Reader's Notes

Branch Retinal Artery Occlusion (secondary branch retinal vein involvement)

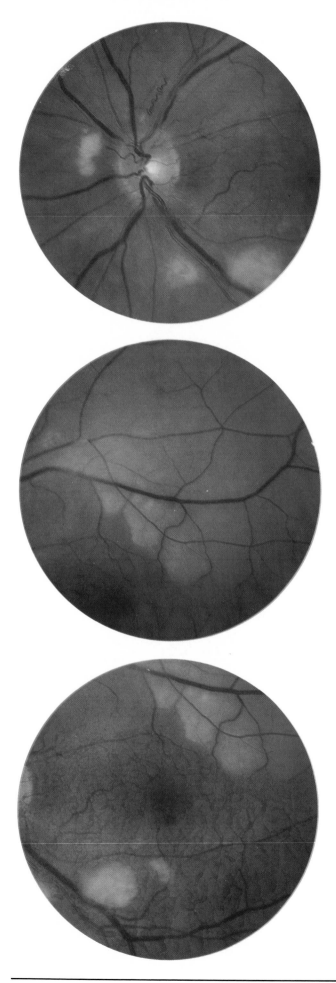

Multiple areas of cotton-wool spots can be seen. Irregular, tortuous, fine vessels are seen superior to the optic nerve and inferior temporal to the optic nerve along the inferior temporal arcade.

A definite embolus can be seen at the bifurcation of the superior temporal branch artery. Definite ischemic retinal whitening is present in the superior temporal quadrant.

The foveal region is spared as far as the occlusion is concerned.

The vessels in the papillomacular bundle show filling with the fluorescein dye. There is irregular filling of the superior temporal artery. The normal patchy choroidal filling can be seen. Areas of nonperfusion blocking the background fluorescence correspond to the cotton-wool spots seen on the color photograph or clinically.

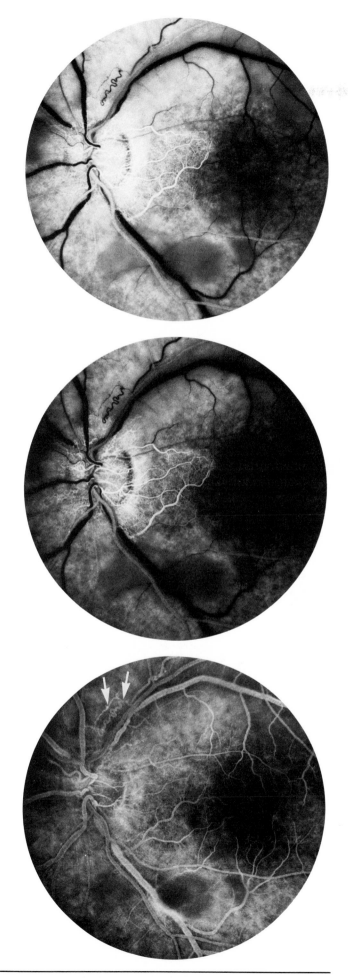

The superior temporal vein shows an irregular caliber. The fine tortuous vessels superior to the optic nerve do not fill with fluorescein dye during the arterial phase of the angiogram.

The areas of nonperfusion persist late in the angiogram. There is some staining of the wall of the inferior temporal vein adjacent to the area of nonperfusion. The fine tortuous vessels superior to the optic nerve are filled with fluorescein dye but do not leak. These vessels are compatible with collaterals (arrows).

AUTHOR'S NOTE

This patient shows definite retinal arterial occlusive disease with what appear to be secondary venous changes as evidenced by the irregularity of the superior temporal vein with collateralization around the arterio-venous crossing site. This patient had severe carotid artery disease and underwent endarterectomy.

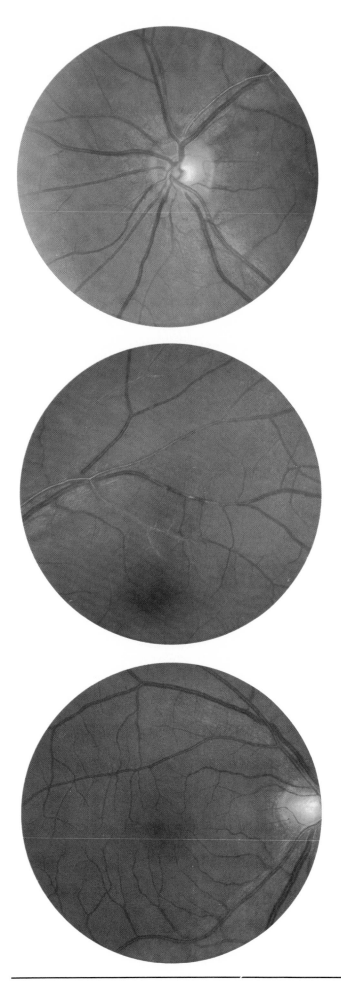

Possible Vasculitis—Etiology Unknown (with negative fluorescein angiographic findings)

The left optic nerve appears normal. The superior temporal branch artery shows an increased light reflex characteristic of what is referred to as "copper wiring." The remainder of the branches of the central retinal artery and central retinal vein appear normal.

The first two branches of the superior temporal retinal artery reveal marked narrowing and what appears to be almost complete occlusion with what is referred to as "silver wiring." The accompanying superior temporal vein reveals abnormal deposition of material on the surface of the venous wall which could be referred to as early "sheathing."

The right optic nerve, macular region, and retinal vasculature appear normal.

During the laminar phase of the angiogram, there is no evidence of abnormality in filling of the branch retinal arteries. The perifoveal capillaries appear to be intact.

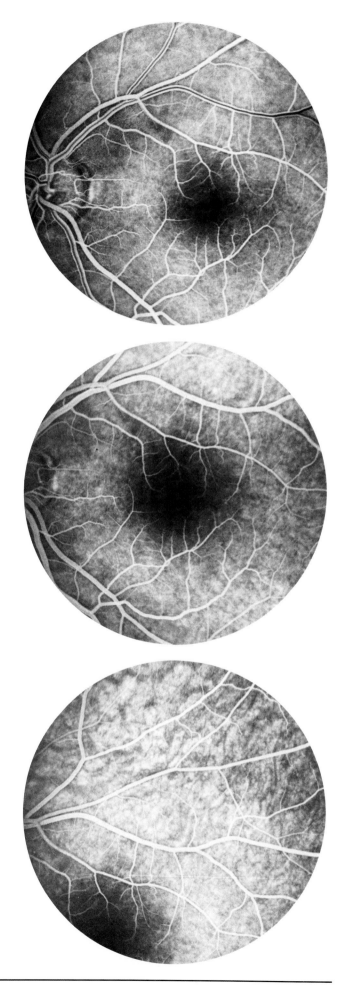

Later in the angiogram, there is a normal filling pattern of the retinal veins. There is no evidence of fluorescein leakage.

The late angiogram shows no staining of the vessel walls, either on the arterial or venous side of the circulation.

AUTHOR'S NOTE

This 35-year-old white male complained of intermittent changes of vision which appeared to be gray in color. Extensive medical work-up with particular attention being paid to hematologic, cardiovascular, and collagen vascular disorders was negative. The patient's vision was always 20/20 in the left eye. A scotoma could be mapped out corresponding to the area of retina associated with the vascular abnormality. However, fluorescein angiography has always been negative.

Branch Retinal Artery Occlusion (incomplete)

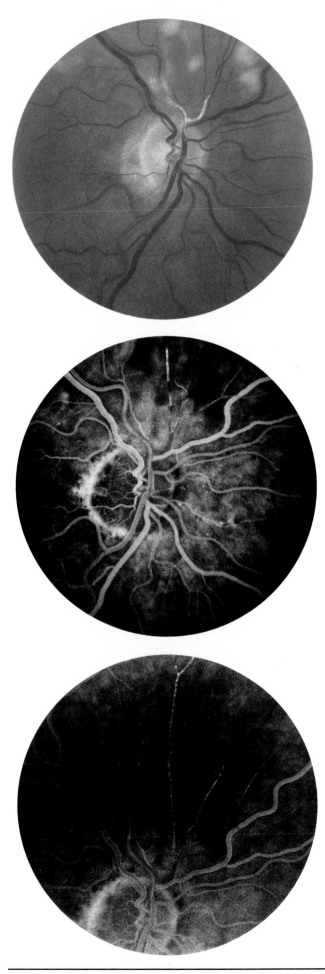

Embolization is present along the superior branch of the central retinal artery occlusion. Just distal to the embolization, areas of cotton-wool spots, or soft exudates, can be seen.

During the venous phase of the angiogram, there is delayed filling of the arterial branches superior to the optic nerve.

Very late in the angiogram there is blockage of the background choroidal fluorescence by the areas of nonperfusion corresponding to the soft exudates seen clinically. The more peripheral branches of the arterial tree show irregular filling with fluorescein dye, while some have no fluorescein molecules at all.

AUTHOR'S NOTE

Clinically, the changes in this patient resemble platelet embolization.

Retinal Arteriosclerosis

Arteriosclerosis is a general term referring to thickening and hardening of the arteries. Arteriolosclerosis and intimal atherosclerosis are the two most common types of arteriosclerosis affecting the retinal vessels. Arteriolosclerosis is related to systemic hypertension. Histologically, there is endothelial hyperplasia, intimal hyalinization, and medial hypertrophy.

In atherosclerosis, there is an atheroma, which is secondary to accumulation of fat-laden cells between the intimal elastic lamella and the endothelium of the arterial wall. Usually, the atheromas form in the retinal artery where the artery penetrates the dura on the optic nerve and in the cribriform lamella.

Hypertensive Retinopathy

Hypertensive retinopathy affects the retinal arteries, and different degrees of retinopathy develop depending on the severity of the hypertensive disease. The changes involving the artery consist primarily of generalized narrowing, focal constriction, and generalized sclerosis. Frequently, arterio-venous crossing changes are seen due to the common adventitial sheath around the artery and vein. Gunn's sign consists of an apparent compression of the vein by the overlying artery, and the Salus sign consists of a deflection in the course of the vein. The retinopathy changes vary depending upon the degree of hypertension.

Hypertensive Retinopathy

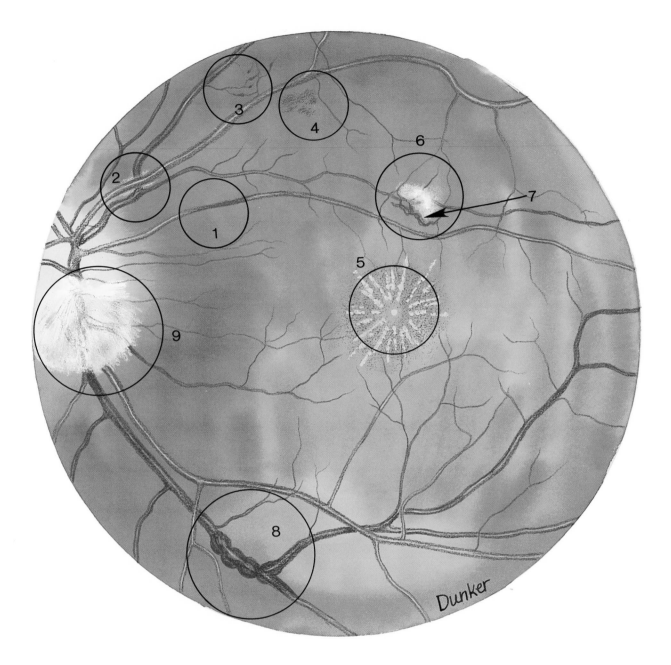

Clinical Groupings

Group I	1. Arterial narrowing 2. Arterio-venous nicking	Group IV	8. Venous engorgement 9. Disc edema
Group II	3. Microaneurysms 4. Intraretinal hemorrhage (splinter, dot, blotch) 5. Hard exudate		
Group III	6. Soft exudate 7. Intraretinal microvascular abnormalities (IRMA)		

AUTHOR'S NOTE

The above groups have been found to be useful in describing hypertensive retinopathy in terms of its minimal to its most severe presentation. These groupings are artificial, and frequently there is some overlap between the findings in the different groups.

Reader's Notes

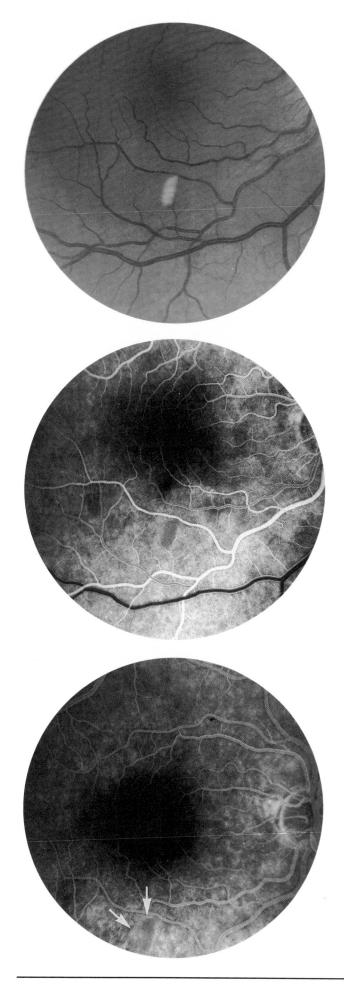

Hypertension (involvement at the capillary level)

A single area of soft exudate is present inferior to the macula. There does not appear to be any retinal vascular disease.

During the early laminar phase, there is an area of nonperfusion corresponding to the soft exudate seen clinically. This soft exudate appears to be secondary to a small capillary occlusion.

Late in the angiogram there is still an area of nonperfusion surrounded by some increased hyperfluorescence (*arrows*).

AUTHOR'S NOTE

Frequently, the walls of vessels adjacent to areas of capillary nonperfusion will stain with fluorescein, indicating a secondary effect on the vessel wall and the blood-retinal barrier. This patient is being treated for systemic hypertension.

Hypertension (splinter hemorrhages)

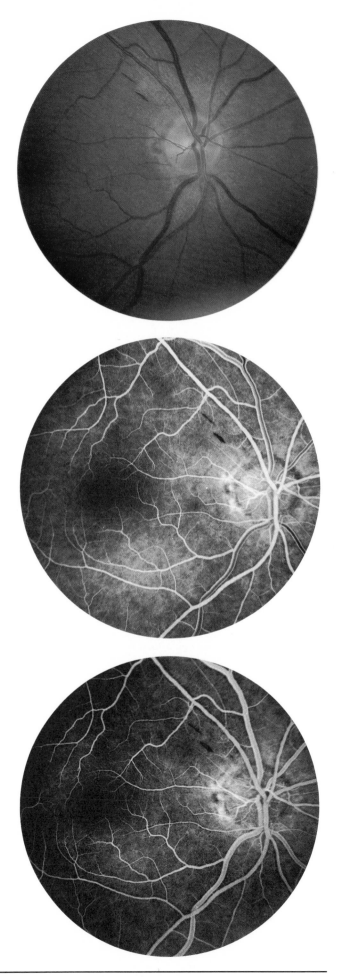

The retinal arteries appear slightly narrowed with an increased light reflex. Two splinter intraretinal hemorrhages are present along the superior temporal artery.

During the laminar phase of the angiogram the two splinter hemorrhages block the background choroidal fluorescence.

Late in the angiogram there is continued blockage of the background choroidal fluorescence by the intraretinal hemorrhage. No other significant retinal vascular disease appears to be present.

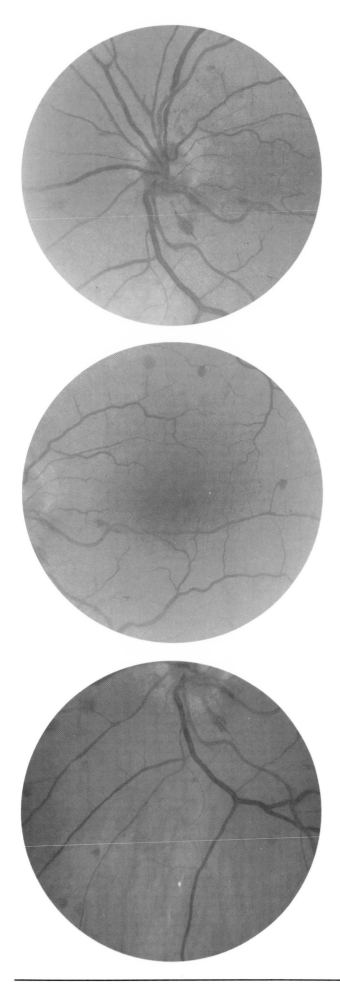

Hypertension (intraretinal hemorrhages, arterial changes, arterio-venous nicking changes)

The optic nerve is slightly hyperemic. Splinter hemorrhages can be seen. The retinal veins are slightly engorged.

Intraretinal blotch hemorrhages are present. The retinal artery passing through the posterior pole shows narrowing and irregularity.

Along the inferior temporal arcade there is significant arterio-venous nicking change. The more peripheral branches of the retinal artery are markedly attenuated and irregular.

The intraretinal hemorrhages in the posterior pole block the background choroidal fluorescence. The retinal artery passing inferior to the macula is irregular in caliber.

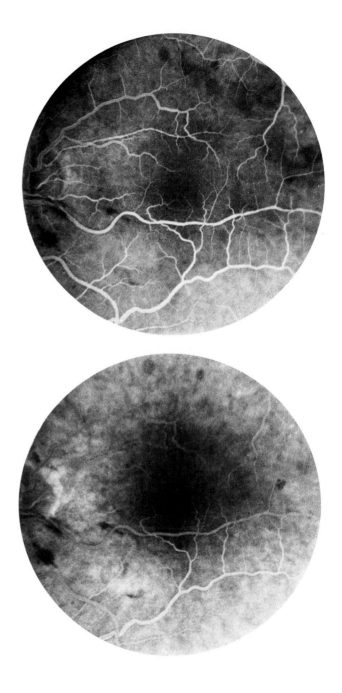

The late angiogram shows continued blockage of the background choroidal fluorescence by the intraretinal hemorrhages. These areas of blockage correspond to the hemorrhages seen clinically. There do not appear to be any areas of nonperfusion.

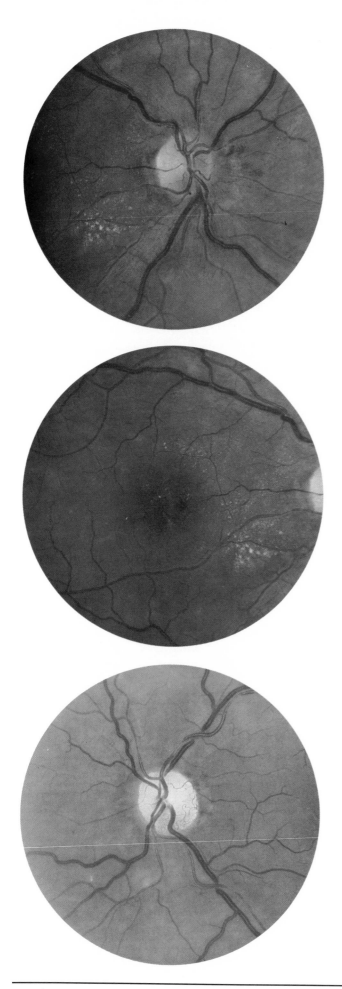

Hypertension (hard exudate, microaneurysms, marked arterial narrowing)

Branches of the central retinal artery are markedly narrowed and irregular. Nasal to the optic nerve are a few intraretinal hemorrhages.

In the papillomacular bundle there is intraretinal deposition of hard exudate.

The left eye shows evidence of optic atrophy with narrowing of the retinal arteries.

During the laminar phase of the fluorescein angiogram, the irregularity of the inferior temporal artery is obvious. The intraretinal hard exudates seen clinically have no effect on the fluorescein pattern.

There is dilatation of the capillary bed with micro-aneurysmal change inferior to the fovea.

The left eye shows staining of the atrophic optic nerve.

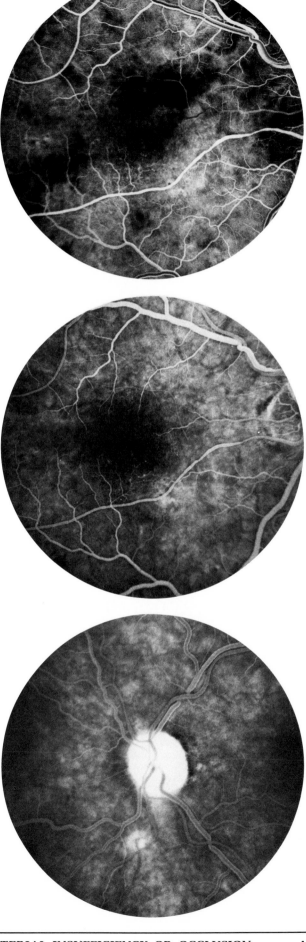

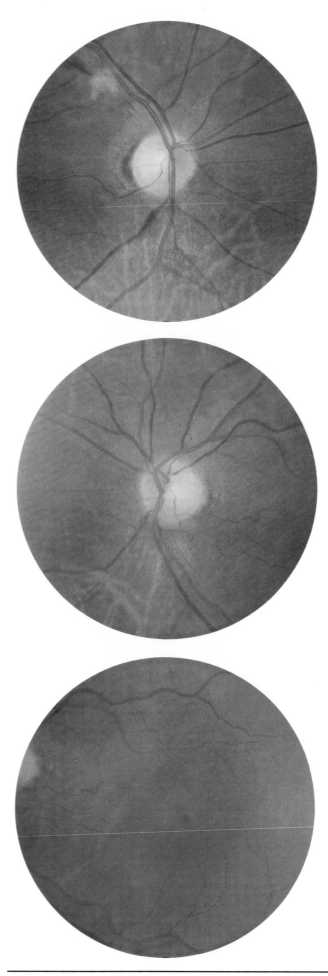

Hypertension (intraretinal hemorrhages, cotton-wool spots, macular edema)

Intraretinal hemorrhages and cotton-wool spots are evident in the right eye.

The retinal arteries are slightly narrowed in the left eye.

No significant abnormality appears to be present in the posterior pole of the left eye.

The intraretinal hemorrhages along the superior and inferior temporal arcades block the background choroidal fluorescence. There is dilatation of the capillary bed along the superior temporal arcade, near the splinter hemorrhage.

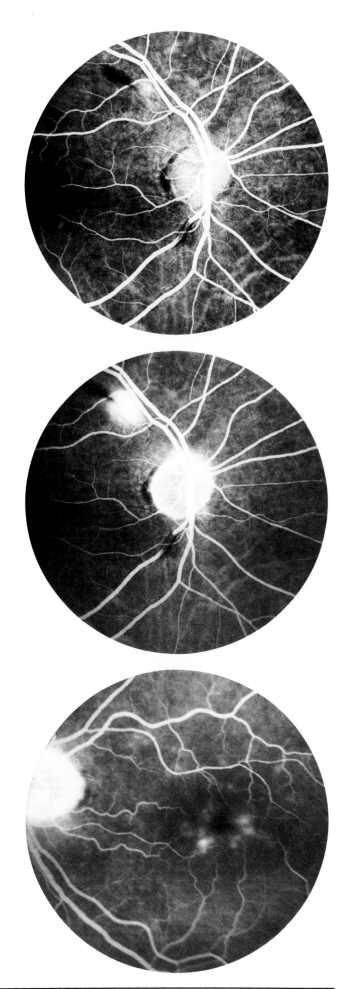

Later in the angiogram there is hyperfluorescence along the superior temporal arcade from the intraretinal microvascular abnormalities around the area of soft exudate. The intraretinal hemorrhages continue to block the background fluorescence.

The left eye shows leakage of fluorescein in the perifoveal region, indicating macular edema.

AUTHOR'S NOTE

The value of fluorescein angiography in this patient is clearly evident. Clinically, the left macular region appeared normal, although the vision was reduced to 20/60. The fluorescein angiogram of the left eye substantiates the presence of macular edema. Frequently, intraretinal microvascular abnormalities form around areas of nonperfusion or soft exudate.

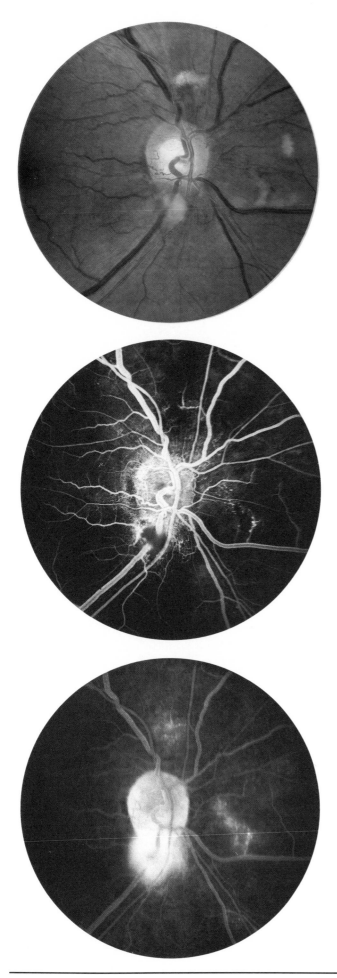

Hypertension (cotton-wool spots, marked arterial narrowing, IRMA, microaneurysms)

Multiple areas of soft exudate can be seen surrounding the optic nerve. The retinal arteries are markedly narrowed. Nasal to the optic nerve there are a few scattered microaneurysms and fine intraretinal microvascular abnormalities (IRMA).

The venous phase of the angiogram shows areas of nonperfusion corresponding to the soft exudates clinically. A few scattered microaneurysms and IRMA are seen in the vicinity of the areas of nonperfusion, especially nasally and at the inferior edge of the optic nerve.

Late in the angiogram there is leakage of fluorescein with hyperfluorescence from the microaneurysms and IRMA.

Reader's Notes

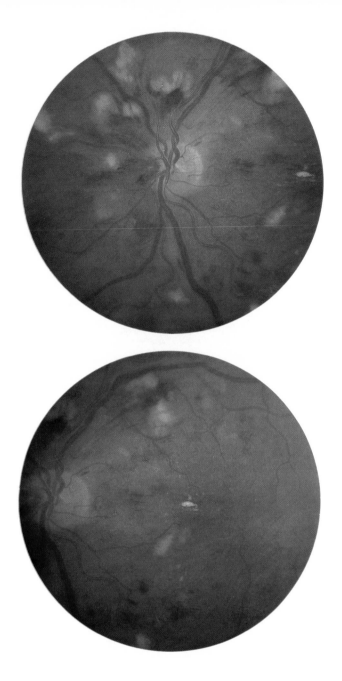

Hypertension (multiple hemorrhages and soft exudates, hard exudate, arterial narrowing, venous changes, microaneurysms, and IRMA)

Multiple intraretinal blotch and splinter hemorrhages are present. There are numerous cotton-wool spots or soft exudate. The retinal arteries are narrowed, and the retinal veins show some engorgement with "sausaging" changes. This is apparent along the superior temporal vein.

Intraretinal hard exudate can be seen in the perifoveal region. Scattered microaneurysms are present.

During the laminar phase of the fluorescein angiogram there are multiple areas of nonperfusion corresponding to the soft exudates clinically. There are numerous microaneurysms and IRMA throughout the posterior pole and surrounding the zones of nonperfusion.

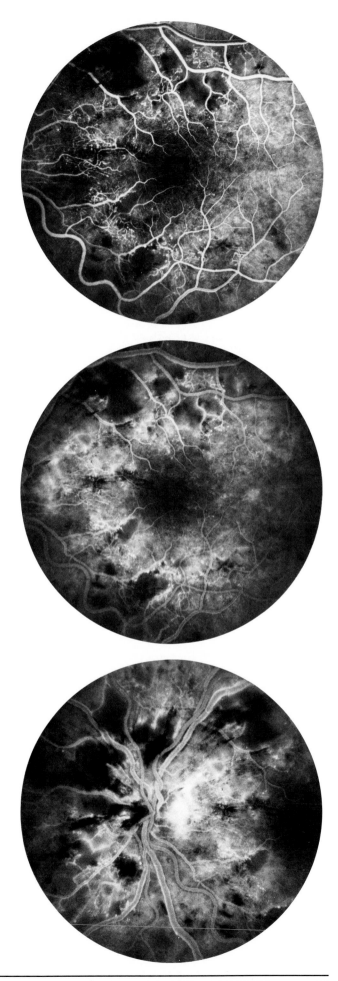

Later in the angiogram there is intraretinal leakage of fluorescein in the posterior pole from the microaneurysms and IRMA.

Late venous phase of the optic nerve area shows staining of the venous walls due to a breakdown of the blood-retinal barrier. There is diffuse intraretinal accumulation of the fluorescein dye from leaking microaneurysms and IRMA. The intraretinal hemorrhages block the background choroidal fluorescence, and many areas of nonperfusion persist.

AUTHOR'S NOTE
This patient had severe systemic hypertension, untreated, at the time of ophthalmic evaluation.

Hypertension (soft exudates, intraretinal hemorrhages, IRMA microaneurysms, and intraretinal hard exudate)

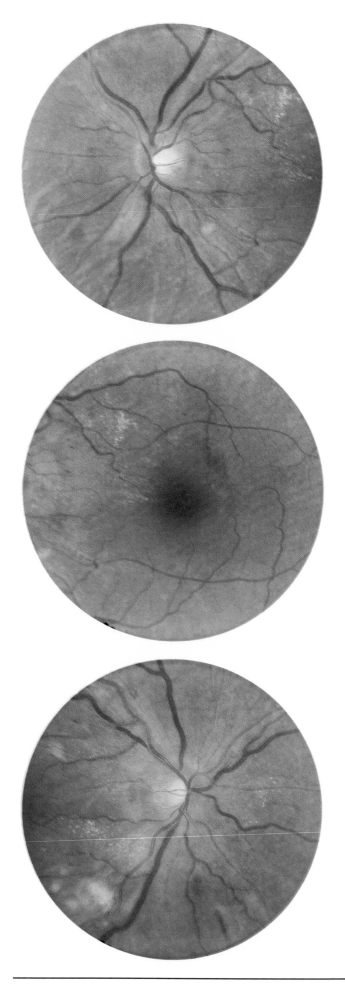

Surrounding the left optic nerve are a few scattered areas of soft exudate. Surrounding the areas of soft exudate are intraretinal microvascular abnormalities. Inferior nasal to the optic nerve there is intraretinal hemorrhage. The retinal arteries are definitely narrowed with arterio-venous (A-V) nicking changes.

Nasal to the macula is deposition of intraretinal hard exudate. A few scattered microaneurysms can also be seen in the posterior pole.

Branches of the central retinal artery in the right eye are narrowed with A-V nicking changes. There is deposition of intraretinal hard exudate both nasal and temporal to the optic nerve. Along the inferior temporal arcades are areas of soft exudate surrounded by IRMA. There are scattered areas of intraretinal splinter and blotch hemorrhages.

During the laminar phase of the fluorescein angiogram in the left eye there is dilatation of the capillary bed. There are areas of capillary dropout and nonperfusion. Along the inferior temporal artery there is evidence of intraretinal microvascular abnormalities.

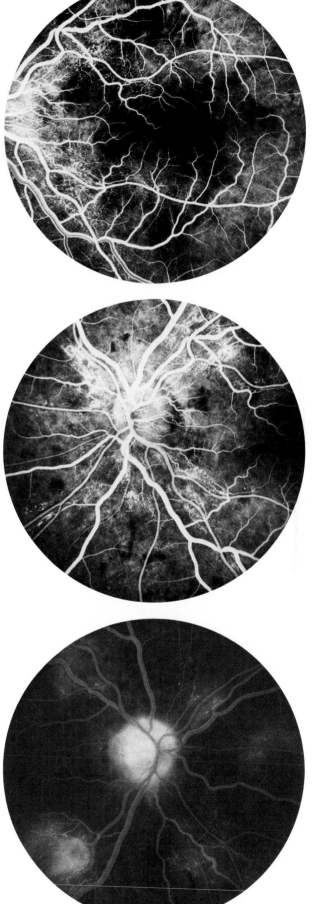

Later in the angiogram the IRMA surrounding the optic nerve are clearly visible. There is some very slight leakage from some of the microaneurysms, IRMA, and dilated capillaries. The intraretinal hemorrhages block the background choroidal fluorescence.

The late angiogram of the right optic nerve shows some staining of the optic nerve tissue secondary to dilated leaking capillaries. A few scattered microaneurysms can also be seen. Along the inferior temporal arcade there is an area of increased hyperfluorescence from IRMA surrounding an area of soft exudate seen clinically.

Hypertension (disc edema)

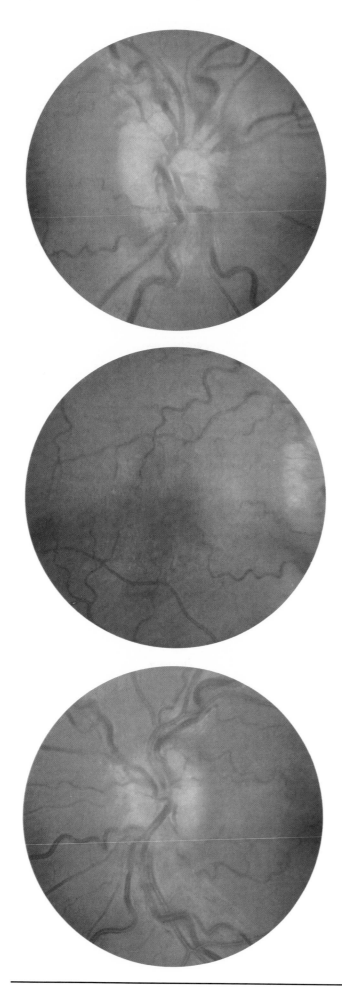

The right optic nerve shows a pale disc edema with blurred disc margins.

In the posterior pole the retinal arteries are narrowed. Pigment epithelial mottling change is also present.

The left optic nerve shows blurred disc margins with a pale disc edema. The retinal arteries are slightly narrowed with slight engorgement of the retinal veins.

The capillaries on the surface of the right optic nerve are dilated.

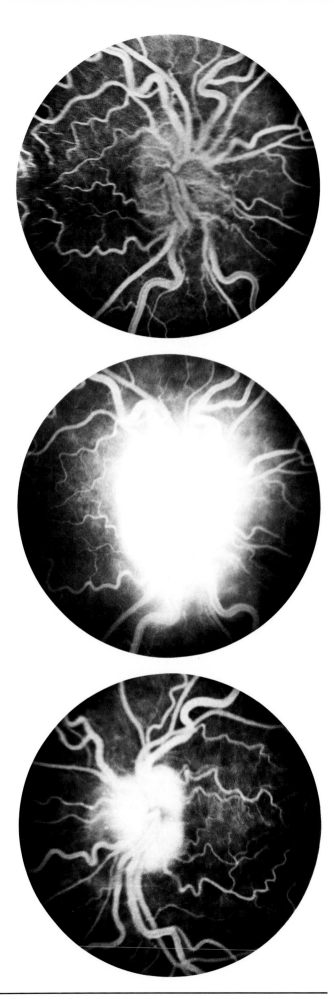

Late in the angiogram there is diffuse leakage of fluorescein and staining of the optic nerve tissue, indicating disc edema.

The left optic nerve also shows marked hyperfluorescence due to leakage of the capillaries, indicating disc edema.

AUTHOR'S NOTE
This patient had severe hypertension and underwent a renal transplant.

Hypertension (pretreatment)

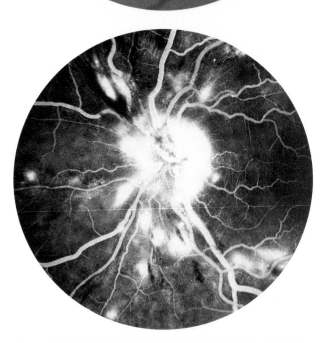

The left optic nerve is hyperemic with blurred disc margins. There are multiple intraretinal hemorrhages surrounding the nerve. The retinal veins are engorged, and the retinal arteries are attenuated. Significant arterio-venous nicking changes are present.

There is thickening of the sensory retina secondary to intraretinal edema with deposition of hard exudate encroaching toward the fovea.

The intraretinal hemorrhages block the background choroidal fluorescence. There is diffuse leakage of fluorescein from the dilated capillaries on the surface of the nerve, indicating disc edema. Late leakage from scattered microaneurysms is also present.

Hypertension (post-treatment)

The optic nerve shows sharp disc margins with normal color. The retinal veins are less engorged. The retinal arteries are not as attenuated as in the pretreatment state.

There is less retinal edema and, therefore, less sensory retinal thickening. There is residual intraretinal hard exudate.

The fluorescein angiogram shows virtually no significant retinal vascular disease. There is no significant leakage from dilated capillaries on the surface of the nerve or microaneurysmal change.

AUTHOR'S NOTE

The post-treatment color photographs and fluorescein angiogram were done 6 weeks after intensive antihypertensive treatment.

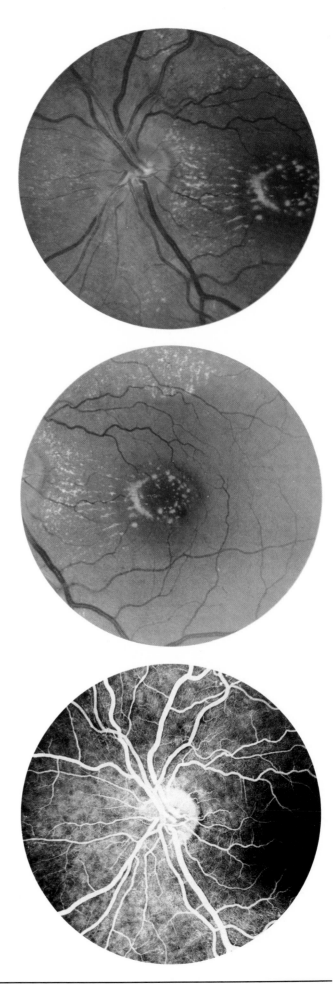

Hypertension (pretreatment)

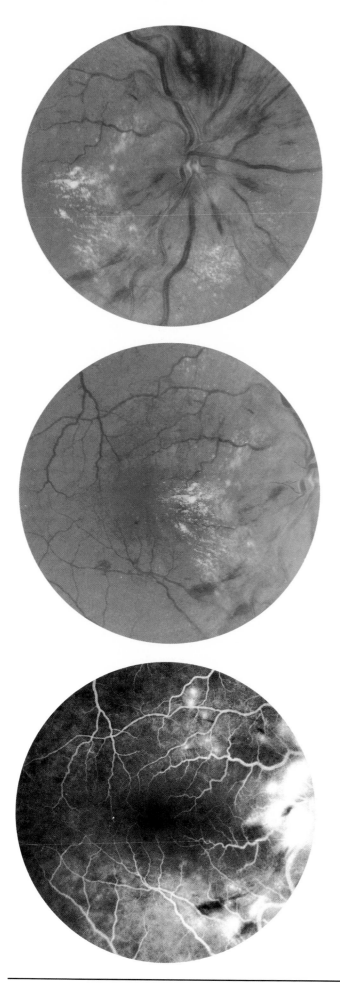

The right optic nerve is hyperemic with blurred disc margins. There are multiple intraretinal hemorrhages surrounding the nerve. The retinal veins are engorged and show some sausaging changes. The retinal arteries are narrowed with prominent A-V nicking changes.

Sensory retinal edema with deposition of hard exudate extending toward the fovea is present. There are scattered intraretinal blotch and splinter hemorrhages.

There is diffuse leakage of fluorescein from dilated capillaries on the surface of the nerve with staining of the optic nerve tissue, indicating disc edema. Intraretinal hemorrhage blocks the background choroidal fluorescence. There are scattered areas of microaneurysmal change and intraretinal microvascular abnormalities which diffusely leak fluorescein intraretinally.

Hypertension (post-treatment)

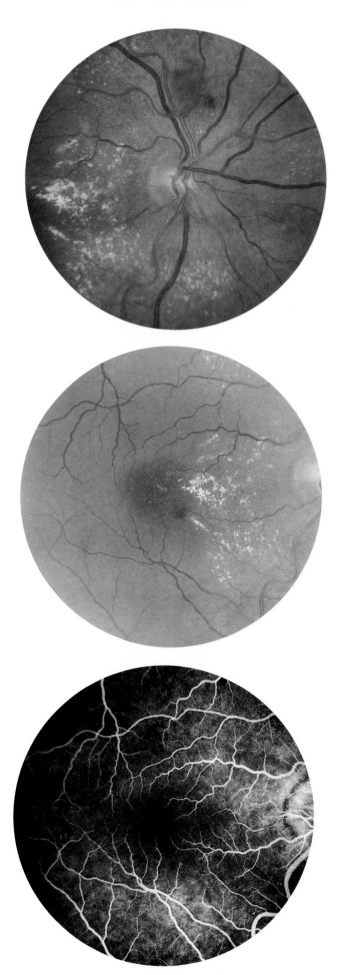

The optic nerve shows sharp disc margins with normal color. The retinal veins are of normal caliber. There is some slight narrowing of the retinal arteries with A-V nicking changes.

Residual hard exudate can be seen in the posterior pole and paramacular region. There is essentially no thickening of the sensory retina from retinal edema.

The fluorescein angiogram shows no significant leakage from the optic nerve. The retinal vascular changes are very minimal with a few scattered microaneurysms being present.

AUTHOR'S NOTE

There was significant improvement in visual acuity in both eyes of this patient due to the reduction of macular edema and disc edema secondary to aggressive antihypertensive treatment.

Reader's Notes

Giant Cell Arteritis (temporal arteritis)

Visual loss in this disorder results from involvement of the ophthalmic artery and its branches. Frequently, there is simultaneous involvement of the temporal artery or other branches of the carotid system. Many investigators feel that the internal elastic lamina must be present for the vessels to be affected in this inflammatory process. Therefore, the retinal arteries frequently are not directly involved. Often, elderly patients develop ischemic optic neuropathy. In a significant number of cases, there may be no evidence of temporal artery involvement, but there is an elevated erythrocyte sedimentation rate.

Therefore, all elderly patients with ischemic optic neuropathy or central retinal artery occlusion with an elevated sedimentation rate should be considered as having giant cell arteritis until proven otherwise.

Three of the more common disorders in which ischemic optic neuropathy is seen are:

1. Giant cell arteritis
2. Diabetes mellitus
3. Systemic hypertension

Normal Optic Nerve

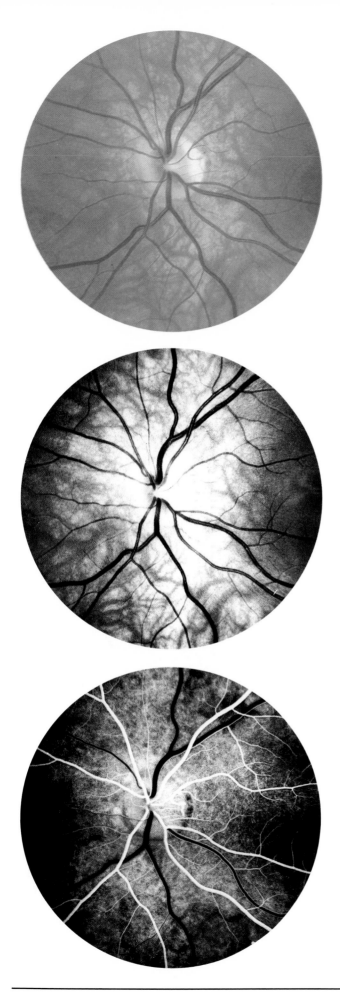

There is evidence of peripapillary atrophy. Therefore, the disc margins do not appear very sharp. There is a normal arterio-venous ratio.

The red-free photograph shows the lack of pigmentation of the pigment epithelium surrounding the optic nerve with the peripapillary atrophy being quite evident. The larger choroidal vessels can also be seen.

The normal patchy choroidal phase can be seen with the retinal arteries filling in a normal fashion.

The laminar phase of the angiogram shows no significant abnormalities of the retinal vessels. The normal optic nerve capillaries are filled with fluorescein.

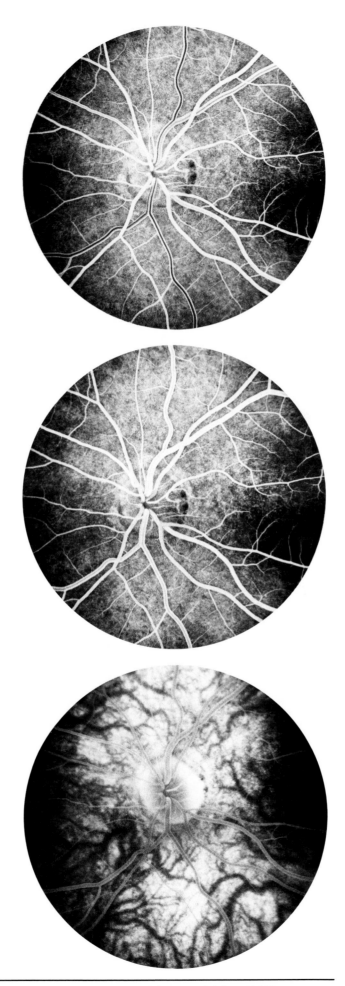

The arterio-venous phase of the angiogram shows increased hyperfluorescence from the choroid in the vicinity of the optic nerve due to lack of pigmentation of the pigment epithelium. The disc margin appears relatively sharp.

The late phase of the angiogram shows the larger choroidal vessels. There is a ring of hyperfluorescence surrounding the optic nerve corresponding to the peripapillary atrophy. However, there is no leakage of fluorescein dye or staining of the optic nerve tissue.

AUTHOR'S NOTE

A normal nerve with peripapillary atrophy is demonstrated to point out the confusion that frequently exists between hyperfluorescence around the nerve and hyperfluorescence due to disc edema and staining of the optic nerve tissue.

Ischemic Optic Neuropathy
(secondary to giant cell arteritis)

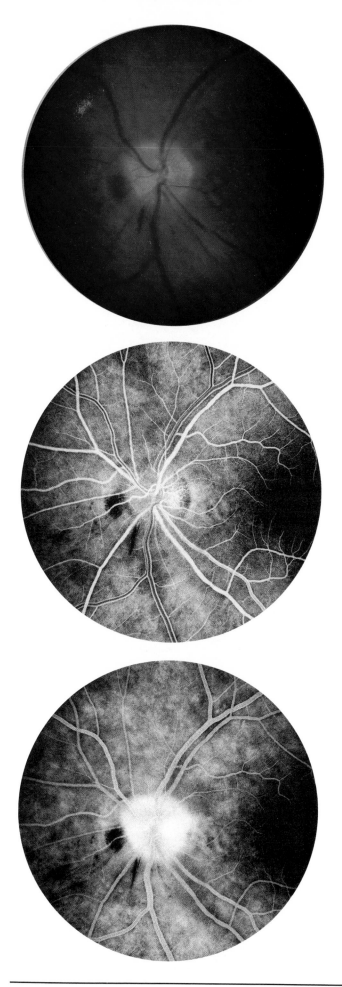

The optic nerve shows a pale disc edema with blurred disc margins. The retinal arteries are markedly attenuated and irregular. Scattered blotch and splinter hemorrhages are present. Temporal to the optic nerve there is intraretinal deposition of hard exudate.

During the laminar phase of the angiogram there is blockage of the background choroidal fluorescence by the intraretinal hemorrhages on the nasal aspect of the optic nerve. The capillaries on the surface of the nerve are dilated.

There is leakage of fluorescein from the dilated optic nerve capillaries with staining of the optic nerve tissue, indicating disc edema. The intraretinal hemorrhages continue to block the background choroidal fluorescence.

AUTHOR'S NOTE

This patient was 75 years of age with a markedly elevated sedimentation rate and a positive temporal artery biopsy for giant cell arteritis.

Optic Atrophy (secondary to ischemic optic neuropathy in association with giant cell arteritis)

The optic nerve shows definite atrophy. There is some slight narrowing and irregularity of the retinal arteries.

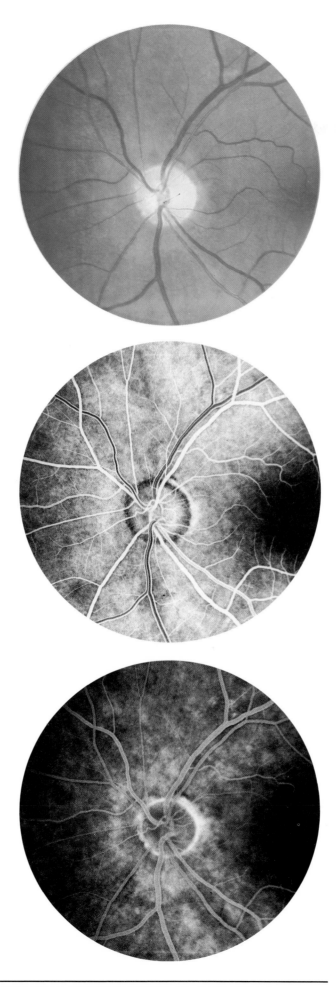

During the laminar phase of the angiogram the disc margin appears sharp. The retinal arteries are slightly narrowed.

The late angiogram shows some hyperfluorescence surrounding the optic nerve due to a rim of peripapillary atrophy. There appears to be a lack of normal staining of the optic nerve tissue due to a lack of capillaries in association with optic atrophy.

AUTHOR'S NOTE

This is the picture of the previous patient with ischemic optic neuropathy 3 months after onset of symptoms.

Ischemic Optic Neuropathy
(progression from a stage of venous stasis retinopathy)

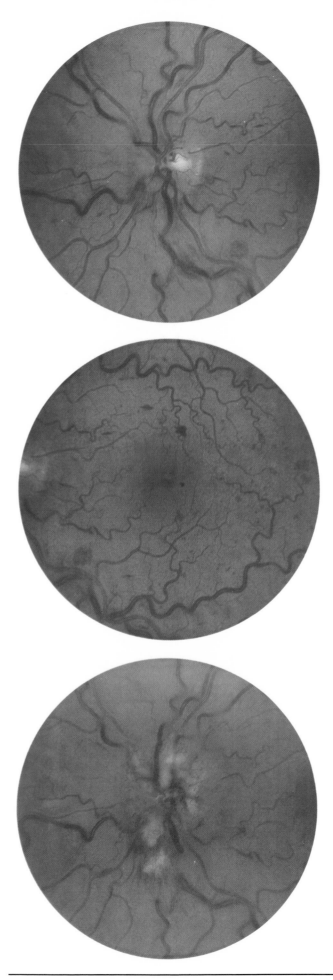

The optic nerve is slightly hyperemic with slightly blurred disc margins. The retinal veins are significantly tortuous and engorged. A-V nicking changes are prominent.

Branches of the retinal vein are markedly tortuous. Multiple intraretinal dot and blotch hemorrhages are present. There is no significant macular edema.

One year later the disc margins are definitely blurred with a pale disc edema. The optic nerve is surrounded by soft exudate. The retinal veins are engorged and tortuous.

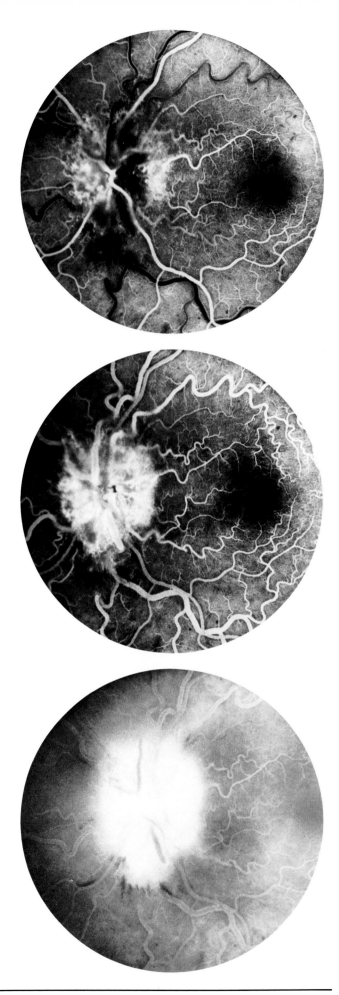

Capillaries on the surface of the optic nerve are significantly dilated. There are areas of nonperfusion on the surface of the nerve and inferior to the nerve, corresponding to the soft exudate seen clinically.

There is leakage of fluorescein from the dilated capillaries on the surface of the nerve. In the posterior pole there are punctate areas of blocked hyperfluorescence due to the small intraretinal dot hemorrhages.

The late angiogram shows diffuse leakage of fluorescein from the dilated optic nerve capillaries with staining of the optic nerve tissue.

AUTHOR'S NOTE

This patient was found to have severe carotid artery disease on the left side, and endarterectomy was recommended.

Ischemic Optic Neuropathy
(secondary to generalized arteriosclerosis and carotid artery disease)

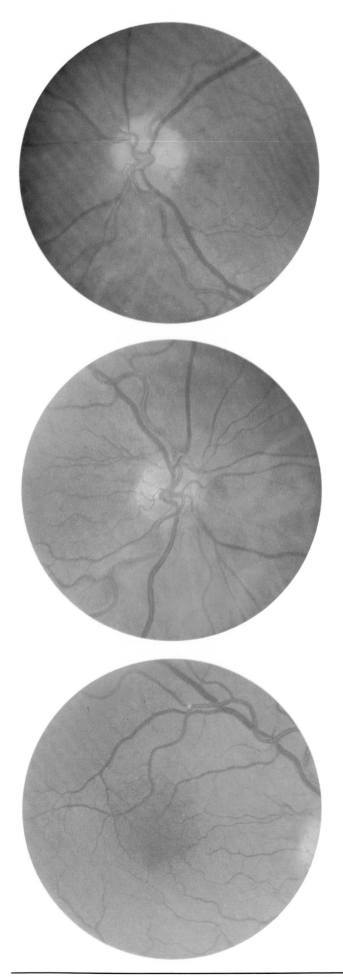

The optic nerve shows some blurriness of the disc margins with a pale disc edema at the superior pole and hyperemia secondary to dilated capillaries at the inferior pole. The retinal arteries are slightly narrowed.

The right eye shows a normal optic nerve with sharp disc margins.

In the right eye there is a glistening embolus at the bifurcation of the superior temporal artery.

AUTHOR'S NOTE

Ischemic optic neuropathy frequently presents clinically with a segment of the optic nerve appearing hyperemic while the remaining part of the nerve appears pale.

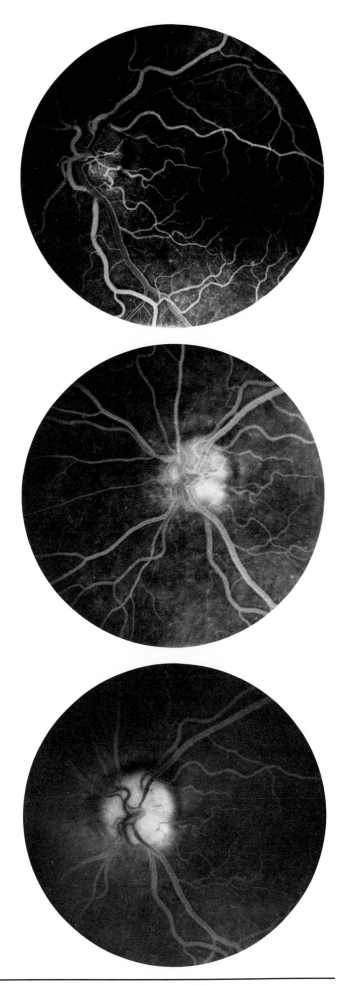

Fluorescein angiography during the early laminar phase of the left eye shows dilatation of the capillaries at the inferior pole of the optic nerve with lack of capillary filling on the superior aspect of the nerve.

During the venous phase of the angiogram there is diffuse leakage of fluorescein from the dilated capillaries.

The late angiogram shows diffuse hyperfluorescence and leakage of fluorescein with staining of the optic nerve tissue, indicating disc edema.

AUTHOR'S NOTE

On angiography this clinical finding is substantiated by dilated capillaries corresponding to the hyperemic aspect of the nerve and lack of capillary filling corresponding to the atrophic portion of the nerve. Invariably, patients with ischemic optic neuropathy have a prominent afferent pupillary defect on the side of the ischemic optic neuropathy.

Ischemic Optic Neuropathy
(secondary to diabetes mellitus)

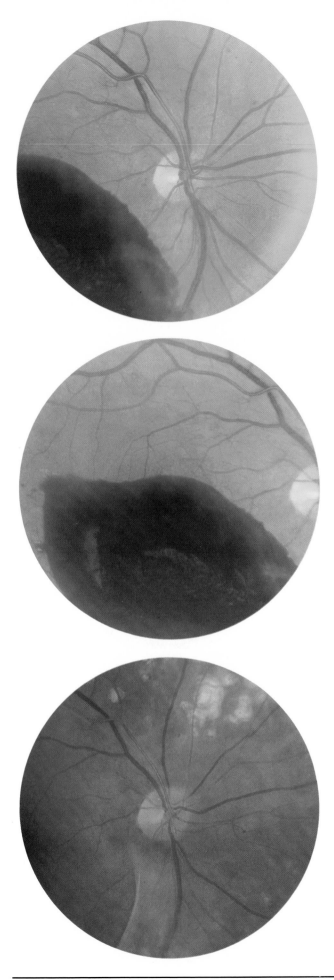

The optic nerve appears normal. Superior nasal to the optic nerve are punctate microaneurysms and a few scattered intraretinal dot hemorrhages.

A preretinal hemorrhage obscures the macula.

The optic nerve appears normal. Panretinal photocoagulation scars can be seen. Fibrous tissue extends from the inferior pole of the optic nerve along the inferior temporal arcade.

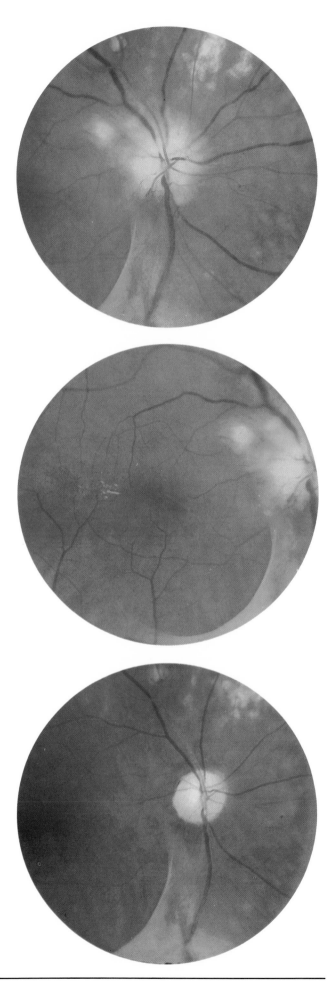

A pale disc edema with blurred disc margins can be seen. The retinal arteries are narrowed.

A few scattered microaneurysms and intraretinal hard exudate are present in the posterior pole. Fibrous tissue extends from the inferior pole of the ischemic optic nerve along the inferior temporal arcade.

Three months later there is optic atrophy with a very attenuated retinal artery.

AUTHOR'S NOTE

This 32-year-old juvenile-onset diabetic presented with finger-counting vision due to a preretinal hemorrhage overlying the macula. Vision improved to 20/20 after panretinal photocoagulation and absorption of the preretinal and vitreous hemorrhage. The vision eventually dropped to light perception secondary to optic atrophy in association with ischemic optic neuropathy. The course from initial examination to the stage of optic atrophy was 24 months.

Bibliography

Acacio I, Goldberg MF: Peripapillary and macular vessel occlusions in sickle cell anemia. *Am J Ophthalmol* 75:861–866, 1973.

Anderson B, Vallotton W: Etiology and therapy of retinal vascular occlusions. *Arch Ophthalmol* 54:6, 1955.

Anderson JD, Lubow M: Atrial myxoma as a source of retinal embolism. *Am J Ophthalmol* 76:769, 1973.

Anderson RG, Gray EB: Spasm of the central retinal artery in Raynaud's disease: Report of a case. *Arch Ophthalmol* 17:662, 1937.

Appen RE, Wray SH, Cogan DG: Central retinal artery occlusion. *Am J Ophthalmol* 79:374, 1975.

Arden GB, Greaves DP: The reversible alterations of the electroretinogram of the rabbit after occlusion of the retinal circulation. *J Physiol (Lond)* 133:266, 1956.

Ashton N: The eye in malignant hypertension. *Trans Am Acad Ophthalmol Otolaryngol* 76:17, 1972.

Atlee WE Jr: Talc and cornstarch emboli in eyes of drug abusers. *JAMA* 219:49, 1972.

Augsburger JJ, Magargal LE: Visual prognosis following treatment of acute central retinal artery obstruction. *Br J Ophthalmol* 64:913–917, 1980.

Ball CJ: Atheromatous embolism to the brain, retina and choroid. *Arch Ophthalmol* 76:690, 1966.

Boeck J: Ocular changes in periarteritis nodosa. *Am J Ophthalmol* 42:567, 1956.

Breshin DJ, Gifford RW, Fairbairn JF, et al: Prognostic importance of ophthalmoscopic findings in essential hypertension. *JAMA* 195:91, 1966.

Brown GC, Magargal LE, Shields JA, et al: Retinal arterial obstruction in children and young adults. *Ophthalmology* 88:18–25, 1981.

Brown GC, Shields JA: Cilioretinal arteries and retinal arterial occlusion. *Arch Ophthalmol* 97:84–92, 1979.

Brucker AJ: Disk and peripheral retinal neovascularization secondary to talc and cornstarch emboli. *Am J Ophthalmol* 88:864, 1979.

Byers B: Blindness secondary to steroid injections into the nasal turbinates. *Arch Ophthalmol* 97:79, 1979.

Chopdar A: Multiple major retinal vascular occlusions in sickle cell haemoglobin C disease. *Br J Ophthalmol* 59:493, 1975.

Coverdale HV: The cause and results of obstruction of the central artery of the retina: A study of eleven cases. *Br J Ophthalmol* 13:529–571, 1929.

David NJ, Norton EWD, Gass JDM, et al: Fluorescein angiography in central retinal artery occlusion. *Arch Ophthalmol* 77:619–629, 1967.

David NJ, Norton EWD, Gass JDM, et al: Fluorescein retinal angiography in carotid occlusion. *Arch Neurol* 14:281, 1966.

Delaney WV Jr, Torrisi PE: Occlusive retinal vascular disease and deafness. *Am J Ophthalmol* 82:232, 1976.

Dunphy EB: Ocular manifestations of Raynaud's disease. *Trans Am Ophthalmol Soc* 30:420, 1932.

Ellis PP: Occlusion of the central retinal artery after retrobulbar corticosteroid injection. *Am J Ophthalmol* 85:352, 1978.

Friberg TR, Gragoudas ES, Regan CDJ: Talc emboli and macular ischemia in intravenous drug abuse. *Arch Ophthalmol* 97:1089, 1979.

Gass JD: A fluorescein angiography study of macular dysfunction secondary to retinal vascular disease. III. Hypertensive retinopathy. *Arch Ophthalmol* 80:569, 1968.

Givner E, Jaffee N: Occlusion of the central retinal artery following anesthesia. *Arch Ophthalmol* 43:197, 1950.

Godfrey RC: Occlusion of the retinal artery in two cases of orbital granuloma. *Br J Ophthalmol* 53:703, 1969.

Gold D: Retinal arterial occlusion. *Trans Am Acad Ophthalmol Otolaryngol* 83:392–408, 1977.

Gresser EB: Partial occlusion of retinal vessels in a case of thromboangitis obliterans. *Am J Ophthalmol* 15:235, 1932.

Hamasaki DI, Kroll AJ: Experimental central retinal artery occlusion: An electrophysiological study. *Arch Ophthalmol* 80:243, 1968.

Hayreh SS: Pathogenesis of visual field defects: Role of the ciliary circulation. *Br J Ophthalmol* 54:289–311, 1970.

Hayreh SS, Kolder HE, Weingeist TA: Central retinal artery occlusion and retinal tolerance time. *Ophthalmology* 87:75–78, 1980.

Henkes HE: Electroretinography in circulatory disturbances of the retina. II. The electroretinogram in cases of occlusion of the central retinal artery or one of its branches. *Arch Ophthalmol* 51:42–53, 1954.

Hollenhorst RW: Significance of bright plaques in the retinal arterioles. *Trans Am Ophthalmol Soc* 59:252, 1961.

Hollenhorst RW: Carotid and vertebral-basilar arterial stenosis and occlusion: Neuro-ophthalmologic considerations. *Trans Am Acad Ophthalmol Otolaryngol* 66:166, 1962.

Hollenhorst RW, Lesink ER, Whisnant JP: Experimental embolization of retinal arterioles. *Trans Am Ophthalmol Soc* 60:316, 1962.

Honour AJ, Russell RR: Intra-arterial embolism in response to injury. *Trans Ophthalmol Soc U K* 81:451, 1961.

Ide CH, Almond CH, Hart WM, et al: Hematogenous dissemination of microemboli: Eye findings in a patient with Starr-Edwards aortic prosthesis. *Arch Ophthalmol* 76:769, 1973.

Inkeles DM, Walsh JB: Retinal fat emboli as a sequela to acute pancreatitis. *Am J Ophthalmol* 80:935, 1975.

Irinoda K: *Colour Atlas and Criteria of Fundus Changes in Hypertension.* Philadelphia, Lippincott, 1970.

Jampol LM, Condon P, Dizon-Moore R, et al: Salmon-patch hemorrhages after central retinal artery occlusion in sickle cell disease. *Arch Ophthalmol* 99:237–240, 1981.

Jampol LM, Wong AS, Albert DL: Atrial myxoma and central retinal artery occlusion. *Am J Ophthalmol* 75:242, 1973.

Karjalainen K: Occlusion of the central retinal artery and retinal branch arterioles. A clinical, tonographic, and fluorescein angiographic study of 175 patients. *Acta Ophthalmol (Suppl)* 109:1971.

Keith NM, Wagener HP, Barker NW: Some different types of essential hypertension: Their course and prognosis. *Am J Med Sci* 197:332, 1939.

Kelley JS, Randall HG: Peripheral retinal neovascularization in rheumatic fever. *Arch Ophthalmol* 97:81, 1979.

Kollarits CR, Lubow M, Hissong SL: Retinal strokes. *JAMA* 222:1273, 1972.

Krapin D: Occlusion of the central retinal artery in migraine. *N Engl J Med* 270:359, 1964.

Kraushar MF, Seelenfreund MH, Freilich DB: Central retinal artery closure during orbital hemorrhage from retrobulbar injection. *Trans Am Acad Ophthalmol Otolaryngol* 78:65–70, 1974.

Kresca LJ, Goldberg MF, Jampol LM: Talc emboli and retinal neovascularization in a drug abuser. *Am J Ophthalmol* 87:334, 1979.

Kroll AJ: Experimental central retinal artery occlusion. *Arch Ophthalmol* 79:453, 1968.

Lee J, and Sapira J: Retinal and cerebral microembolization of talc in a drug abuser. *Am J Med Sci* 265:75, 1973.

Leffertstra LJ: Results of early treatment in a case of spasm of the central retinal artery. *Ophthalmologica* 144:433, 1962.

Leishman R: The eye in general vascular disease: Hypertension and arteriosclerosis. *Br J Ophthalmol* 41:641, 1957.

Liversedge LA, Smith VH: Neuromedical and ophthalmic aspects of central retinal artery occlusion. *Trans Ophthalmol Soc U K* 82:571, 1962.

Lorentzen SE: Occlusion of the central retinal artery: A follow-up. *Acta Ophthalmol* 47:690–703, 1969.

Magargal LE, Goldberg RE: Anterior chamber paracentesis in the management of acute central retinal artery obstruction. *Br J Ophthalmol* 64:913–917, 1980.

McLeod D: Cilioretinal arterial circulation in central retinal vein occlusion. *Br J Ophthalmol* 60:419–427, 1976.

CHAPTER 2

Venous Insufficiency or Occlusion

Differential Diagnosis

A. ARTERIOSCLEROSIS
B. HYPERTENSION
C. DIABETES MELLITUS
D. OPEN ANGLE GLAUCOMA
E. HYPERVISCOSITY
F. SUDDEN DECREASE IN BLOOD PRESSURE
G. SEVERE BLOOD LOSS

H. BLOOD DYSCRASIAS
I. INFLAMMATION (EALES' DISEASE; SARCOIDOSIS; BEHÇET'S SYNDROME; PAPILLOPHLEBITIS, ETC.)
J. VENOUS STASIS RETINOPATHY
K. SECONDARY TO METASTATIC FUNGAL CHORIORETINITIS

Retinal Vein Occlusion

Occlusion, or obstruction, of the retinal venous side of the circulation can be conveniently divided into central retinal vein occlusions and branch retinal vein occlusions. Patients who develop a central retinal vein occlusion usually are aware of a sudden, painless loss of vision in the involved eye. However, some patients may be unaware of the obstruction if the macular area has been spared. In these patients, the vision may be normal or minimally affected. The exact mechanism of central retinal vein occlusions still remains in question. There seem to be numerous factors which can give the clinical funduscopic appearance of what we term a central retinal vein occlusion.

Equally as confusing as the mechanism of occlusion is the different terminology used over the years to define this particular retinal vascular disorder. Hemorrhagic retinopathy, venous stasis retinopathy, impending central retinal vein occlusion, and partial central retinal vein occlusion are just some of the terms which appear in the literature. At this point in time, a definite clinical classification upon which all agree is not available. It seems that the best way to clinically classify central retinal vein occlusion is to consider this entity along a spectrum of clinical severity, depending on the extent of venous obstruction.

If the degree of outflow obstruction is mild and retinal ischemia is very minimal or nonexistent, edema and hemorrhage may be unassociated with permanent retinal damage. Resolution of the fundus changes and return to almost normal vision occur following re-establishment of the venous outflow.

In venous occlusive disease with a moderate degree of outflow obstruction, permanent damage to the vascular endothelium may occur secondary to mechanical dilatation. In these cases, even when the venous outflow returns to normal, serous exudation from the damaged or dilated retinal capillaries persists with resultant macular edema, retinal pigment epithelial disruption, and, in many cases, retinal atrophy. These changes, if they involve the center of the macula, can result in a decrease of visual acuity.

When the outflow obstruction is of a high degree, significant retinal ischemia can result and can be severe. There is frequently extensive central and peripheral destruction of the capillary bed with severe decrease in central and peripheral vision. This can be carefully documented with visual fields. The damage is frequently permanent. Eyes with severe retinal ischemia are at risk for developing secondary proliferative changes such as rubeosis iridis with resultant neovascular glaucoma or proliferative retinopathy with possible vitreous hemorrhage and/or tractional retinal detachment.

In discussing the ophthalmoscopic features and fluorescein angiographic findings of central retinal vein occlusions, it is helpful to divide the findings into acute and chronic stages.

The funduscopic picture of acute central retinal vein occlusion (CRVO) presents along a spectrum of clinical findings. Acute CRVO is characterized by dilated, engorged, and tortuous retinal veins filled with darkened deoxygenated blood (figure). There is a variable amount of retinal hemorrhage, ranging from a few flame-shaped or punctate hemorrhages to extensive large intraretinal blotch hemorrhages

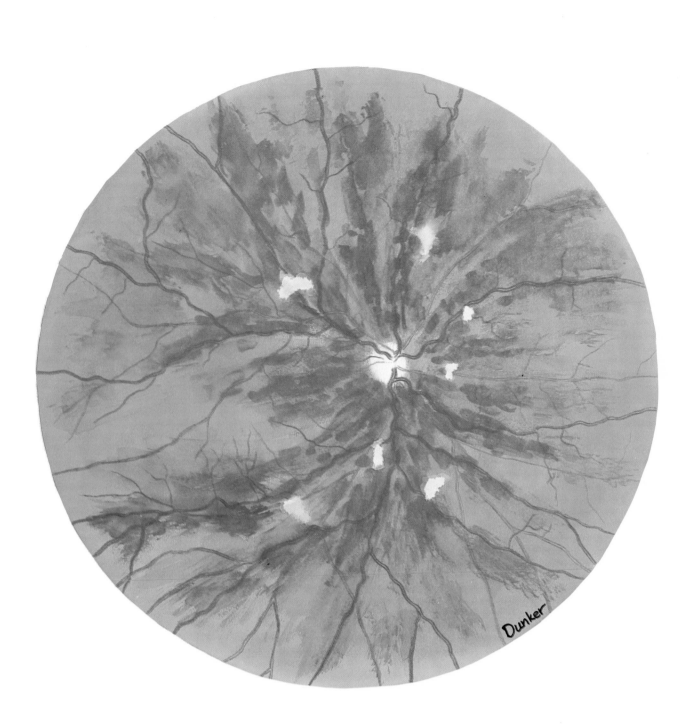

in all the quadrants of the retina. In the more severe types of occlusion where there is extensive intraretinal hemorrhage, the normal retinal architecture is obscured. The retina can be edematous, particularly in the posterior pole. Cotton-wool spots or soft exudates are frequently present in varying numbers, depending on the extent of the retinal ischemia. The disc margin is usually slightly blurred or may be obscured by hemorrhages on the surface of the disc. The retinal arteries are usually sclerotic.

The fundus appearance of chronic central retinal vein occlusions may take months to develop. The hemorrhages gradually disappear over the months, although a few scattered flame-shaped or dot hemorrhages may persist, particularly in the periphery (figure). Cotton-wool spots usually are not present. Microaneurysms and venous loops are visible. Collateral and shunt vessels on the disc margin are a common finding. Chronic macular edema may be visible, or the macula may be atrophic with diffuse pigment epithelial mottling change. Intraretinal hard exudates are frequently prominent. Neovascularization of the iris, disc, or retina sometimes occurs. Preretinal macular fibrosis is also a possible long-standing complication. The veins appear to be less engorged, and some may be occluded or sheathed. The disc may be normal or atrophic. The fluorescein angiographic findings can vary from the acute to the chronic stage of CRVO.

Listed below are some of the fluorescein angiographic findings of an acute CRVO:

1. The retinal venous circulation time may be prolonged.

2. In some cases, the arterial inflow transit time is also delayed.

3. The intraretinal hemorrhages block the background choroidal fluorescence. Leakage of fluorescein can be seen from dilated capillaries on the surface of the optic nerve and throughout the posterior pole. Hypofluorescent areas secondary to capillary dropout and retinal nonperfusion can be seen.

4. Frequently there is destruction of the perifoveal capillary net.

5. Late in the angiogram there can be intraretinal accumulation of fluorescein dye from dilated capillaries, intraretinal microvascular abnormalities, and microaneurysms, indicating retinal edema. The retinal venous walls sometimes stain with fluorescein dye, indicating a breakdown in the blood-retinal barrier and loss of integrity of the tight endothelial junctions.

Listed below are fluorescein angiographic findings in chronic central retinal vein occlusion:

1. Collateral and shunt vessels at the disc margin

2. Microaneurysms leaking fluorescein

3. Areas of capillary nonperfusion appearing as hypofluorescent areas

4. Persistent macular edema as evidenced by diffuse intraretinal accumulation of fluorescein dye

5. Staining of the venous walls with fluorescein dye

6. Leaking dilated capillaries and venules

7. Fluorescein leakage from neovascularization of the disc, elsewhere in the retina, or on the surface of the iris

As far as management is concerned, there has been no evidence in a prospective, randomized fashion with a significant number of patients that shows any specific treatment to be better than the natural history of the disease. There has been some recent evidence that perhaps photocoagulation treatment may be of some benefit in preventing, or at least controlling, the more serious secondary complications of CRVO, such as rubeosis iridis with neovascular glaucoma and proliferative retinopathy with possible subsequent vitreous hemorrhage.

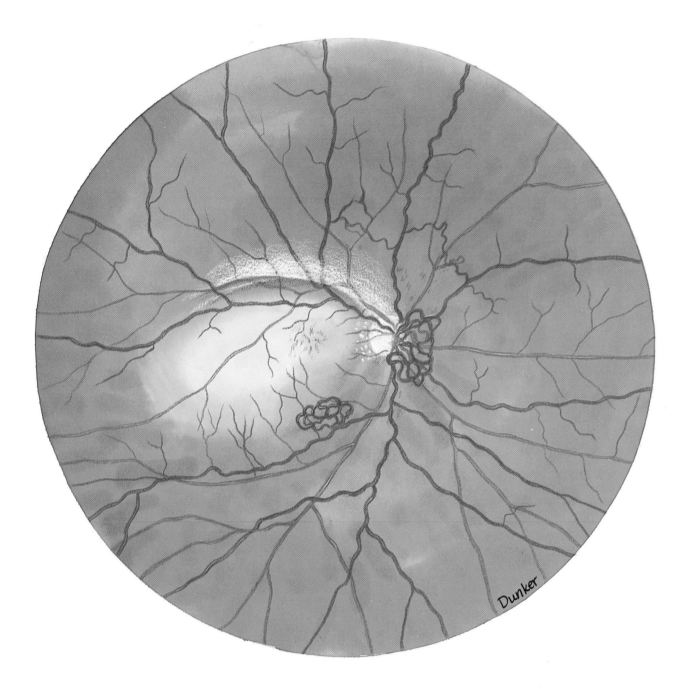

Venous Occlusive Disease

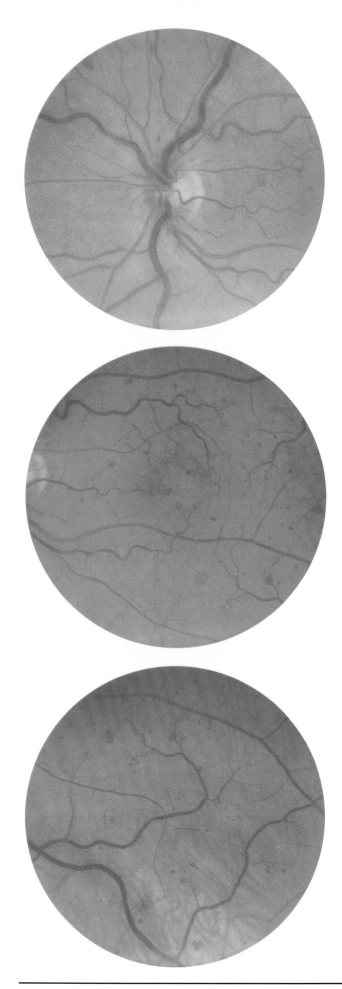

The optic nerve is slightly hyperemic. The retinal veins are slightly engorged.

Multiple intraretinal dot and blotch hemorrhages are present. There is slight mottling of the retinal pigment epithelium in the macular region.

Beyond the arcades are scattered intraretinal dot and blotch hemorrhages.

During the arterial phase of the angiogram there is blockage of the background choroidal fluorescence by the intraretinal hemorrhages. There is increased hyperfluorescence in the perifoveal region secondary to atrophy of the retinal pigment epithelium.

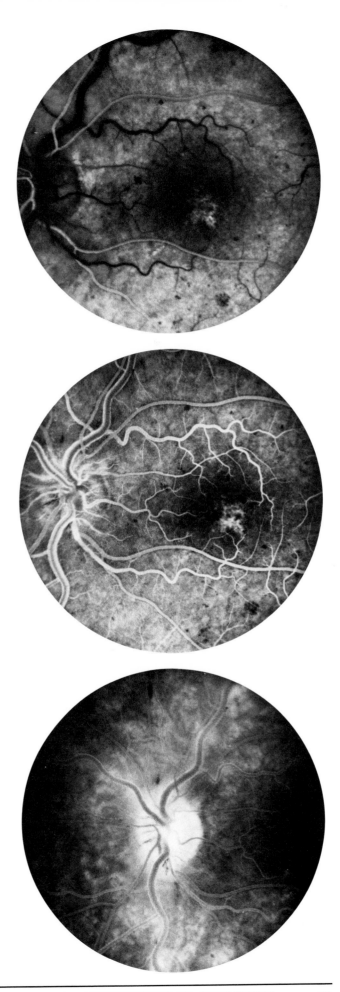

During the laminar phase of the angiogram there is still blockage of the background fluorescence by the intraretinal dot and blotch hemorrhages. There is slight staining of the venous walls, indicating some loss of endothelial integrity. The pigment epithelial window defects in the perifoveal region remain the same.

The late angiogram shows some slight staining of the optic nerve. There is also minimal staining of the retinal venous walls.

AUTHOR'S NOTE

This patient was found to have significant narrowing of the carotid artery on the left side, i.e. the same side as the minimal venous occlusive disease.

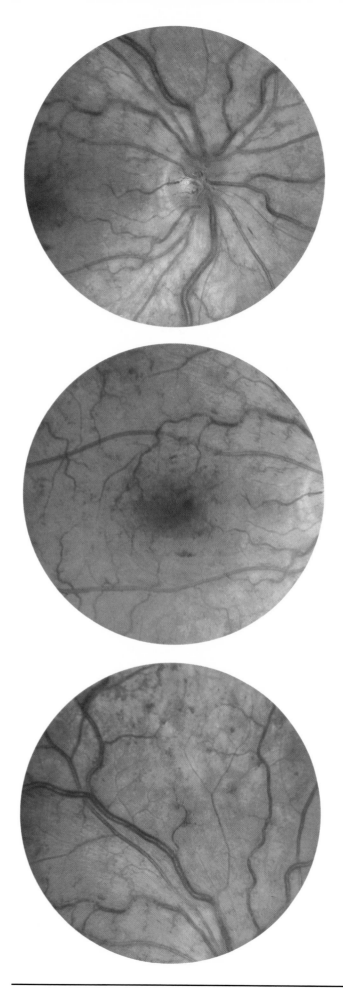

Venous Occlusive Disease
(probable papillophlebitis—
pre- and post-treatment)

The optic nerve of the right eye is slightly hyperemic. The branches of the central retinal vein are definitely engorged. Surrounding the optic nerve are multiple intraretinal dot and blotch hemorrhages. There appears to be dilatation of the capillaries on the surface of the nerve.

In the posterior pole the retinal veins show some irregularity. There are multiple intraretinal dot and blotch hemorrhages.

Beyond the arcades there are intraretinal dot and blotch hemorrhages.

During the early laminar phase of the angiogram, there is dilatation of the capillaries on the surface of the nerve. There is also extensive dilatation of the intraretinal capillaries surrounding the nerve and extending along all the retinal vessels.

During the venous phase of the angiogram there is intraretinal leakage of fluorescein from the dilated capillary bed. The walls of the smaller branched veins stain with fluorescein dye. The intraretinal hemorrhages block the background choroidal fluorescence.

The late angiogram shows diffuse intraretinal leakage of fluorescein dye, indicating diffuse retinal edema. The intraretinal hemorrhages continue to block the background choroidal fluorescence throughout the angiogram.

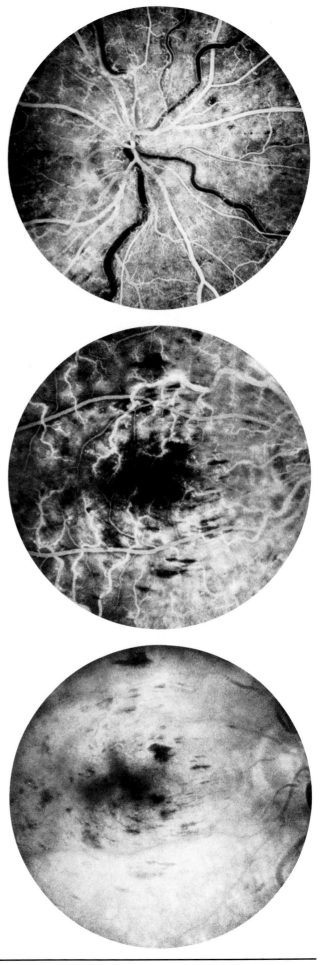

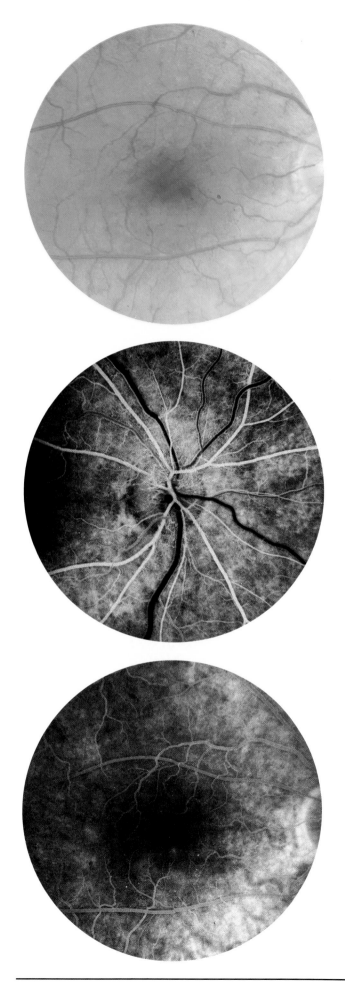

Color photograph of the right posterior pole shows some very faint punctate intraretinal hemorrhages.

The early laminar phase of the angiogram shows dilated capillaries on the surface of the nerve and surrounding the nerve intraretinally. However, this dilatation is much less than during the acute stage.

The late angiogram of the posterior pole shows some subtle fluorescein leakage intraretinally.

AUTHOR'S NOTE

This is the post-treatment appearance of a patient with venous occlusive disease, most likely secondary to papillophlebitis. This was a 22-year-old white female with vision reduced in the right eye to 20/200. After 2 weeks of systemic steroids, the patient's vision improved to 20/25 with a marked improvement in the clinical picture. There are other patients with the presumptive diagnosis of papillophlebitis who have improved spontaneously without any specific treatment.

Reader's Notes

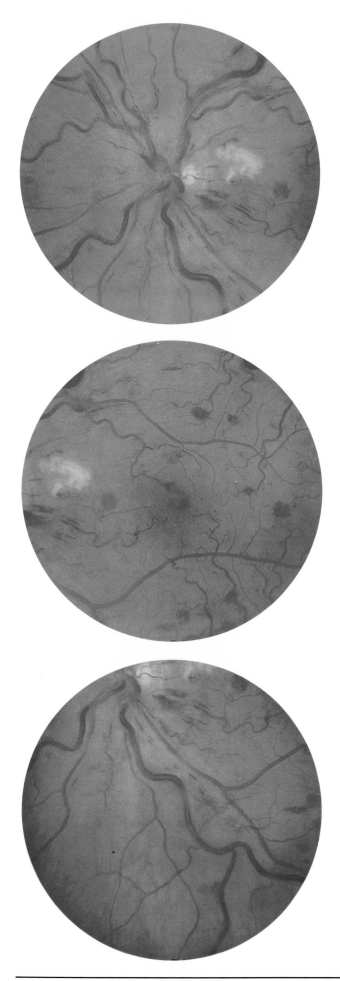

Venous Occlusive Disease
(probable papillophlebitis with soft exudate—spontaneous improvement)

The optic nerve of the left eye is hyperemic with slight blurriness of the margins. There are several intraretinal hemorrhages overlying the nerve. The branches of the central retinal vein are definitely engorged and slightly tortuous.

In the papillomacular bundle there is an area of soft exudate. Throughout the posterior pole are multiple intraretinal dot and blotch hemorrhages.

Beyond the temporal arcades there are intraretinal dot and blotch hemorrhages.

Standard 30° color photograph of the posterior pole.

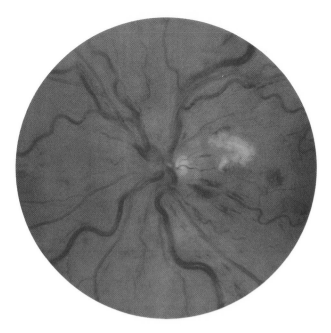

Sixty degree photograph of the posterior pole.

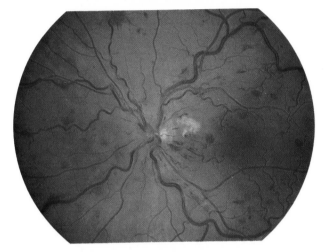

Comparison of the 30° and 60° photographs. The *black arrows* indicate the extent of the 30° field as compared to the now available 60° photograph.

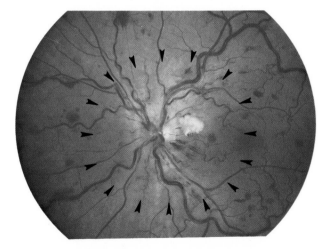

AUTHOR'S NOTE

The capability of now taking 60° or wide angle photographs permits a panoramic view of pathology without the necessity of taking numerous photographs.

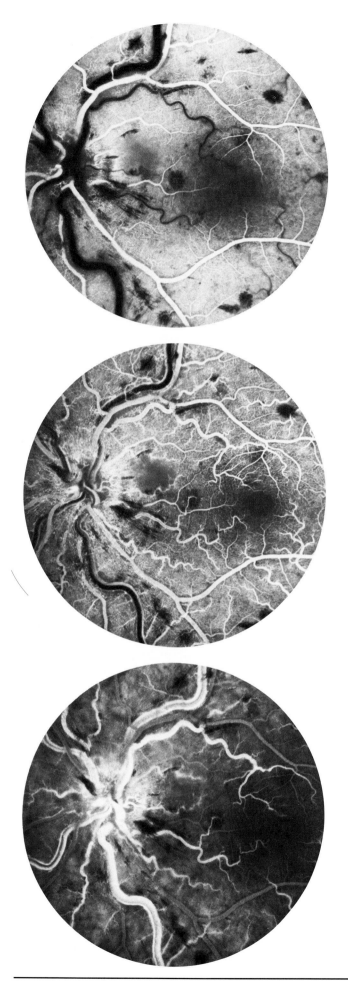

During the arterial phase of the angiogram there is blockage of the background choroidal fluorescence by the intraretinal hemorrhages. There is dilatation of the capillaries along the edge of the optic nerve and overlying the inferior nasal portion of the nerve.

During the laminar phase of the angiogram the perifoveal capillaries are well visualized. There is dilatation of the capillary bed surrounding the optic nerve and throughout the posterior pole. An area of nonperfusion can be seen just temporal to the optic nerve corresponding to the soft exudate seen clinically.

Later in the angiogram there is some leakage of fluorescein from the dilated capillaries on the optic nerve. The capillaries surrounding the area of nonperfusion slightly leak fluorescein. The intraretinal hemorrhages continue to block the background fluorescence.

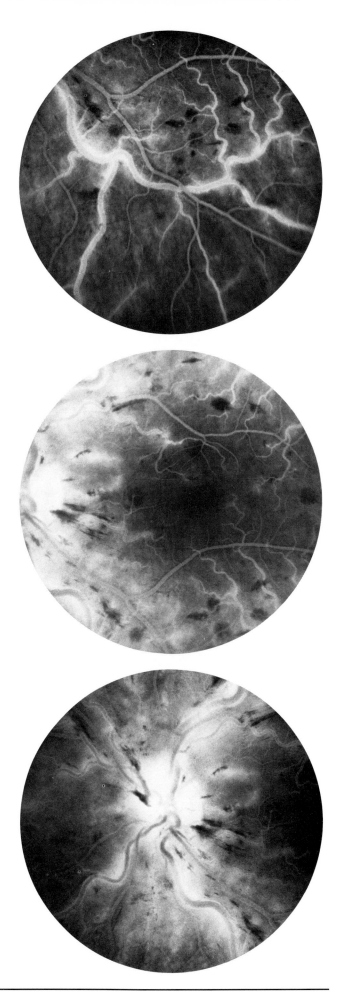

There is obvious staining of the inferior temporal vein and its branches. This is due to slight leakage of fluorescein dye from a breakdown in the blood-retinal barrier. Intraretinal hemorrhages continue to block the background choroidal fluorescence.

The late angiogram shows diffuse intraretinal accumulation of fluorescein, indicating retinal edema. There is slight increased leakage of fluorescein from the capillaries surrounding the area of nonperfusion in the papillomacular bundle.

The late angiogram shows leakage of fluorescein from dilated capillaries on the surface of the nerve and staining of the optic nerve tissue. Intraretinal leakage of fluorescein also extends along the branches of the central retinal vein. Even very late in the angiogram the intraretinal hemorrhages and hemorrhages overlying the nerve block the background fluorescence.

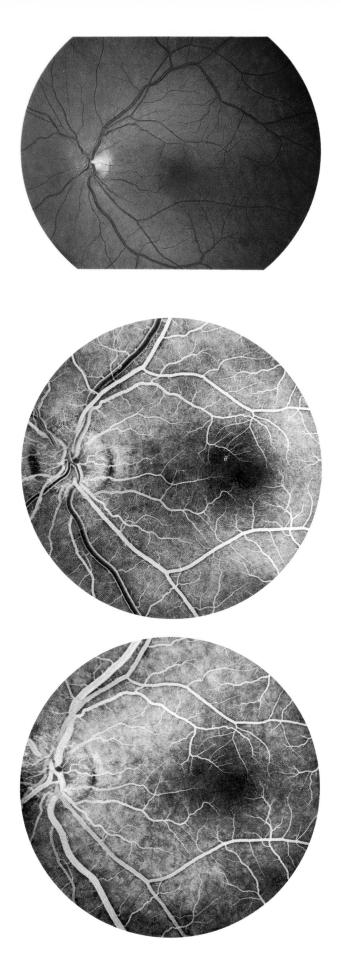

The 60° photograph of the left eye shows some very slight hyperemia of the optic nerve. The retinal veins appear of normal caliber. There is marked resolution of the soft exudate in the papillomacular bundle.

The laminar phase of the fluorescein angiogram shows some dilatation of the capillaries on the surface of the optic nerve. The retinal veins appear normal. There does not appear to be any significant blockage by intraretinal hemorrhage. No areas of capillary dropout or nonperfusion can be seen.

Later in the angiogram the dilated capillaries on the surface of the nerve are still visible. The retinal veins appear to be of normal caliber.

AUTHOR'S NOTE

This 26 year-old white female had spontaneous improvement as far as the intraretinal hemorrhages, soft exudate, and venous engorgement were concerned. A complete systemic work-up was done and was negative. The only residual finding was some capillary dilatation on the surface of the left optic nerve. Vision improved from 20/60 to 20/20 with no specific treatment.

Reader's Notes

Central Retinal Vein Occlusion
(with intact perifoveal capillary net)

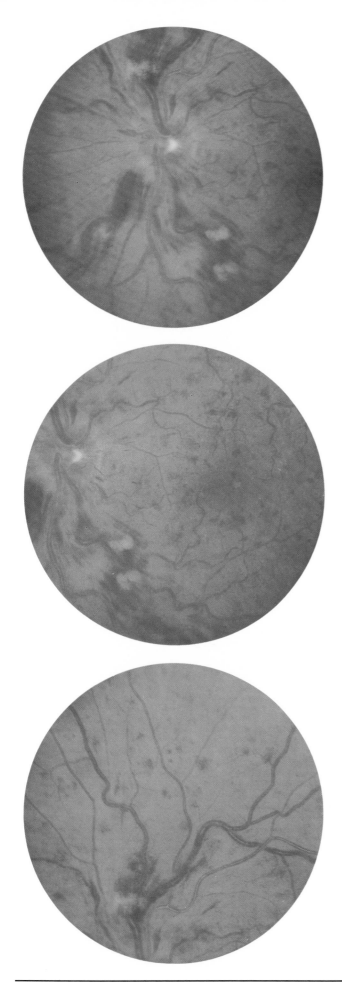

The left optic nerve is slightly hyperemic with blurred disc margins. Branches of the central retinal vein are markedly engorged and tortuous. Surrounding the optic nerve and along the course of the veins are multiple intraretinal hemorrhages with scattered areas of soft exudate.

The posterior pole shows multiple intraretinal dot and blotch hemorrhages.

Beyond the temporal arcades are intraretinal dot and blotch hemorrhages. Arterio-venous nicking changes are evident.

The fluorescein angiogram of the posterior pole shows integrity of the perifoveal capillaries. There is some microaneurysmal formation along the inner capillary ring of the avascular zone. Dilatation of the capillaries throughout the posterior pole with microaneurysmal change is also present. The intraretinal hemorrhages block the background choroidal fluorescence. There is dilatation of the capillaries on the surface of the optic nerve. Along the inferior temporal arcade are several areas of nonperfusion corresponding to the soft exudate seen clinically.

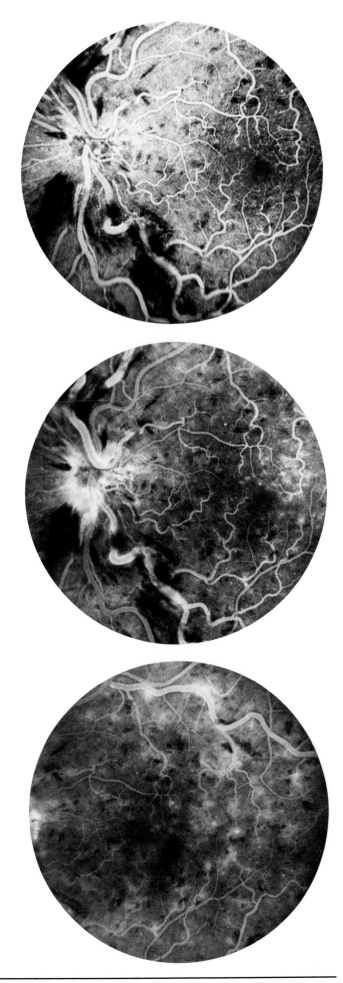

Later in the angiogram there is leakage of fluorescein from the dilated capillaries on the surface of the nerve. There is also leakage of fluorescein from the microaneurysms in the macular region. The intraretinal hemorrhages continue to block the background choroidal fluorescence.

The late angiogram shows staining the superior temporal branch vein due to a breakdown in the blood-retinal barrier. There is intraretinal accumulation of fluorescein dye from leaking microaneurysms indicating retinal edema.

AUTHOR'S NOTE

The maintenance of a good perifoveal capillary net and minimal macular edema permitted the vision in this eye to be recorded at the 20/25 level.

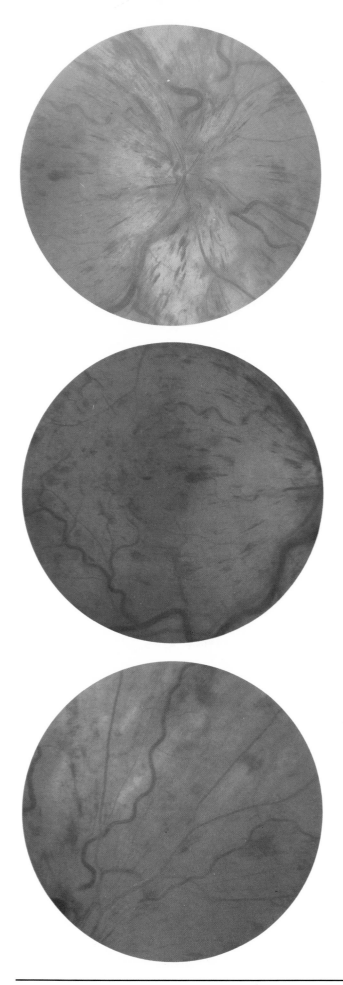

Central Retinal Vein Occlusion
(disrupted perifoveal capillary net)

The right optic nerve is hyperemic with blurred margins. Surrounding the optic nerve and along the branches of the central retinal vein are multiple intraretinal dot, blotch, and splinter hemorrhages. The retinal veins are definitely engorged and tortuous.

In the posterior pole there are scattered intraretinal dot and blotch hemorrhages. Many of the hemorrhages extend along the nerve fiber layer.

The superior nasal quadrant of the right eye shows multiple intraretinal hemorrhages with increased tortuosity of the retinal veins.

The intraretinal hemorrhages block the background choroidal fluorescence. There is marked disruption of the perifoveal capillaries. Multiple microaneurysms can be seen. There is dilatation of the capillaries both intraretinally in the posterior pole and overlying the optic nerve.

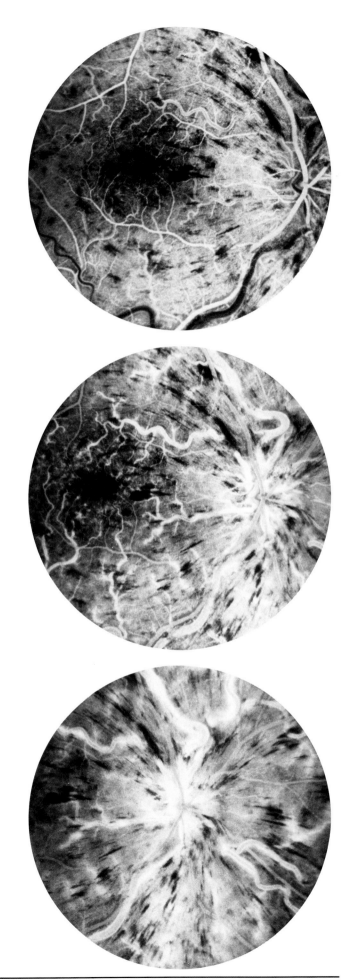

The capillaries on the surface of the nerve leak fluorescein. The microaneurysms in the posterior pole diffusely leak fluorescein. The intraretinal hemorrhages continue to block the background choroidal fluorescence.

The late angiogram shows diffuse staining of the walls of the branches of the central retinal vein. There is also diffuse intraretinal accumulation of fluorescein dye from dilated capillaries and microaneurysms. The intraretinal hemorrhages continue to block the background choroidal fluorescence.

AUTHOR'S NOTE

This patient's vision was 20/200 even though the macular edema was not very extensive. The vision was probably reduced due to marked disruption of the perifoveal capillary net.

Central Retinal Vein Occlusion
(foveal hemorrhage)

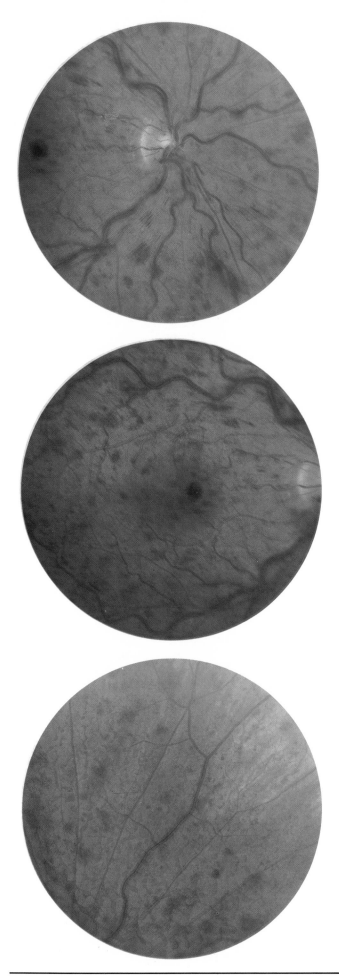

The optic nerve is slightly hyperemic. The retinal veins are engorged and slightly tortuous. Surrounding the optic nerve are multiple intraretinal dot, blotch, and splinter hemorrhages. The hemorrhages extend along all the branches of the central retinal vein.

In the posterior pole there is a fairly dense hemorrhage directly in the fovea. Additional intraretinal dot and blotch hemorrhages are present. The inferior temporal branch vein shows marked irregularity throughout its course.

In the superior nasal quadrant of the right eye there are scattered intraretinal hemorrhages. These hemorrhages extend 360° around the mid-periphery.

There is dilatation of the capillaries on the surface of the nerve. Microaneurysmal changes and dilated capillaries can be seen throughout the macular region. The intraretinal hemorrhages throughout the posterior pole block the background choroidal fluorescence. The foveal hemorrhage is slightly larger than the normal retinal avascular zone and blocks part of the background choroidal fluorescence.

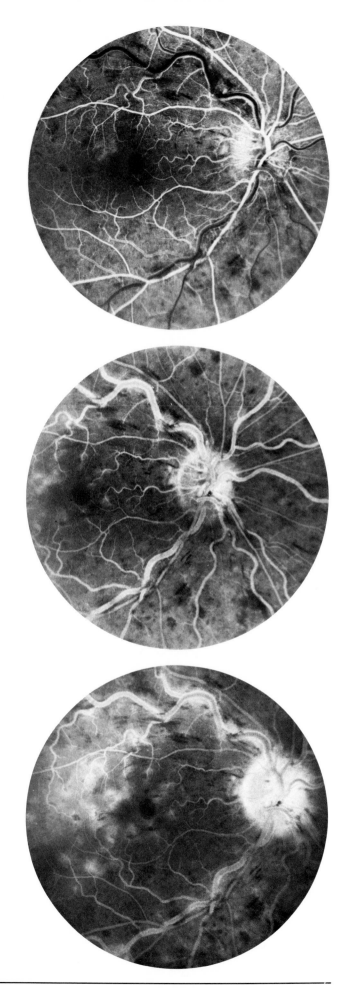

There is slight leakage of fluorescein from the dilated capillaries on the surface of the nerve. The foveal hemorrhage, with blockage of the background fluorescence, is more apparent.

There is diffuse leakage of fluorescein intraretinally temporal to the foveal hemorrhage. This leakage is from microaneurysms, dilated capillaries, and intraretinal microvascular abnormalities. There is staining of the optic nerve tissue due to leakage from dilated capillaries. There is also staining of the retinal venous walls due to a breakdown in the blood-retinal barrier and loss of endothelial integrity.

AUTHOR'S NOTE

This patient's vision was reduced to 20/200, most likely secondary to the foveal hemorrhage. There is evidence of retinal edema temporal to the foveal region involving the temporal macula. This type of venous occlusion could be considered a venous stasis retinopathy. This patient had severe carotid artery disease on the right side. This could also be considered a type of nonischemic central retinal vein occlusion.

Central Retinal Vein Occlusion
(cystoid macular edema)

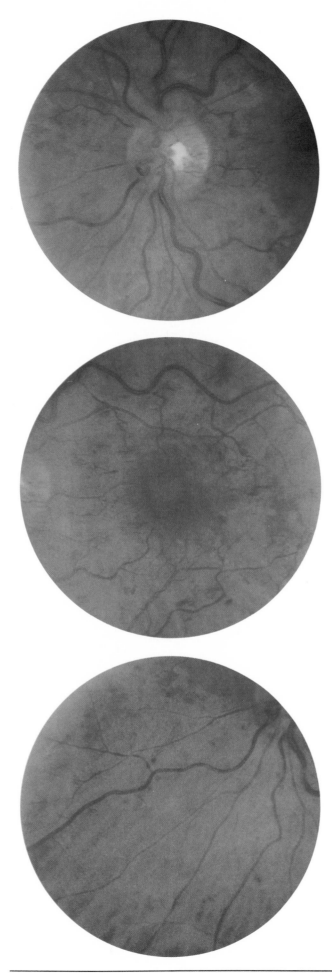

The optic nerve of the left eye is hyperemic. There appear to be dilated capillaries on the surface of the nerve. The retinal veins are slightly engorged.

In the macular region there are multiple intraretinal dot and blotch hemorrhages. Several splinter hemorrhages can be seen. There is some slight thickening of the sensory retina in the macular region. (The grayish color directly in the fovea is artifact.)

In the inferior nasal quadrant of the left eye intraretinal dot and blotch hemorrhages can be seen. These hemorrhages extend 360° around the mid-periphery.

The laminar phase of the angiogram shows dilatation of the capillaries on the surface of the nerve. There is also dilatation of the perifoveal capillaries. Microaneurysmal changes can be seen in the macular region. The intraretinal hemorrhages block the background choroidal fluorescence.

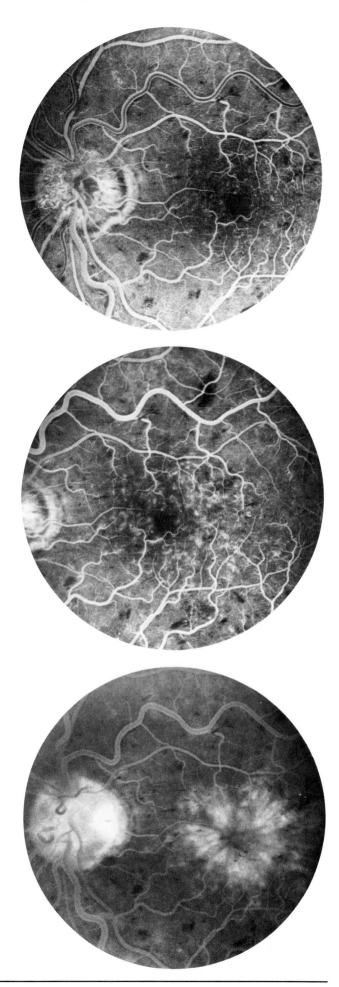

During the venous phase of the angiogram, there is increased leakage of fluorescein from the microaneurysms and the dilated capillaries. The deep intraretinal hemorrhages and superficial hemorrhages continue to block the background choroidal fluorescence.

Late in the angiogram there is a classic cystoid macular edema pattern.

AUTHOR'S NOTE
This 65-year-old white male had a clinically apparent bruit over the left carotid artery.

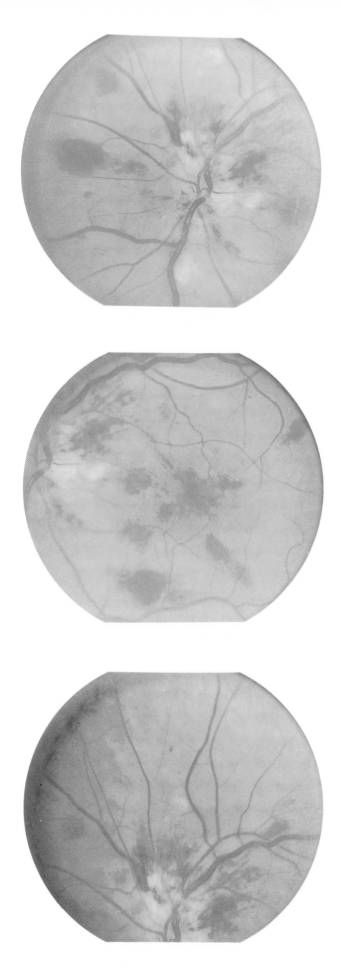

Central Retinal Vein Occlusion
(blotch hemorrhage with soft exudate)

The optic nerve of the left eye is slightly hyperemic. There is some dilatation of the capillaries on the surface of the nerve. The major branches of the central retinal vein are engorged. Surrounding the optic nerve are multiple intraretinal blotch hemorrhages and areas of soft exudate.

In the macular region there are large blotch hemorrhages with hemorrhages in the perifoveal region.

Small dot and blotch hemorrhages extend into the mid-periphery.

The laminar phase of the angiogram shows definite dilatation of the capillaries on the surface of the nerve. The intraretinal blotch hemorrhages surrounding the optic nerve block the background choroidal fluorescence. There are several areas of nonperfusion corresponding to the soft exudate seen clinically.

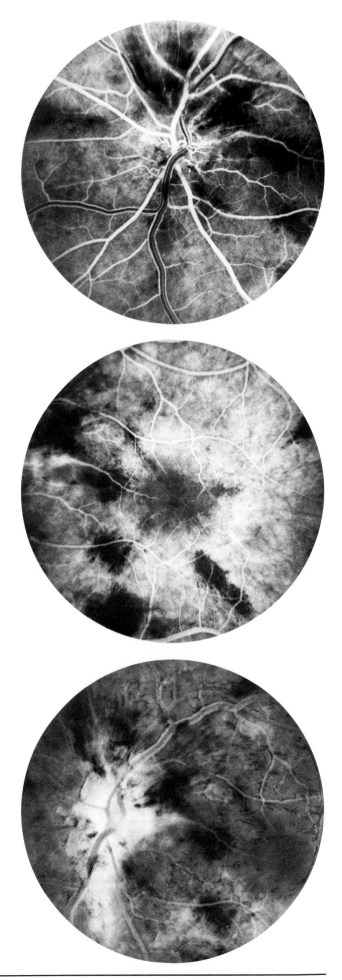

Fluorescein angiography of the macular region shows intraretinal dot and splinter hemorrhages in the perifoveal region. These hemorrhages plus the larger blotch hemorrhages block the background choroidal fluorescence. Temporal to the optic nerve is an area of nonperfusion surrounded by leaking capillaries.

The late angiogram shows staining of the optic nerve tissue due to the leaking capillaries. There is slight staining of the venous walls due to a breakdown in the integrity of the blood-retinal barrier.

Central Retinal Vein Occlusion
(partial disruption of the perifoveal capillary net)

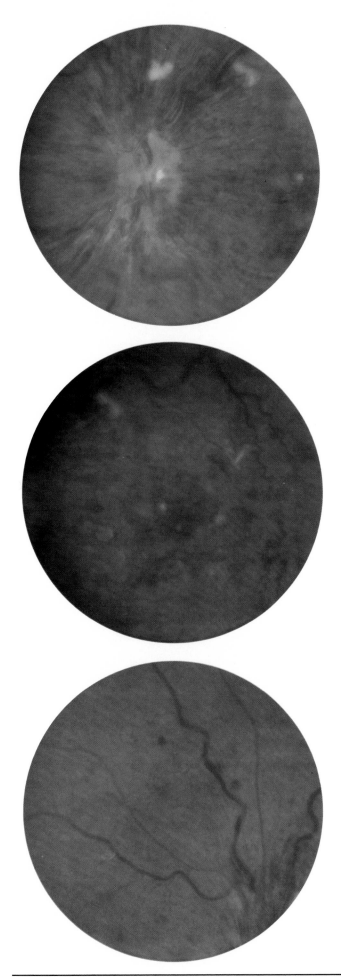

The left optic nerve is definitely hyperemic. The retinal veins are engorged and tortuous; 360° around the optic nerve are multiple intraretinal hemorrhages. There are several areas of soft exudate.

There is thickening of the sensory retina in the macular region. Scattered areas of soft exudate and multiple intraretinal dot and blotch hemorrhages are evident.

Superior nasal to the optic nerve there are dot and blotch hemorrhages.

The laminar phase of the angiogram shows disruption of the perifoveal capillary net primarily at its nasal aspect. There are multiple microaneurysms with dilatation of the capillary bed throughout the posterior pole. The capillaries on the temporal aspect of the optic nerve are also dilated. The intraretinal hemorrhages block the background choroidal fluorescence.

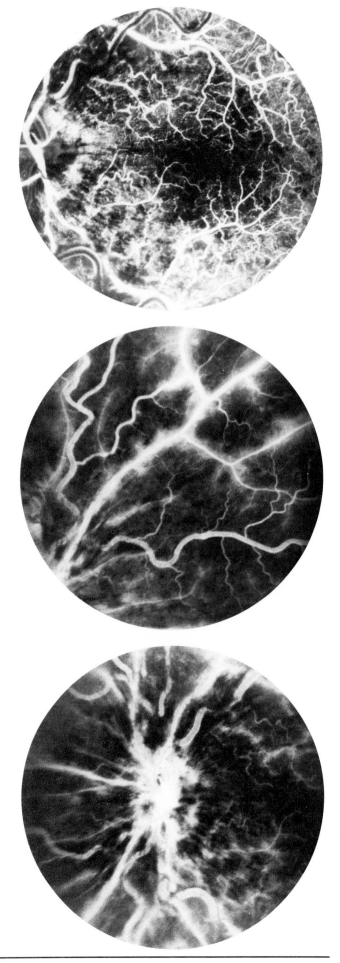

Branches of the central retinal vein stain brightly with fluorescein. The intraretinal hemorrhages continue to block the background choroidal fluorescence.

Later in the angiogram there is leakage of fluorescein on the optic nerve from the dilated capillaries with staining of the optic nerve tissue. The major branches of the central retinal vein stain with fluorescein dye. There is diffuse intraretinal leakage of fluorescein from the dilated capillary bed.

Acute Central Retinal Vein Occlusion (hemorrhagic)

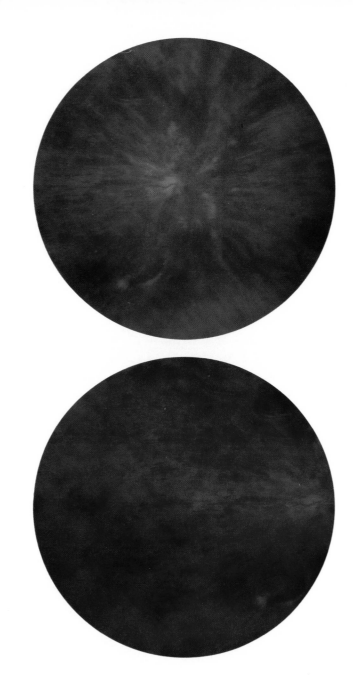

The optic nerve is hyperemic with blurred disc margins. There are punctate hemorrhages overlying the nerve with diffuse intraretinal hemorrhages surrounding the nerve. The retinal veins are engorged and tortuous. There are several areas of soft exudate.

The macular region shows multiple intraretinal dot and blotch hemorrhages. There is thickening of the sensory retina.

During the arterial phase of the angiogram there is blockage of the background choroidal fluorescence by the intraretinal hemorrhages. There is some dilatation of the capillaries on the temporal aspect of the nerve.

During the laminar phase of the angiogram there is intraretinal leakage of fluorescein, indicating retinal edema. There is still extensive blockage of the background choroidal fluorescence by the diffuse intraretinal hemorrhages.

The late angiogram shows diffuse intraretinal leakage of fluorescein. There is also staining of the optic nerve tissue due to leakage of the dilated capillaries on the surface of the nerve. The retinal venous walls stain with fluorescein, indicating a breakdown in the blood-retinal barrier.

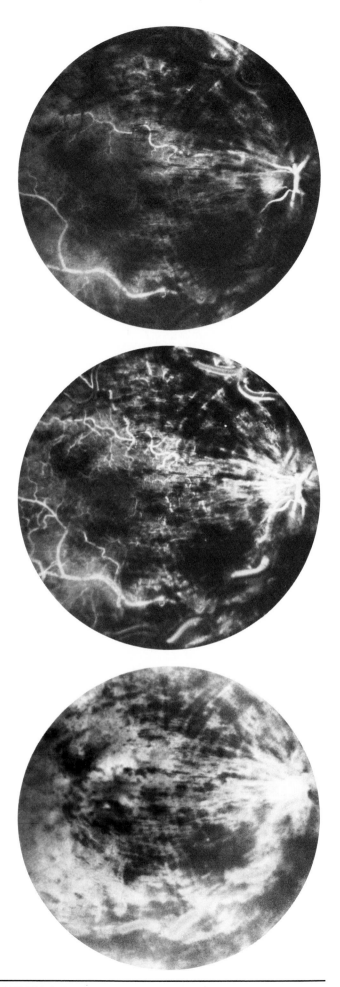

AUTHOR'S NOTE

One cannot determine the extent of nonperfusion and ischemia until there is significant clearing of the intraretinal hemorrhages.

Acute Central Retinal Vein Occlusion (hemorrhagic)

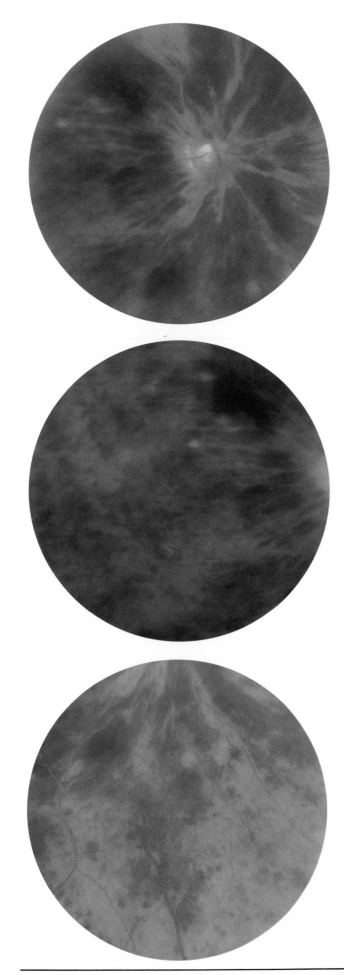

The right optic nerve is slightly hyperemic. There are hemorrhages overlying the nerve in addition to multiple blotch hemorrhages 360° around the optic nerve.

In the posterior pole and macular region there is diffuse intraretinal hemorrhage, obscuring the smaller caliber vessels. The retinal arteries appear to be slightly narrowed. There are small areas of soft exudate.

Beyond the arcades, extending into the mid-periphery, are multiple intraretinal dot and blotch hemorrhages.

During the arterial phase of the angiogram there is extensive blockage of the background choroidal fluorescence by the intraretinal blotch hemorrhages.

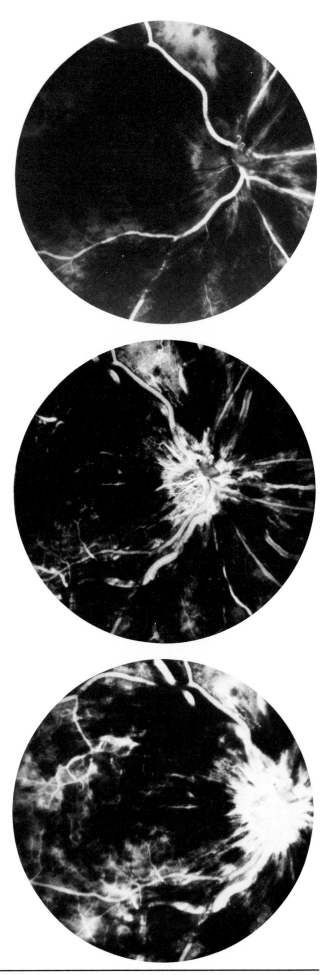

Later in the angiogram dilatation of the capillaries on the surface of the nerve is evident. There is increased hyperfluorescence from the choroid in areas not obscured by intraretinal blotch hemorrhages. There are areas where the intraretinal capillaries are dilated.

The late angiogram shows leakage of fluorescein from dilated optic nerve capillaries and staining of optic nerve tissue. There is also staining of the branches of the central retinal vein. There is intra retinal accumulation of the fluorescein dye from the dilated capillary bed and microaneurysmal formation.

Central Retinal Vein Occlusion (predominant optic nerve involvement)

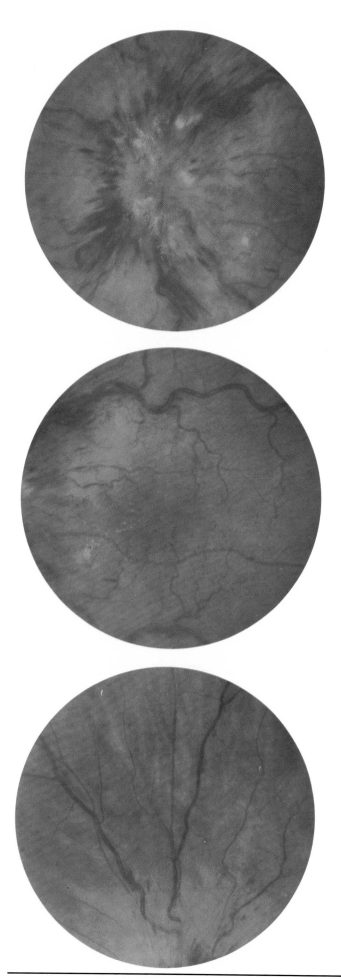

The left optic nerve is edematous with blurred disc margins. There are multiple areas of soft exudate surrounding the nerve and intraretinal peripapillary blotch hemorrhages. The retinal veins are engorged and tortuous.

There are a few scattered dot and blotch hemorrhages in the macular region. There is some deposition of hard exudate nasal to the fovea.

Superior to the optic nerve are a few scattered intraretinal dot and blotch hemorrhages. The retinal veins are slightly engorged.

There is extensive dilatation of the capillaries on the surface of the nerve. There are also areas of nonperfusion overlying the optic nerve corresponding to the soft exudate seen clinically. The peripapillary intraretinal hemorrhages block the background choroidal fluorescence.

There is minimal intraretinal leakage of fluorescein. There is some staining of the retinal venous walls.

The late stage of the angiogram shows diffuse leakage of the fluorescein from the dilated optic nerve capillaries and staining of the optic nerve tissue, indicating disc edema. There is very minimal intraretinal leakage of fluorescein in the macular region.

AUTHOR'S NOTE

This clinical picture could be termed papillophlebitis. However, the patient was 67 years old, and the term "papillophlebitis" is usually reserved for younger patients. Complete medical workup on this patient was negative.

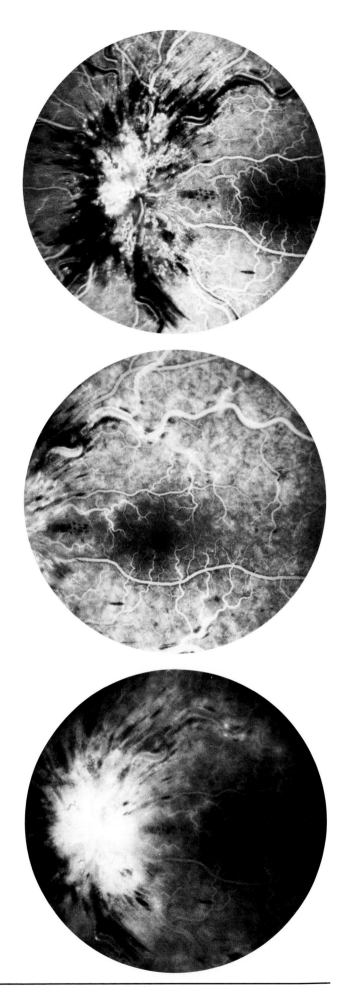

Central Retinal Vein Occlusion
(chronic with collaterals)

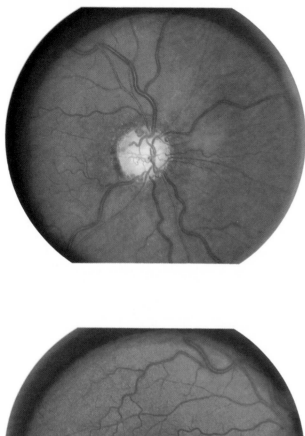

Collateralization can be seen on the surface of the nerve. A collateral vessel is clearly evident between the branches of the central retinal vein at the 4 o'clock and 5 o'clock positions on the edge of the optic nerve. In the center of the cup, dilated capillaries are clearly visible. The retinal veins are slightly engorged.

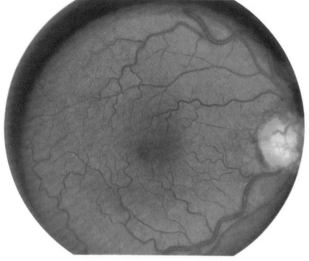

The posterior pole and macular region show no significant abnormality. Very small drusen are visible.

During the arterial phase of the angiogram a cilio-retinal vessel can be seen extending from the temporal aspect of the nerve toward the macula. The vessels within the center of the disc, which appear as capillaries clinically, have not yet filled with the fluorescein dye.

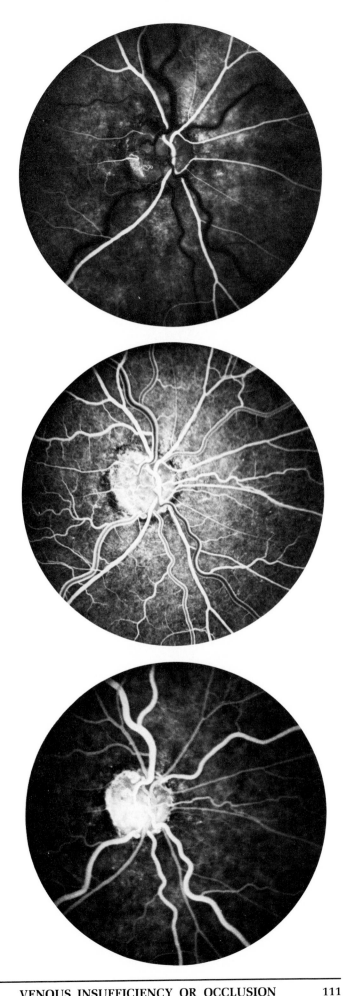

During the laminar phase of the angiogram all of the collaterals have filled with the fluorescein dye. There is no evidence of any significant leakage.

The later stages of the angiogram show some very subtle leakage of fluorescein from the fine collaterals on the surface of the nerve.

AUTHOR'S NOTE

Fluorescein angiography is important in differentiating disc neo-vascularization from collaterals after a vein occlusion. With disc neovascularization there is early hyperfluorescence of the newly formed vessels with diffuse leakage of fluorescein. Collaterals, on the other hand, fill with fluorescein during the laminar or venous phase of the angiogram and only very subtly leak the fluorescein dye.

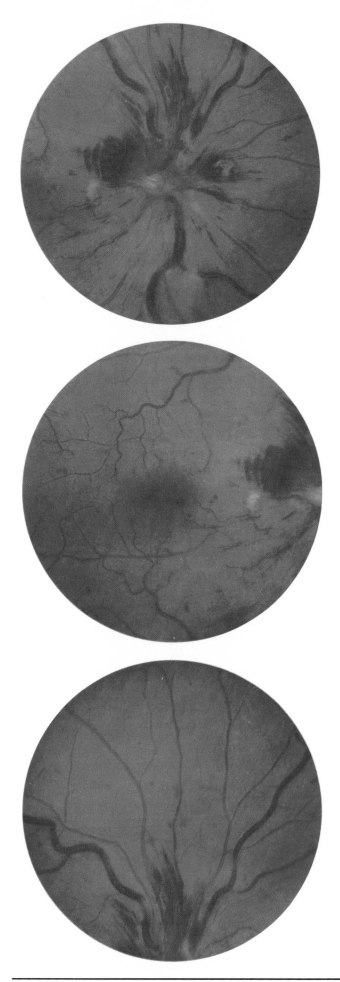

Venous Occlusive Disease
(acute stage with spontaneous resolution)

The right optic nerve is markedly hyperemic with blurred disc margins. Several portions of the nerve are obscured by overlying blotch hemorrhage. There are intraretinal blotch, dot, and splinter hemorrhages surrounding the nerve. The retinal veins are markedly engorged. In the peripapillary region there are scattered soft exudates.

In the posterior pole there are scattered dot and blotch hemorrhages. The retinal arteries appear to be slightly narrowed.

Superior to the optic nerve are scattered intraretinal hemorrhages. These hemorrhages are scattered 360° around the mid-periphery.

During the laminar phase of the angiogram there is blockage of the background choroidal fluorescence by the intraretinal hemorrhages in the peripapillary region. There are several small areas of nonperfusion in the papillomacular bundle and in the peripapillary region corresponding to the soft exudate seen on the color photographs (preceding page).

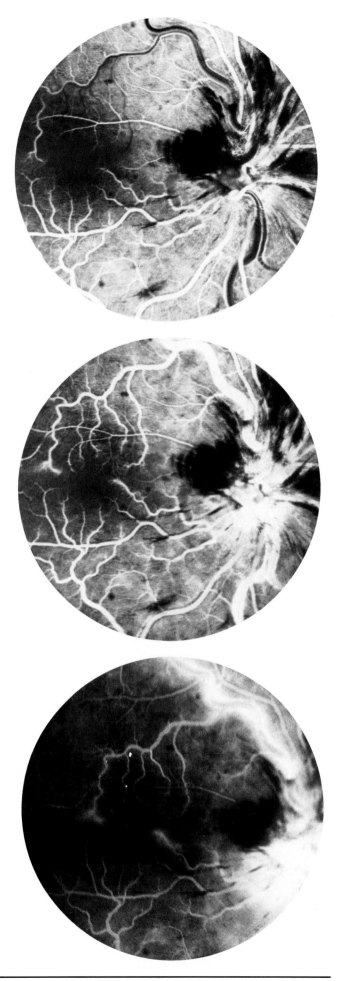

Later in the angiogram the marked engorgement of the retinal veins is obvious. The intraretinal hemorrhages continue to block the background choroidal fluorescence. There is leakage of fluorescein from the dilated capillaries on the surface of the optic nerve.

The late angiogram shows diffuse leakage of fluorescein from the dilated capillaries on the optic nerve with staining by the optic nerve tissue. There is also leakage and staining of the fluorescein dye along the superior temporal vein, indicating a breakdown in the blood-retinal barrier. There is some very faint perifoveal intraretinal leakage of fluorescein from the small caliber venules.

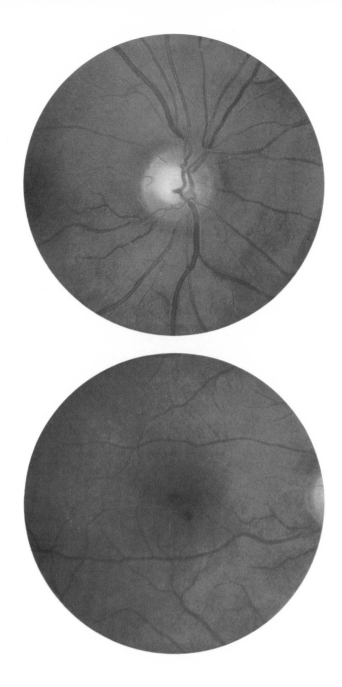

The right eye shows increased visibility of the capillaries on the nasal surface of the optic nerve. The retinal veins are of normal caliber. There are no intraretinal hemorrhages or soft exudate.

The posterior pole and macular region appear normal.

AUTHOR'S NOTE

This is a 58-year-old white female whose initial vision was 20/80. In 10 weeks, without any specific treatment, there was complete resolution of the venous occlusive picture with vision improving to the 20/15 level. Complete medical work-up was negative.

During the laminar phase of the angiogram a few dilated capillaries can be seen on the superior nasal surface of the optic nerve. (These correspond to the color photographs on the previous page.)

Later in the angiogram there is very subtle leakage of fluorescein from these dilated capillaries. The retinal veins appear to be of normal caliber.

The late angiogram of the right nerve shows slight staining of the peripheral portions of the optic nerve due to leakage from the dilated capillaries. The retinal veins are essentially normal. There is no evidence of capillary nonperfusion or intraretinal hemorrhage.

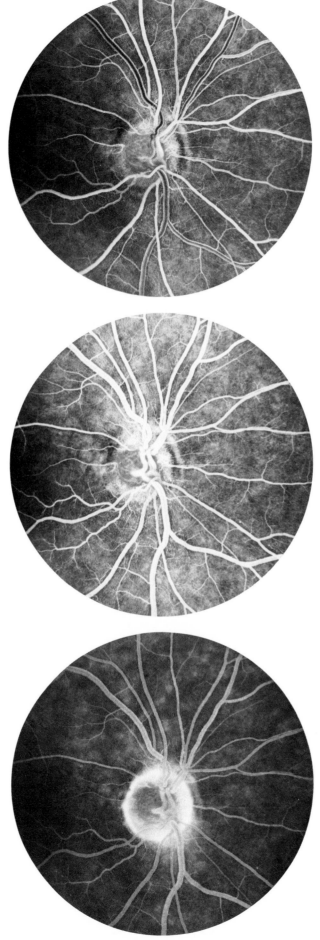

Venous Occlusive Disease
(with significant disc edema)

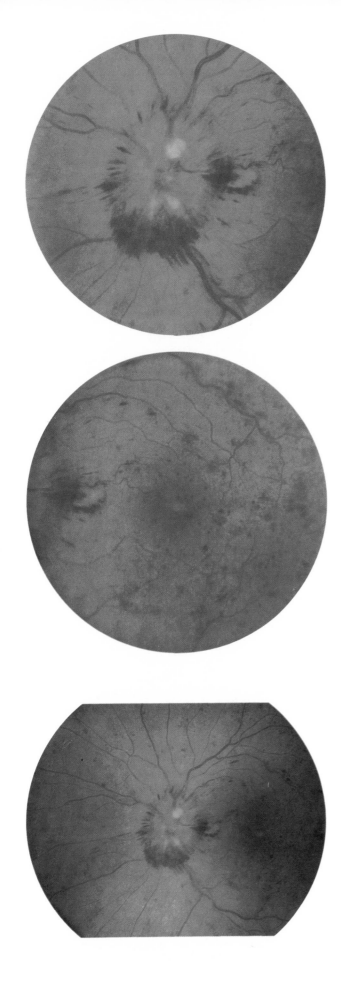

The left optic nerve is markedly edematous with blurred disc margins. Overlying the nerve are soft exudates and scattered hemorrhages. The retinal veins are slightly engorged.

In the posterior pole there are multiple intraretinal dot and blotch hemorrhages.

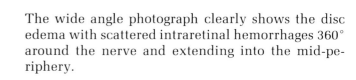

The wide angle photograph clearly shows the disc edema with scattered intraretinal hemorrhages 360° around the nerve and extending into the mid-periphery.

During the arterial phase of the fluorescein angiogram there are multiple dilated capillaries on the surface of the nerve. Part of the fluorescence from the optic nerve is obscured by the soft exudates. In addition, the hemorrhages overlying the periphery of the nerve block the background fluorescence.

In the posterior pole there is slight leakage of fluorescein from the capillary bed. There is some slight staining of the retinal venous walls.

Later in the angiogram there is diffuse leakage of fluorescein from the dilated optic nerve capillaries with staining of the optic nerve tissue. The hemorrhages surrounding the nerve continue to block the background choroidal fluorescence.

AUTHOR'S NOTE

Although this patient showed marked disc edema in the left eye, the vision was 20/30. No systemic disease was found which could be related to this clinical picture. The term papillophlebitis could be used for this particular clinical picture. Terms such as incomplete or partial central retinal vein occlusion have also been used to describe this type of presentation, but they are confusing terms.

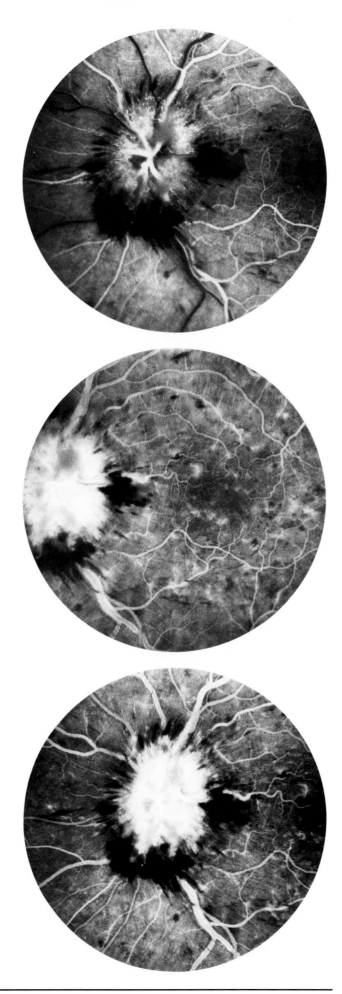

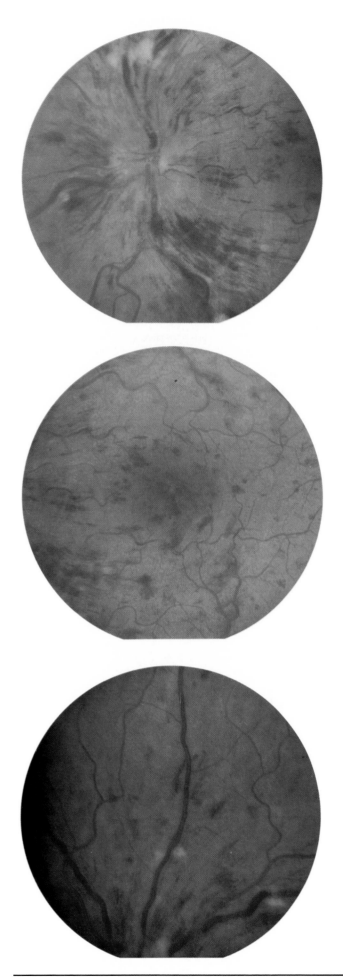

Venous Occlusive Disease
(acute stage with spontaneous resolution)

The left optic nerve is hyperemic with slight blurriness of the disc margins. The branches of the central retinal vein are engorged and slightly tortuous. Intraretinal blotch and splinter hemorrhages are scattered along the branches of the central retinal vein and throughout the peripapillary retina. A few scattered areas of soft exudate can also be seen along the course of the venous branches.

Throughout the posterior pole are scattered intraretinal dot and blotch hemorrhages. Many of the hemorrhages appear to follow the course of the nerve fiber layer. Some of the hemorrhages are in the perifoveal region.

Superior to the optic nerve, dilatation of the retinal veins can be seen. In addition, there are dot and blotch hemorrhages which extend 360° around the mid-periphery.

During the early laminar phase of the angiogram, dilatation of the capillaries on the surface of the nerve can be seen. The intraretinal hemorrhages in the peripapillary region and along the branches of the central retinal vein block the background choroidal fluorescence. Superior to the optic nerve are small areas of capillary dropout or nonperfusion. (These correspond to the soft exudates seen on the color photographs on the previous page.)

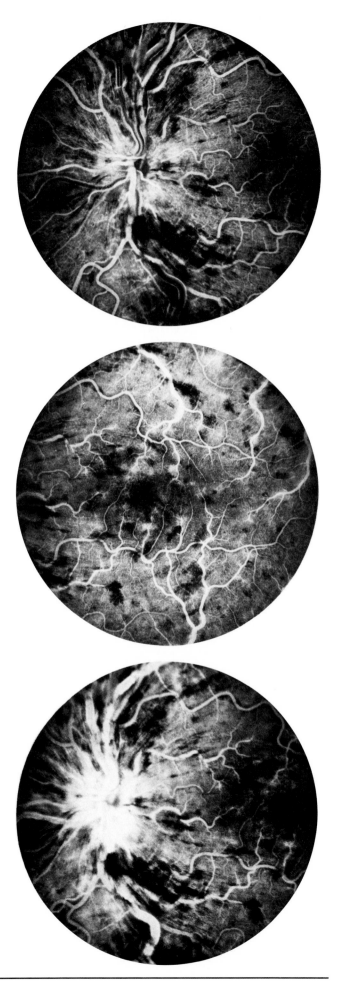

In the posterior pole the small hemorrhages block the background choroidal fluorescence. There is some dilatation of the capillary bed. Subtle leakage of fluorescein can be seen from the smaller branched venules. There is also some slight staining along the venous walls.

There is diffuse leakage of fluorescein dye from the dilated capillaries on the surface of the nerve with staining of the optic nerve tissue. The intraretinal hemorrhages continue to block the background choroidal fluorescence. The engorgement and tortuosity of the major branches of the central retinal vein are evident. In the macular region there is minimal intraretinal leakage of fluorescein.

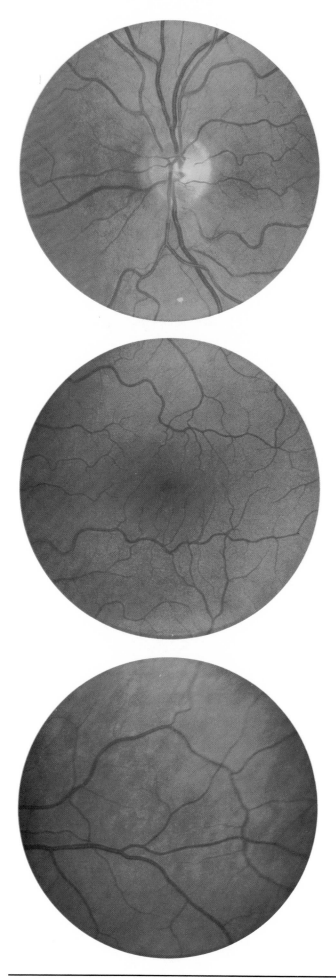

The optic nerve appears normal. The retinal veins are of normal caliber. No peripapillary hemorrhages or soft exudates can be seen.

The posterior pole and macular region show no evidence of intraretinal hemorrhage or evidence of previous venous occlusive disease.

The more peripheral branches of the central retinal vein appear normal. There are no hemorrhages in the mid-periphery.

AUTHOR'S NOTE

This is a case of a 65-year-old white female whose initial vision was 20/60. After 10 weeks of observation without any specific treatment, there was marked improvement in the clinical picture. The patient had clinically detectable bruits over both carotids and a past history of carotid artery disease, verified by carotid angiography.

The optic nerve appears normal. There does not appear to be any significant capillary dilatation. The posterior pole and macular region also appear normal. There is no evidence of intraretinal hemorrhage.

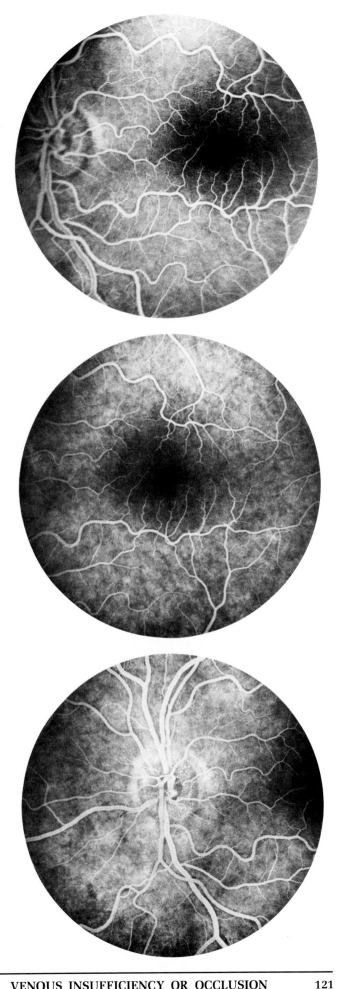

Later in the angiogram the retinal vasculature in the posterior pole is entirely normal. There is no leakage of fluorescein from the smaller branched veins.

The caliber of the retinal veins is normal. The peripapillary retina appears normal without any evidence of intraretinal hemorrhage or soft exudate.

Combined Central Retinal Vein Occlusion and Cilioretinal Arterial Occlusion

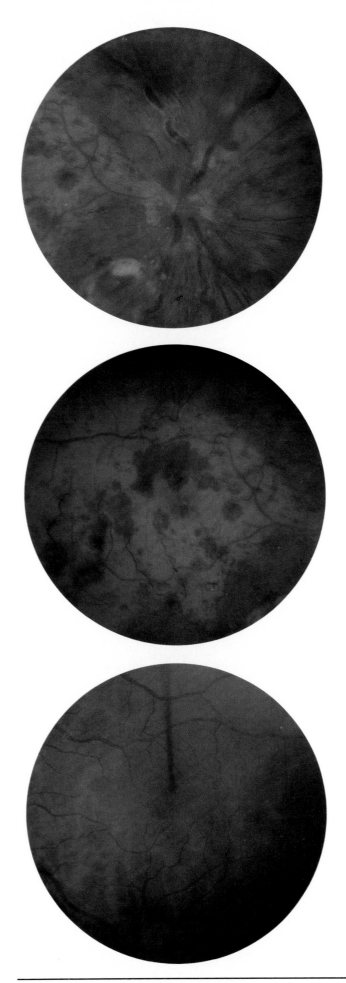

The optic nerve of the right eye shows extensive hyperemia secondary to dilatation of the surface capillaries. Also, surrounding the optic nerve are multiple intraretinal blotch and splinter hemorrhages. The branches of the central retinal vein are markedly engorged and tortuous.

Extending from the temporal edge of the right optic nerve is a large area of ischemic retinal whitening in distribution of a cilioretinal artery. Extensive intraretinal blotch hemorrhages can also be seen.

The left posterior pole is entirely normal.

During the early phases of the fluorescein angiogram, there is marked delay of filling in the posterior pole because of the cilioretinal arterial occlusion. There is some blockage of the background choroidal fluorescence by the intraretinal hemorrhages. Extensive capillary dropout and nonperfusion can be seen throughout the posterior pole, corresponding to the ischemic retinal whitening seen clinically.

Later in the angiogram, there is further filling of the capillary bed along the superior temporal and inferior temporal vessels. There is very sluggish passage of the fluorescein dye through the branches feeding the posterior pole from the cilioretinal artery. The areas of capillary dropout and nonperfusion remain apparent. There is also continuous blockage of the background choroidal fluorescence by the intraretinal hemorrhages.

The late angiogram in the vicinity of the optic nerve shows leakage of fluorescein from the dilated capillaries on the surface of the nerve. There is staining of the engorged branches of the central retinal vein, indicating a breakdown in the blood-retinal barrier. The hemorrhages surrounding the optic nerve continue to block the background choroidal fluorescence.

AUTHOR'S NOTE

This 53-year-old white male presented with an unusual finding of a combined central retinal vein occlusion and cilioretinal artery occlusion. The exact relationship between these two vascular insults is unknown. However, one could hypothesize that the patient's initial blurred vision 2 weeks prior to being seen could indicate the presence of a central retinal vein occlusion and, with engorgement of the optic nerve and pressure on the cilioretinal artery, an additional occlusion of the cilioretinal vessel occurred, which caused the sudden bright flash and drop of vision to the finger-counting level which the patient immediately noticed.

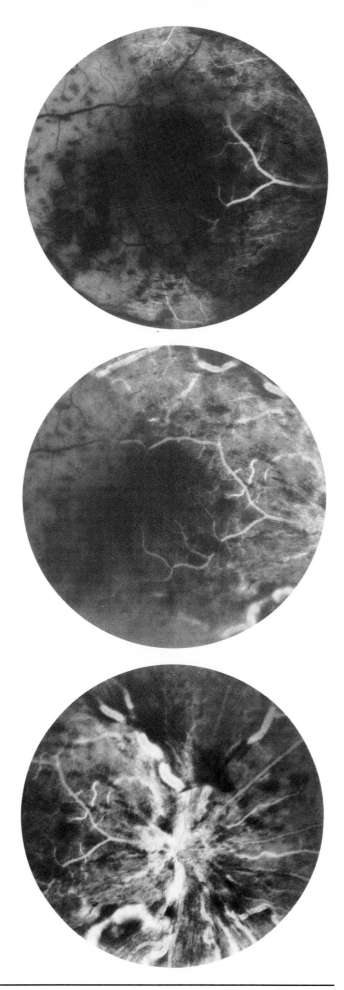

Venous Occlusive Disease
(macroglobulinemia—resolved)

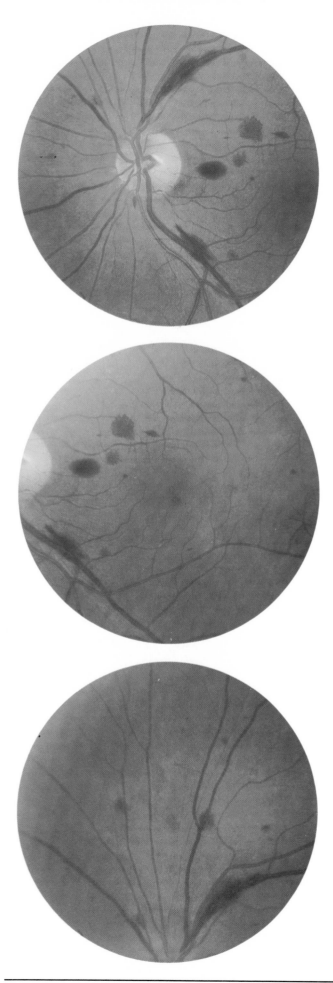

The left optic nerve appears normal. The major branches of the central retinal vein are slightly engorged. Intraretinal dot, blotch, and splinter hemorrhages can be seen.

In the posterior pole, scattered intraretinal hemorrhages are also seen. There was no significant macular edema or evidence of soft exudate.

The hemorrhages extended beyond the posterior pole and major arcades into the mid-periphery.

During the laminar phase of the angiogram the intraretinal hemorrhages along the veins and intraretinally in the posterior pole can be seen blocking the background choroidal fluorescence.

Later in the angiogram there is still blockage of the background choroidal fluorescence by the intraretinal hemorrhages.

The late fluorescein angiogram shows no significant intraretinal leakage of fluorescein dye or staining of the venous walls.

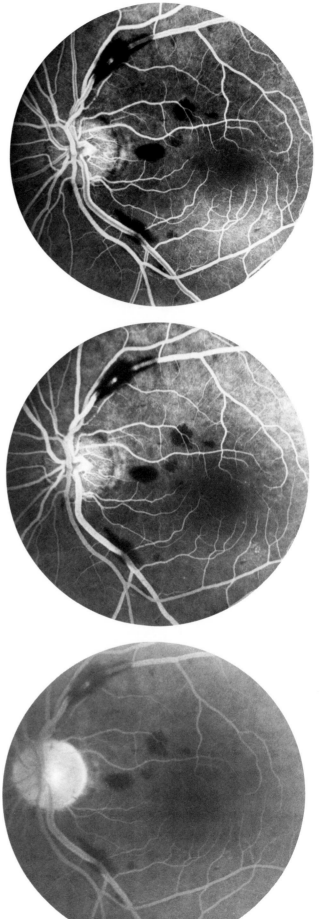

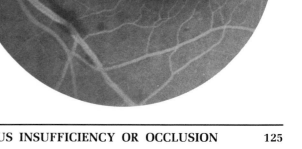

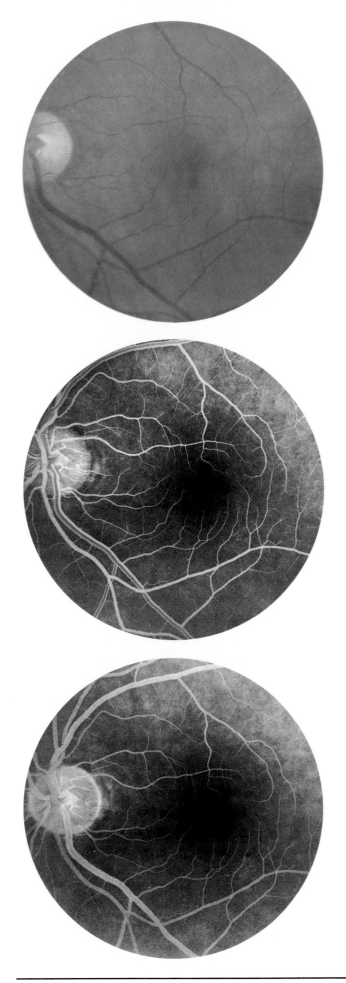

The left posterior pole shows no evidence of intraretinal hemorrhage. The retinal veins appear normal.

During the laminar phase of the fluorescein angiogram, there is no evidence of blocked background choroidal fluorescence from intraretinal hemorrhage.

The late angiogram shows no retinal vascular abnormality. The retinal veins appear entirely normal.

AUTHOR'S NOTE

This patient was diagnosed as having macroglobulinemia. Although his vision with the intraretinal hemorrhage was 20/20, he definitely had symptoms of blurriness. After treatment for his macroglobulinemia, there was an improvement in the funduscopic picture, and the patient's symptoms disappeared.

Branch Retinal Vein Occlusion

The clinical manifestations of hemodynamic changes in retinal branch vein occlusion may vary considerably among individual patients as the disease progresses from an acute to a chronic stage. Therefore, a classification has been devised which takes into account the ophthalmoscopic characteristics and complications which would be secondary to hemodynamic perfusion changes (*figure*).

A. Major branch vein occlusion at disc margin
    1. Without macular edema
    2. With macular edema
B. Major branch vein occlusion away from disc margin
    1. Without macular edema
    2. With macular edema
C. Macular branch vein occlusion
D. Peripheral branch vein occlusion
E. Branch vein occlusion with neovascularization at the disc and elsewhere

Retinal branch vein occlusions always occur at the crossing between an artery and a vein which are joined together by a common adventitial sheath.

The ophthalmoscopic features and fluorescein angiographic findings of branch vein occlusions can conveniently be divided into acute and chronic stages, as with central retinal vein occlusions.

A classic acute branch vein occlusion (BVO) occurs at an arterio-venous crossing. The appearance consists of superficial hemorrhages, retinal edema, and in many cases, soft exudates. The vein beyond the site of occlusion is often dilated. The amount of

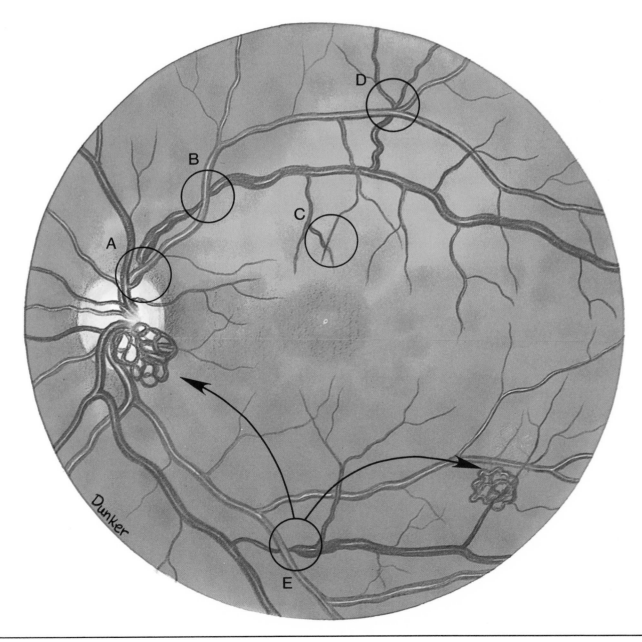

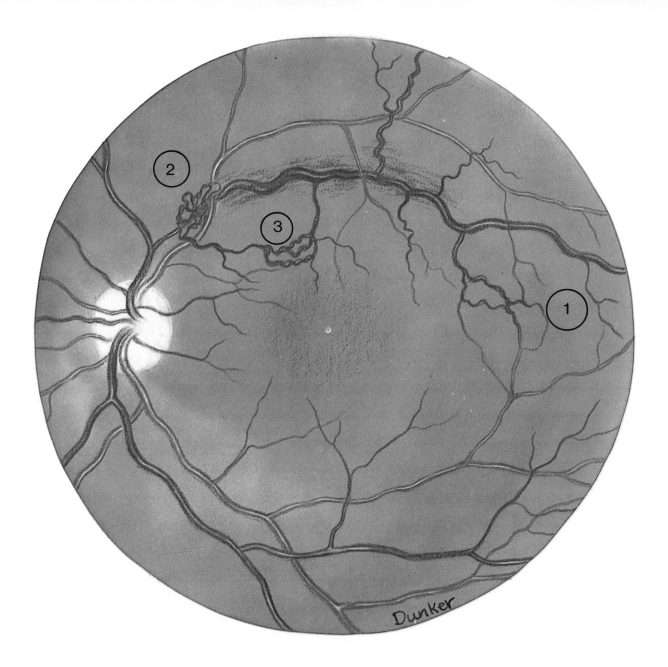

retinal tissue involved depends upon the location of the occlusion. The closer to the disc the occlusion site, the greater the amount of retinal involvement. Characteristically, the changes are limited to one side of the horizontal raphe. The hemorrhage appears as if someone had taken a paint brush and stroked it across the retina; this is because the hemorrhage is most obvious in the nerve fiber layer. There is also some transudation of fluid around the distal vein. Hemorrhage may spare the macular region, involve the macular region, or even appear in small cystoid spaces. One may see marked tortuosity and engorgement of the involved vein, and narrowing of the accompanying artery in the involved quadrant.

The ophthalmoscopic features in the chronic stage of venous occlusion can take several forms. There may be loss of transparency of the involved retina. The retina and involved quadrant may appear edematous and elevated. Invariably, with a major branch vein occlusion, one will see collaterals (*figure*) across the horizontal raphe (1) around the area of the occlusion (2) and in the area of the nasal macula (3). Intraretinal microvascular abnormalities and microaneurysmal formation may also be observed. Depending on the extent and duration of the occlusion, one might appreciate neovascularization either at the disc or elsewhere in the involved quadrant. Macular edema is not an uncommon finding.

Characteristic fluorescein angiographic findings of an acute BVO are:

1. Delay in filling time of the obstructed branch vein

2. Obscuration of the background choroidal fluorescence caused by intraretinal hemorrhage

3. Areas of nonperfusion

4. Diffuse intraretinal leakage of fluorescein dye

5. Staining of the wall of the obstructed branch vein

6. Intraretinal leakage of dye from dilated capillaries, microaneurysms, and intraretinal microvascular abnormalities

Fluorescein angiographic findings which are characteristic of a chronic BVO are:

1. Presence of collaterals and shunt vessels
2. Microaneurysms
3. Areas of capillary loss
4. Macular edema
5. Progressive arteriolar obliteration through nonperfused areas
6. Staining of venous walls with occasional faint leakage into the retina
7. Fluorescein leakage from neovascularization of the disc or elsewhere in the retina
8. Serous detachment of the sensory retina

New diagnostic techniques and more sophisticated equipment developed in recent years now allow us to recognize many previously undiagnosed complications secondary to branch vein occlusions. The following is a list of the more commonly observed complications from branch vein occlusion:

1. Chronic macular edema
2. Neovascularization
3. Vitreous hemorrhage
4. Serous detachments of the sensory retina
5. Rhegmatogenous retinal detachments
6. Internal limiting membrane contraction
7. Abnormal iris vascular patterns
8. Arteriosclerosis

There is agreement that the two most common causes for visual morbidity in BVO are macular edema or nonperfusion and vitreous hemorrhage secondary to neovascularization. Because these complications have responded, at least in part, to argon laser therapy in other conditions, some investigators treat branch vein occlusions with this modality. However, because the pathogenesis and natural history of the disorder have not yet been elucidated by prospective studies, it is not clear whether such treatment is indicated. The national collaborative Branch Vein Occlusion Study is a well controlled, randomized program which will evaluate the natural history of branch vein occlusion and the efficacy of photocoagulation in its treatment.

Branch Retinal Vein Occlusion
(peripheral branch)

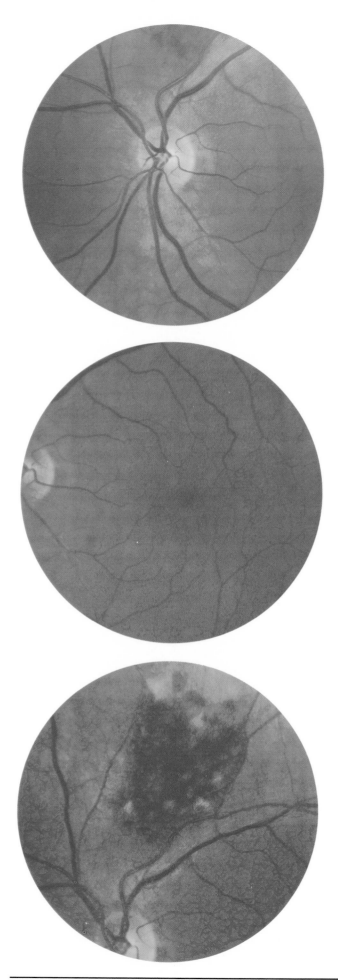

The optic nerve appears normal. The major branches of the central retinal vein appear normal.

The posterior pole and macular region show no significant abnormality.

Superior to the optic nerve and beyond the superior temporal arcades is a wedge-shaped area of intra-retinal hemorrhage and soft exudate.

During the laminar phase of the fluorescein angiogram there is blockage of the background choroidal fluorescence by the intraretinal hemorrhage.

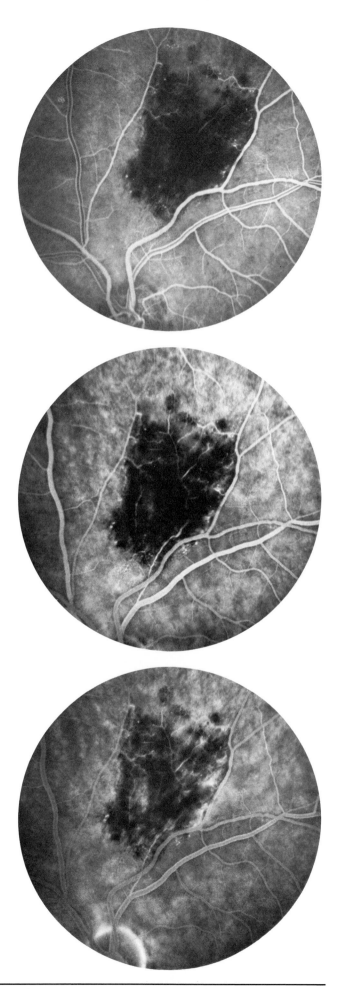

Later in the angiogram the smaller branches of the occluded branch vein can be seen within the hemorrhage. These smaller branches are very irregular. There are areas of capillary dropout and nonperfusion corresponding to the soft exudates seen on the color photographs.

Later in the angiogram there is minimal leakage intraretinally of the fluorescein dye from the small branched veins involved in the occlusion and a few scattered microaneurysms. The site of the occlusion where the superior temporal artery crosses one of the smaller branched veins just inferior to the hemorrhage is obvious.

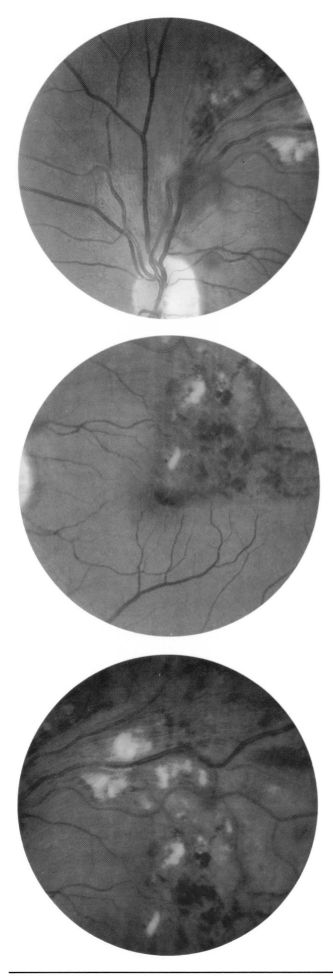

Branch Retinal Vein Occlusion
(major superior temporal occlusion)

The optic nerve appears normal. At the first crossing of the superior temporal artery and vein there is a major branch vein occlusion.

The intraretinal hemorrhage extends into the macular region from the superior temporal branch vein occlusion. Scattered areas of soft exudate can also be seen in the posterior pole. The sensory retina above the horizontal raphe appears to be thickened due to intraretinal edema.

Extending along the superior temporal quadrant and the course of the superior temporal vessels are multiple intraretinal blotch hemorrhages. Scattered areas of soft exudate are also seen within the superior temporal quadrant.

AUTHOR'S NOTE

Frequently one can appreciate thickening of the sensory retina due to intraretinal edema without stereo viewing by a loss in transparency of the portion of the retina which is edematous.

The fluorescein angiogram shows the retinal vascular changes to be limited to the superior portion of the sensory retina above the horizontal raphe. The smaller branches of the superior temporal branch vein are dilated. There is also dilatation of the capillary bed with very fine intraretinal microvascular abnormalities. Areas of blocked fluorescence and nonperfusion appear as black areas on the fluorescein angiogram. These correspond to areas of intraretinal hemorrhage and soft exudate, respectively.

Later in the angiogram there is intraretinal accumulation of fluorescein dye from the dilated capillaries, intraretinal microvascular abnormalities, and leakage from the branches of the superior temporal vein involved in the occlusion.

In the superior temporal quadrant, large areas of nonperfusion and blocked fluorescence from hemorrhage can be seen. There is also staining of the branches of the superior temporal vein due to a breakdown in the blood-retinal barrier.

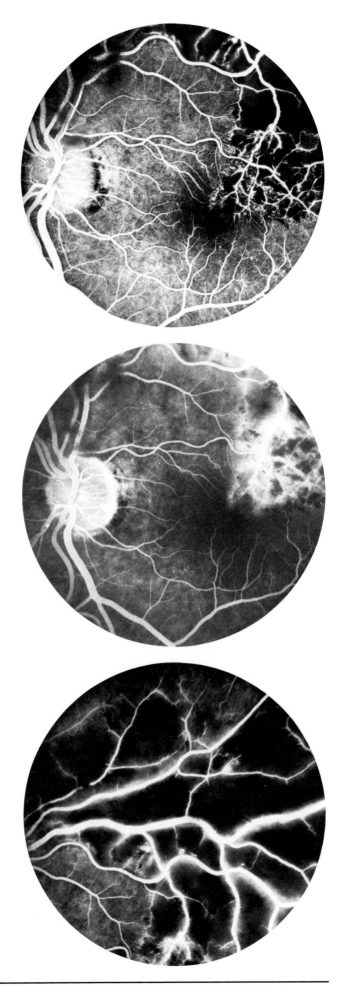

Branch Retinal Vein Occlusion
(multiple areas of collateralization)

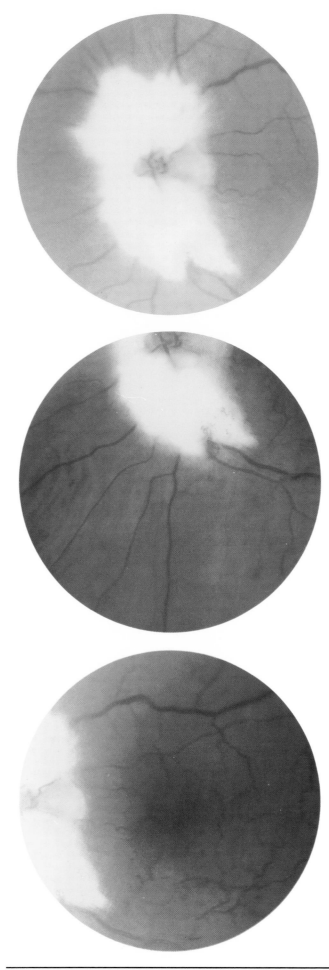

The optic nerve is surrounded by myelinated nerve fibers.

Along the inferior temporal artery and vein, collaterals can be seen. The inferior temporal vein is slightly engorged with the inferior temporal artery appearing irregular and narrowed.

In the posterior pole the retina above the horizontal raphe appears normal. The inferior retina appears to have lost its transparency due to intraretinal edema. Punctate intraretinal hemorrhages are visible.

During the laminar phase of the angiogram, multiple areas of collateralization can be seen both nasal to the fovea and temporal to the fovea across the horizontal raphe. There are also punctate microaneurysms with dilated capillaries and intraretinal microvascular abnormalities in the inferior temporal quadrant.

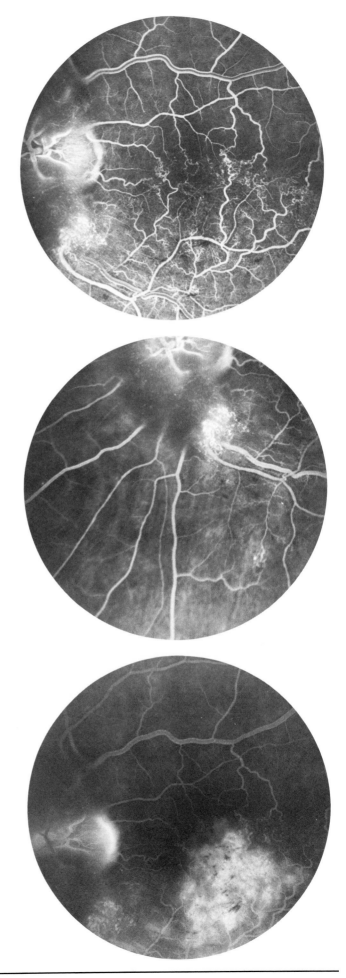

Collaterals without leakage of fluorescein can be seen at the inferior aspect of the myelinated nerve fibers along the inferior temporal arcades. These collaterals surround the occlusion site at the A-V crossing, which is obscured by the myelinated nerve fibers which slightly block the background fluorescence.

Late in the angiogram there is diffuse intraretinal leakage of fluorescein, indicating retinal edema. There is some slight cystoid edema in the perifoveal region. The punctate intraretinal hemorrhages within the edematous retina block the background fluorescence. The superior temporal quadrant is entirely normal.

AUTHOR'S NOTE

This case shows the three classic sites of collaterals in branch retinal vein occlusion: (1) around the occlusion site; (2) draining the nasal macula; (3) temporal to the macula across the horizontal raphe. The myelinated nerve fibers are unrelated to the inferior temporal major branch vein occlusion.

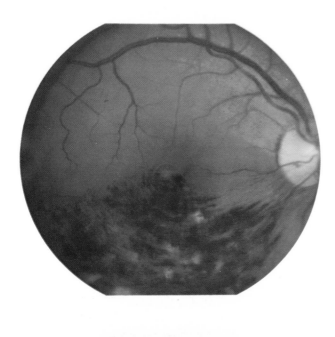

Major Branch Vein Occlusion
(with macular cyst)

A major inferior temporal branch vein occlusion with intraretinal hemorrhage and soft exudate along the course of the inferior temporal vein can be seen. A cystic-like lesion can be seen in the center of the macula.

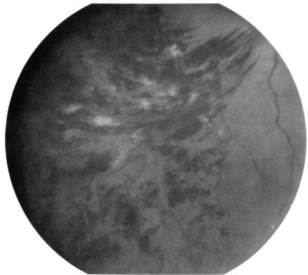

The intraretinal hemorrhage and soft exudate extend into the inferior temporal quadrant.

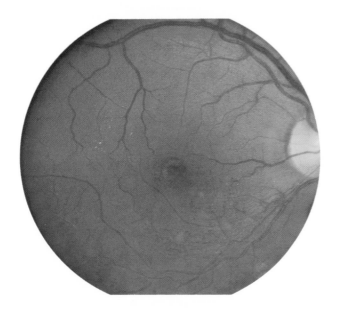

After clearing of the intraretinal hemorrhage, multiple collaterals can be seen across the horizontal raphe temporal to the macula, draining the nasal macula, and around the occlusion site. Pigmentary change is present in the center of the macula.

The red-free photograph clearly shows the hemorrhages and soft exudate along the course of the inferior temporal vein. The cystic lesion involving the center of the macula is also clearly visible.

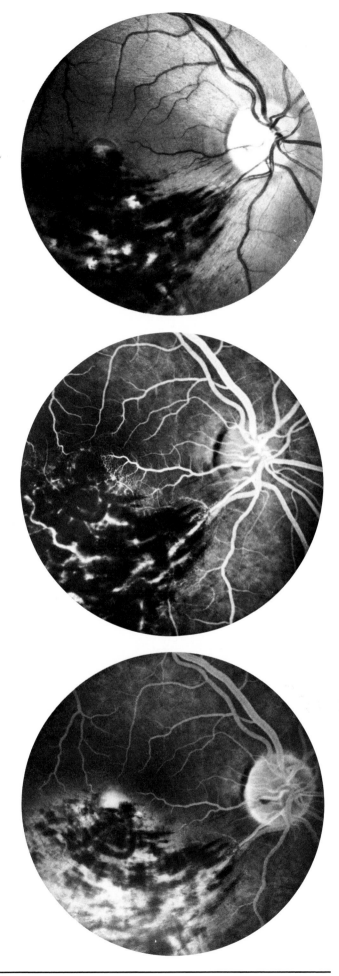

The fluorescein angiogram shows blockage of the background choroidal fluorescence by the intraretinal hemorrhage. There is dilatation of the capillary bed in the perifoveal region.

The late angiogram shows accumulation of the fluorescein dye within the cystic macular lesion. There is diffuse intraretinal accumulation of fluorescein dye from the dilated capillary bed, microaneurysms, and leakage from the retinal veins. The hemorrhages continue to block the background choroidal fluorescence.

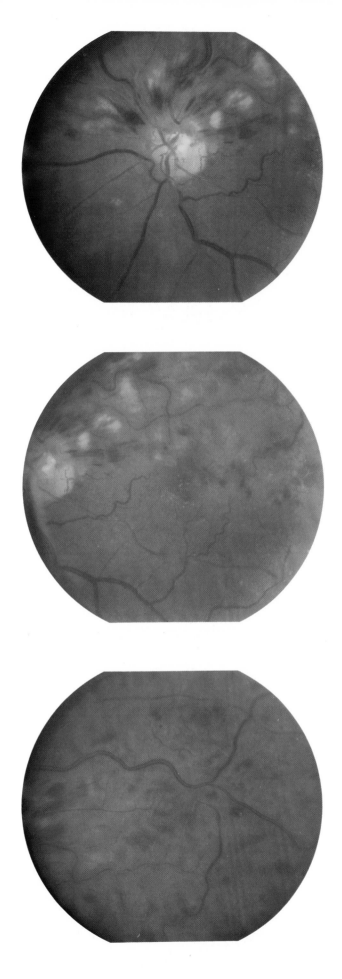

Branch Retinal Vein Occlusion
(hemispheric occlusion with extensive nonperfusion)

A superior hemispheric branch vein occlusion is present. Intraretinal hemorrhage and soft exudate extend into the superior nasal and superior temporal quadrants.

The intraretinal hemorrhage and soft exudate extend toward the center of the macula along the course of the superior temporal vein. Scattered areas of intraretinal hard exudate are also present.

In the superior temporal quadrant a few scattered blotch hemorrhages are present. Many of the smaller caliber venules are occluded.

During the laminar phase of the angiogram there is lack of visibility of the choroidal fluorescent pattern in the superior temporal quadrant. This is due both to intraretinal hemorrhage and because of marked retinal ischemia from capillary dropout and nonperfusion.

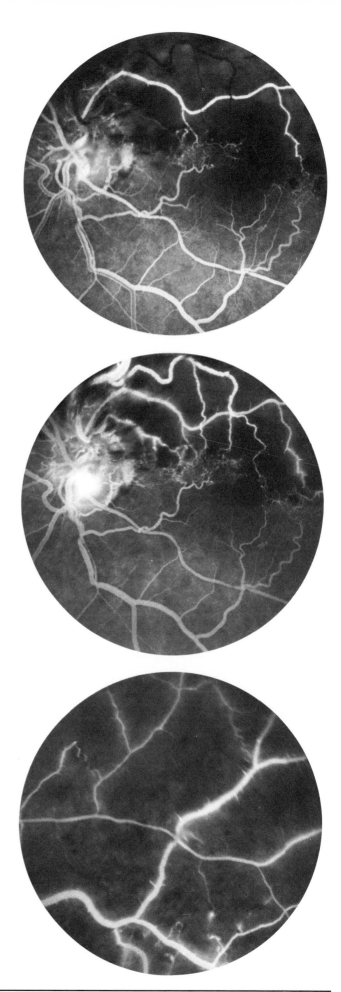

There is slight leakage of fluorescein from dilated capillaries on the surface of the optic nerve. There is some disruption of the perifoveal capillaries at the 12 o'clock position. The vascular changes are limited to the area above the horizontal raphe, which is typical of a branch retinal vein occlusion.

In the superior temporal periphery, there is marked nonperfusion with capillary dropout. There is staining of some of the retinal venous walls, indicating a breakdown in the blood-retinal barrier.

AUTHOR'S NOTE

Patients with extensive areas of capillary dropout and nonperfusion should be followed carefully because there may be an increased risk of proliferative retinopathy.

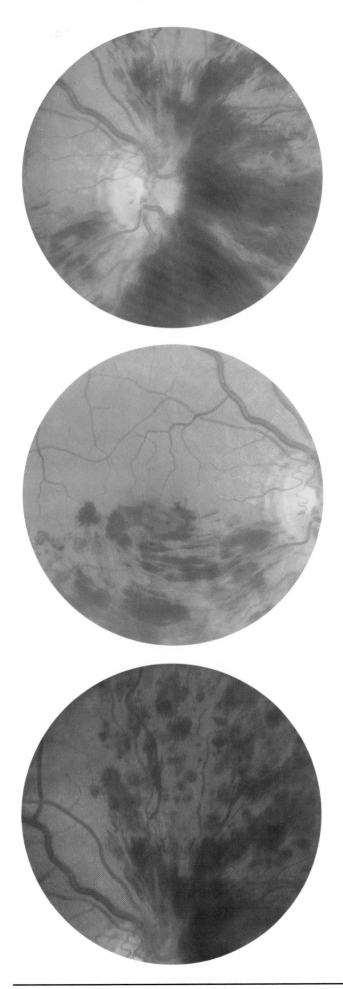

Branch Retinal Vein Occlusion
(three retinal quadrants involved and disc collateralization)

Extensive intraretinal blotch hemorrhages are seen along the nasal aspect of the optic nerve extending from approximately the 11 o'clock to the 8 o'clock position clockwise. Fine collateralization appears to be present on the surface of the nerve.

The hemorrhage extends along the inferior temporal arcade and involves the retina in the posterior pole below the horizontal raphe. The hemorrhage extends into the foveal region.

Involvement of the superior nasal quadrant can be seen. Therefore, the superior nasal, inferior nasal, and inferior temporal quadrants are involved in this occlusion.

Along the inferior temporal arcade there are punctate small hemorrhages, and a few scattered microaneurysms are seen.

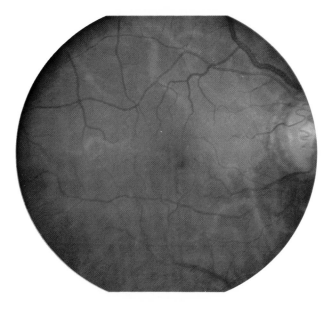

There is almost complete clearing of the hemorrhage surrounding the optic nerve. Fairly large caliber collaterals can be seen on the surface of the nerve.

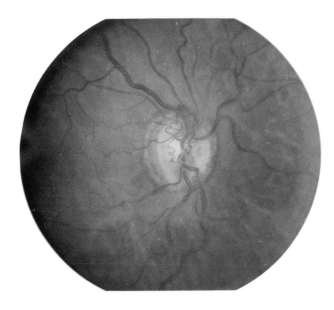

The red-free photograph shows abnormal vessels on the surface of the nerve. Fluorescein angiography will distinguish whether these are collaterals or neovascularization.

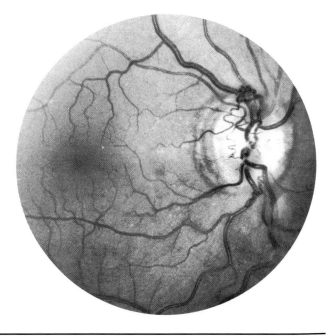

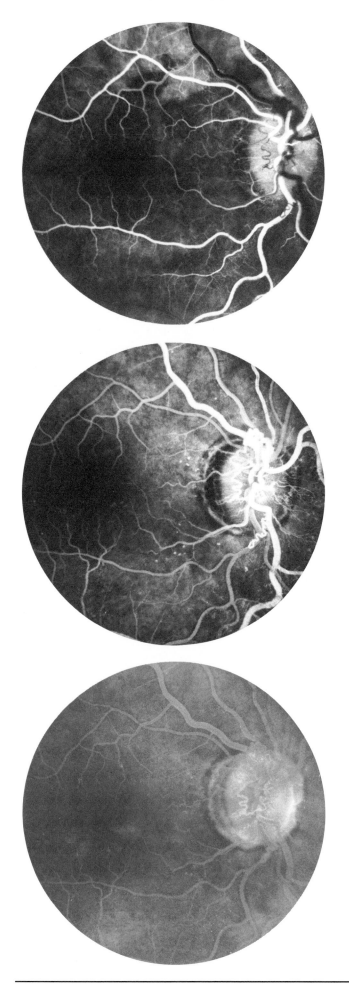

The early laminar phase of the angiogram shows the abnormal vessels on the surface of the nerve to be void of the fluorescein dye. There does not appear to be any significant blockage of the background fluorescence because most of the intraretinal hemorrhage has absorbed.

Later in the angiogram, the collaterals fill with the fluorescein and show no leakage. Scattered punctate hyperfluorescent microaneurysms can be seen temporal to the nerve.

The late angiogram shows no significant leakage of fluorescein, and the collaterals can still be seen. There is very subtle hyperfluorescence in the perifoveal region from the scattered microaneurysms.

AUTHOR'S NOTE

The value of fluorescein angiography can be seen in this case in differentiating disc collaterals secondary to an acute vein occlusion from disc neovascularization. Collaterals, for the most part, do not leak, or only very slightly leak, fluorescein, whereas disc neovascularization will profusely leak fluorescein during the venous phase of the angiogram.

Branch Retinal Vein Occlusion (double macular branch vein occlusion)

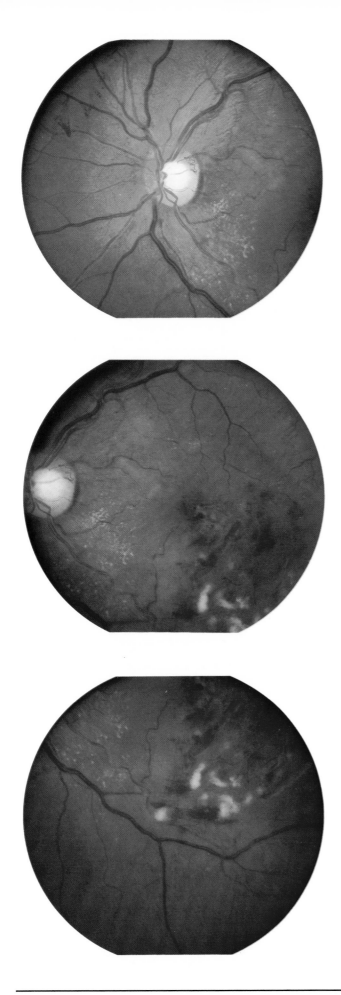

The optic nerve shows fine collaterals at approximately the 2 o'clock position.

Superior to the fovea are punctate microaneurysms with a few scattered intraretinal hemorrhages with some deposition of hard exudate. Along the inferior temporal arcade there is thickening of the sensory retina with intraretinal hemorrhage and soft exudate. Deposition of hard exudate can also be seen. The intraretinal hemorrhage and edema extend into the foveal region.

The intraretinal hemorrhage and soft exudate are secondary to an inferior macular branch vein occlusion.

During the laminar phase of the angiogram there is dilatation of the capillary bed with scattered micro-aneurysms above and below the horizontal raphe.

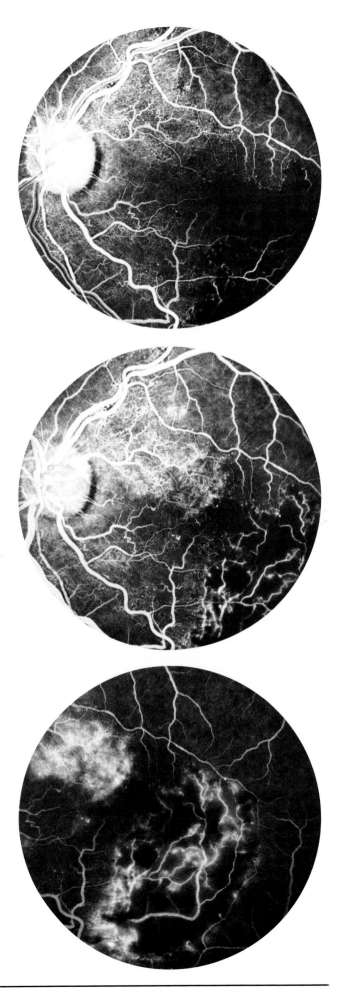

Leakage of fluorescein dye can be seen from the scattered microaneurysms and dilated capillary bed secondary to the superior and inferior temporal macular vein occlusions. The intraretinal hemorrhage secondary to the inferior temporal macular branch vein occlusion blocks the background choroidal fluorescence. There are multiple areas of capillary nonperfusion between the center of the macula and the inferior temporal arcade. These correspond to the soft exudates seen on the color photographs.

The late angiogram shows intraretinal accumulation of fluorescein dye secondary to the superior temporal macular branch vein occlusion and the inferior temporal macular branch vein occlusion. The intra-retinal hemorrhage continues to block the background choroidal fluorescence. The areas of nonperfusion persist in blocking the background fluorescence.

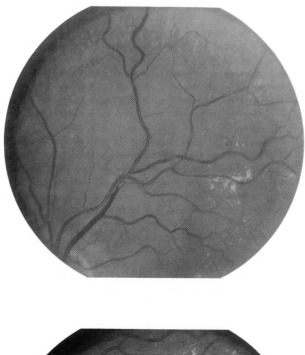

Branch Retinal Vein Occlusion (associated with arterial macroaneurysm)

The site of the superior temporal branch vein occlusion where the artery crosses over the vein is evident. Along the superior temporal arcade there are scattered microaneurysms, a few dot and blotch hemorrhages, and deposition of hard exudate.

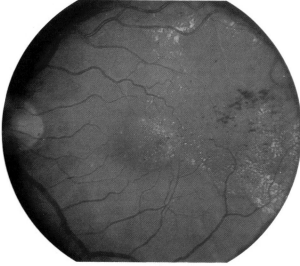

The posterior pole shows hard exudate along the superior temporal arcade. There is thickening of the sensory retina in the macular region secondary to macular edema. There is extensive deposition of hard exudate with intraretinal hemorrhage both in the macular region and temporal to the macula.

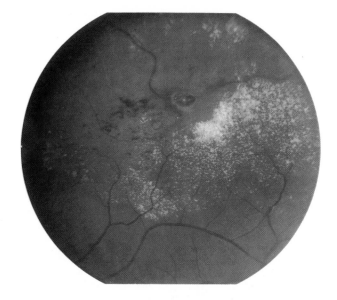

The temporal retina shows an arterial macroaneurysm surrounded by intraretinal hard exudate and a few scattered intraretinal blotch hemorrhages.

During the laminar phase of the angiogram there are scattered microaneurysms with dilatation of the capillary bed along the superior temporal arcade.

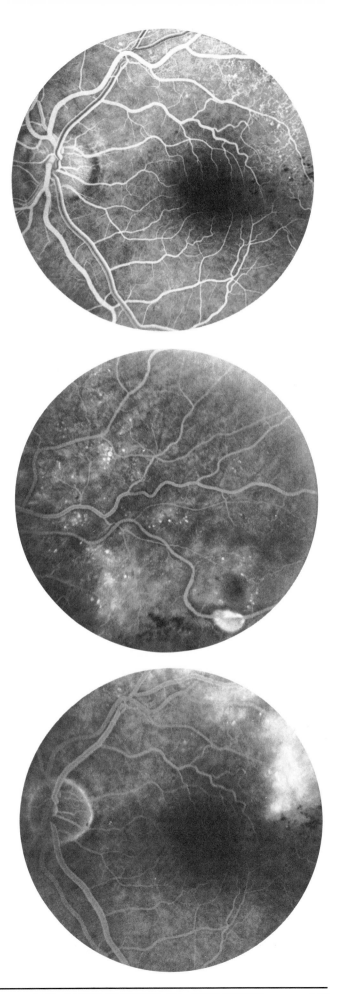

Temporal to the macula there is hyperfluorescence of the arterial macroaneurysm. Multiple small intraretinal microaneurysms which are leaking fluorescein can also be seen. The intraretinal hemorrhage in the vicinity of the arterial macroaneurysm blocks the background choroidal fluorescence.

The late angiogram shows diffuse intraretinal accumulation of fluorescein dye, indicating retinal edema. These changes are limited to the area above the horizontal raphe along the superior temporal arcade.

AUTHOR'S NOTE
Arterial macroaneurysms are not an infrequent finding in patients with retinal branch vein occlusion.

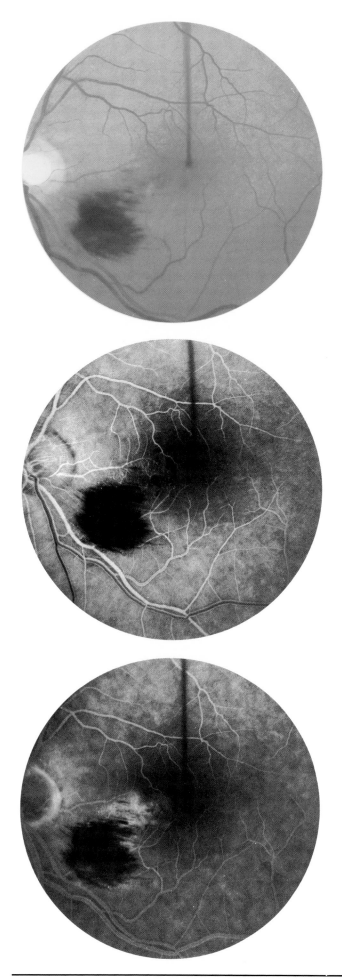

Macular Branch Retinal Vein Occlusion (acute occlusion with sparing of the fovea)

There is evidence of an acute inferior temporal macular branch vein occlusion. The intraretinal hemorrhage is evident. The tip of the fixation pointer is supraimposed over the fovea.

During the laminar phase of the angiogram there is blockage of the background choroidal fluorescence by the intraretinal blotch hemorrhage. The fixation pointer is clearly visible. There is some dilatation of the capillaries and microaneurysmal change superior to the hemorrhage.

The late angiogram shows some slight intraretinal leakage of fluorescein from the dilated capillaries and microaneurysms nasal to the fovea. The foveal region is spared and shows no evidence of fluorescein leakage. The intraretinal hemorrhage continues to block the background choroidal fluorescence.

Macular Branch Retinal Vein Occlusion (acute occlusion with intraretinal hemorrhage, soft exudate, and cystoid edema)

There is intraretinal hemorrhage and soft exudate secondary to an inferior temporal macular branch vein occlusion in the right eye. The abnormalities are confined to the region between the inferior temporal arcade and the center of the macula.

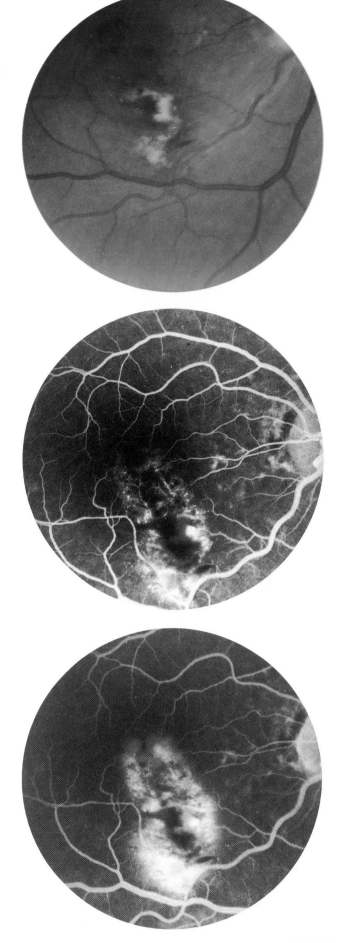

The fluorescein angiogram shows an area of capillary dropout and nonperfusion corresponding to the area of soft exudate. The area of nonperfusion is surrounded by dilated capillaries and microaneurysms.

Later in the angiogram there is leakage of the dye intraretinally with a classic cystoid macular edema pattern. The fluorescein dye leaks into the nonperfused area from the surrounding dilated capillaries and microaneurysms.

Macular Branch Retinal Vein Occlusion

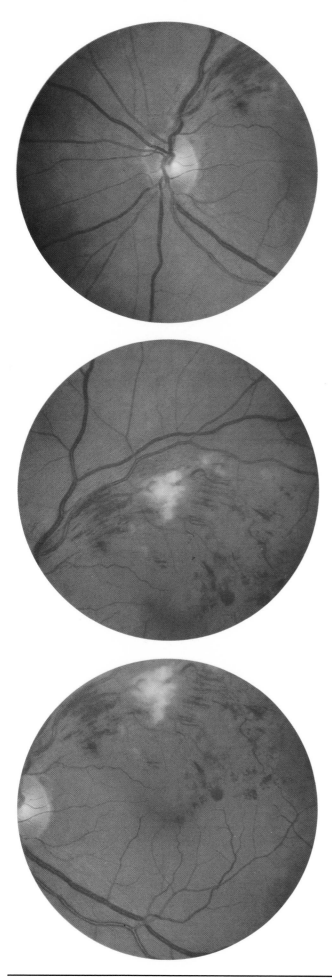

The optic nerve is normal. Along the superior temporal arcade intraretinal splinter and blotch hemorrhages can be seen.

The intraretinal hemorrhages and soft exudates are confined to the area between the superior temporal arcade and the center of the macula.

In the posterior pole there is thickening of the sensory retina between the superior temporal arcade and the center of the fovea, indicating macular edema. Intraretinal hemorrhages and soft exudate are confined to the area superior to the horizontal raphe. The retina along the inferior temporal arcade is entirely normal.

During the arterio-venous phase of the angiogram there is blockage of the background choroidal fluorescence by the intraretinal hemorrhages secondary to the superior temporal macular branch vein occlusion. The areas of soft exudate which were seen on the color photographs appear as areas of nonperfusion. A few scattered microaneurysms and dilatation of the capillary bed are also present.

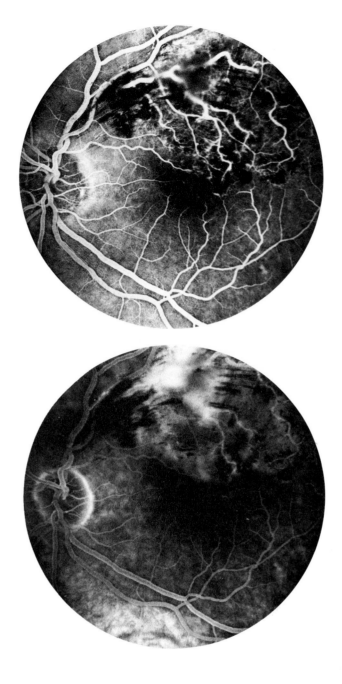

Later in the angiogram there is intraretinal accumulation of fluorescein dye as indicated by the diffuse hyperfluorescence. This indicates intraretinal edema. This intraretinal edema extends toward the foveal region but does not involve the center of the fovea. The intraretinal hemorrhages continue to block the background choroidal fluorescence.

AUTHOR'S NOTE

Clinically, macular retinal branch vein occlusions are characterized as those occlusions which primarily involve the retina from the center of the fovea to either the superior temporal or inferior temporal arcade. If the hemorrhages and retinal changes extend beyond the temporal arcades, the occlusion is then considered a major occlusion. The chances of developing proliferative retinopathy with macular occlusions is less because there is usually less retina involved in the ischemic process.

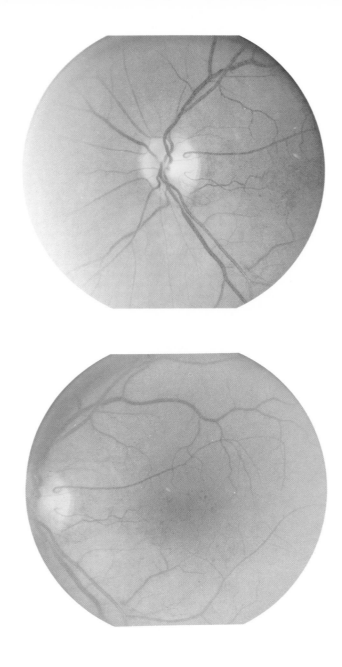

Branch Retinal Vein Occlusion
(old inferior temporal macular occlusion with minimal edema)

The old occlusion site, where the inferior temporal artery crosses the branch of the inferior temporal vein, resulting in the inferior temporal macular branch vein occlusion, is evident.

A few scattered microaneurysms can be seen in the macular region. A single area of hard exudate is also present.

During the venous phase of the angiogram the site of the inferior temporal macular branch vein occlusion can clearly be seen. Fine collaterals surround the occlusion site. The inner perifoveal capillary ring appears intact. However, there are scattered areas of microaneurysms in the perifoveal region which are hyperfluorescent.

Later in the angiogram there is slight leakage of fluorescein from the scattered perifoveal microaneurysms.

The very late stage of the angiogram shows very slight intraretinal accumulation of fluorescein dye in the macular region and perifoveal region, indicating minimal edema.

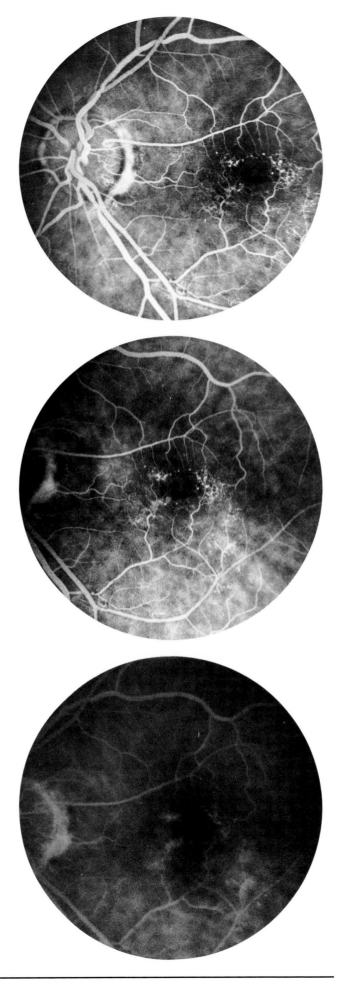

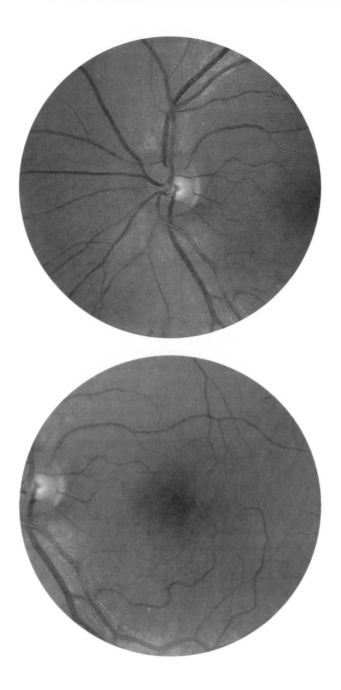

Branch Retinal Vein Occlusion
(inferior temporal macular occlusion with cystoid edema)

The site of the inferior temporal macular branch vein occlusion can be seen where the inferior temporal artery crosses the first branch of the inferior temporal vein.

Along the inferior temporal vessels a few scattered microaneurysms and a few scattered hard exudates are evident.

During the arterio-venous phase of the angiogram there are scattered microaneurysms with dilatation of the capillary bed along the first branch of the inferior temporal vein.

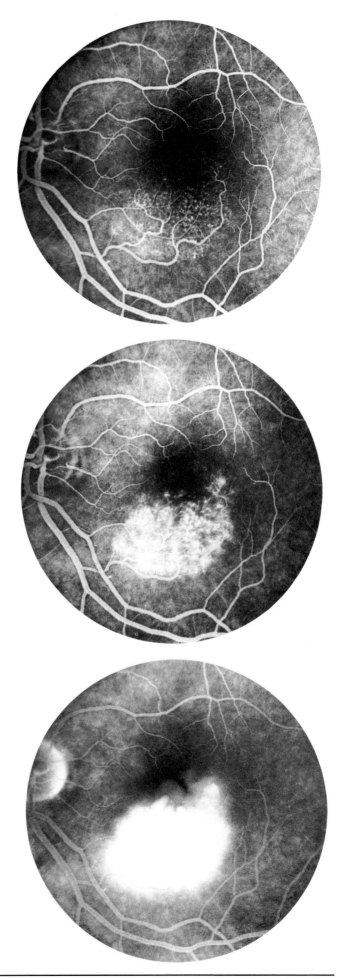

Later in the angiogram there is leakage of fluorescein dye from these dilated capillaries and microaneurysms. These changes are confined to the area between the inferior temporal arcade and the center of the macula. The occlusion site is clearly visible by attenuation of the first branch of the inferior temporal vein under the branch artery.

The late angiogram shows a classic cystoid macular edema pattern with diffuse intraretinal accumulation of fluorescein from the inferior temporal macular branch vein occlusion.

AUTHOR'S NOTE

Clinically, the changes in the posterior pole and macular region were very minimal. However, the patient's vision was reduced to 20/200, and the fluorescein angiogram clearly documented the presence of cystoid macular edema. The value of fluorescein angiography in old macular branch vein occlusions with reduced vision is clearly evident in this particular case.

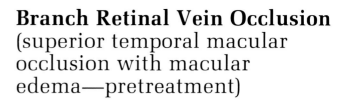

Branch Retinal Vein Occlusion
(superior temporal macular occlusion with macular edema—pretreatment)

There are scattered intraretinal dot and blotch hemorrhages and microaneurysms between the superior temporal arcade and the center of the macula. There are also a few scattered areas of soft exudate in this region.

There are multiple scattered microaneurysms and dilatation of the capillary bed between the center of the fovea and the superior temporal arcade. The small intraretinal blotch hemorrhages block the background choroidal fluorescence. There are several areas of nonperfusion corresponding to the soft exudate seen clinically. The inner perifoveal capillary ring at the 12 o'clock position is dilated and appears more hyperfluorescent.

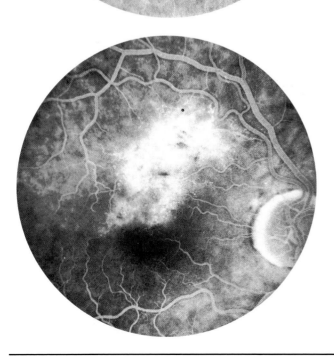

Later in the angiogram there is diffuse leakage of fluorescein intraretinally, indicating macular edema. No definite cystoid pattern is seen. These changes are limited to the superior aspect of the horizontal raphe, and the changes are contained within the area demarcated by the center of the macula and the superior temporal vessels. Therefore, this is a macular branch vein occlusion.

Branch Retinal Vein Occlusion
(superior temporal macular occlusion with macular edema—post-treatment)

Pigmented photocoagulation scars can be seen in the superior and temporal aspects of the macula. The area of soft exudate surrounded by fine microaneurysms and intraretinal microvascular abnormalities is also evident.

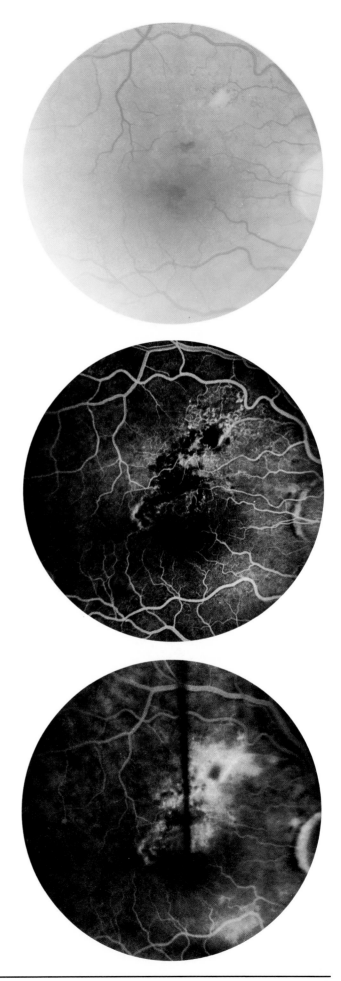

The blocked fluorescence is secondary to the pigmentary change from the photocoagulation to the leaking microaneurysms. The area of soft exudate surrounded by intraretinal microvascular abnormalities causes blockage of the background choroidal fluorescence.

Late in the angiogram there is definitely less leakage in the immediate perifoveal region. The leakage around the soft exudate is evident but had no effect on the visual acuity.

AUTHOR'S NOTE

This is a case of a surgeon whose vision was reduced to 20/80 for 6 months after the acute macular branch vein occlusion. Two weeks after treatment, vision improved to 20/30 and the patient's symptoms were markedly reduced. It is well recognized that there may have been spontaneous improvement in the macular edema without treatment. Hopefully, the national collaborative Branch Vein Occlusion Study will determine the efficacy of treatment as compared to the natural history in patients with macular edema from macular branch vein occlusions.

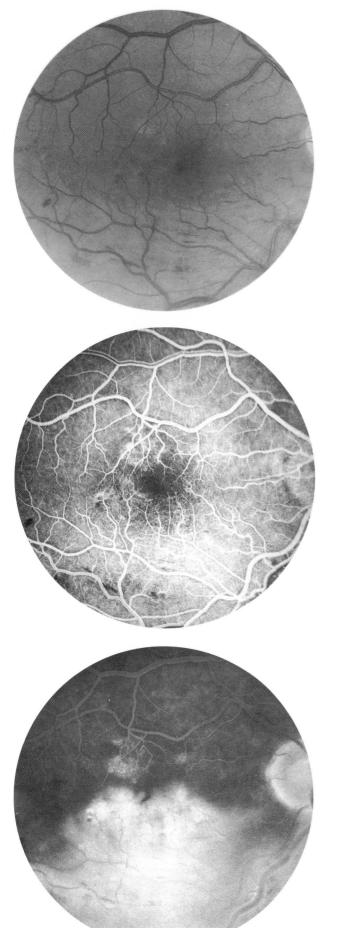

Branch Retinal Vein Occlusion
(inferior temporal macular occlusion with extensive macular and cystoid edema— pretreatment)

Intraretinal hemorrhages and microaneurysms can be seen between the macula and inferior temporal arcade. Just superior to the fovea there is some hypopigmented change at the level of the pigment epithelium.

During the laminar phase of the angiogram there is dilatation of the capillary bed below the horizontal raphe. There are also multiple small scattered microaneurysms. Just superior to the fovea there is an area of increased hyperfluorescence due to atrophy of the retinal pigment epithelium.

Late angiogram shows diffuse leakage of fluorescein intraretinally, indicating retinal edema. Obvious cystoid macular edema can also be seen. The pigment epithelial window defect above the fovea is evident. The diffuse leakage of the fluorescein dye is limited to the area between the center of the macula and the inferior temporal arcade.

Branch Retinal Vein Occlusion
(inferior temporal macular occlusion with extensive macular and cystoid edema— post-treatment)

The atrophic and hyperpigmented changes secondary to argon laser photocoagulation can clearly be seen. There is no evidence of intraretinal hemorrhage. The area of pigment epithelial atrophy above the fovea has not changed.

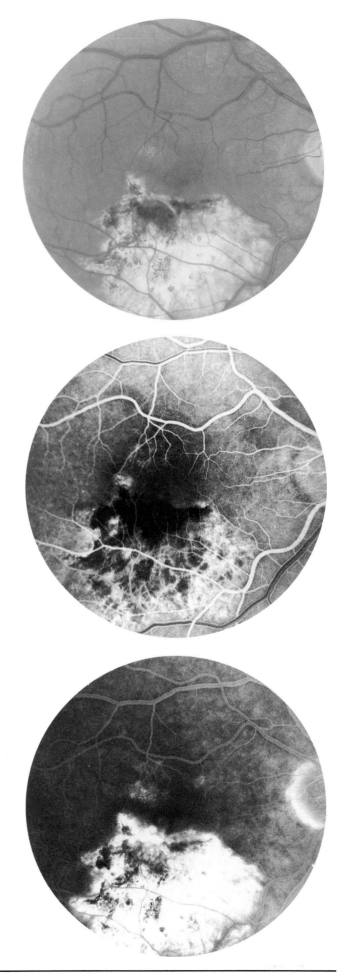

During the laminar phase of the angiogram there is both blockage and hyperfluorescent change from the photocoagulation treatment for the extensive edema.

The late frame of the angiogram shows staining of the photocoagulation scar with continued blockage by the hyperpigmentary change within the photocoagulation area. There does not appear to be any significant leakage of fluorescein in the macula or perifoveal region.

AUTHOR'S NOTE

This is a case of an artist whose vision was reduced to 20/200 for 8 months. Photocoagulation treatment, which was done in four separate sessions, resulted in marked reduction of the edema and improvement of the vision to 20/25.

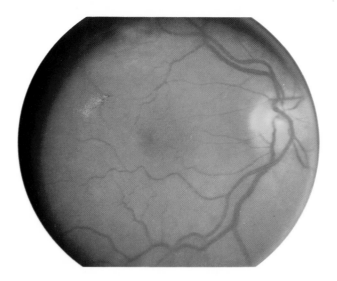

Branch Retinal Vein Occlusion
(associated with probable *Trichosporon* chorioretinitis)

The optic nerve and macular region of the right eye appear normal.

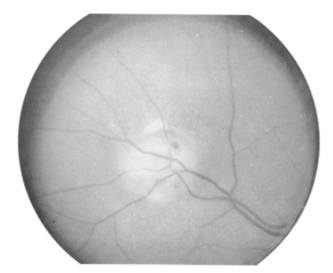

Along the superior temporal arcade there is a slightly elevated disc-like lesion at the level of the choroid which extends into the subretinal space. Overlying the lesion are punctate hemorrhages. Surrounding the lesion are subretinal hard exudates. The branches of the superior temporal artery overlying the lesion are markedly attenuated.

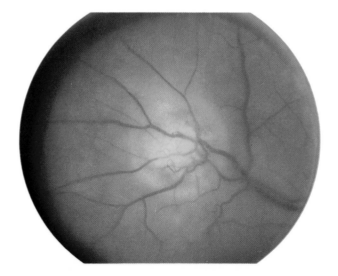

Six months later the disc-like lesion has increased in size and is more vascular. Overlying the lesion, fine vessels can be seen. There appears to be a branch retinal vein occlusion with some collateralization developing.

During the laminar phase of the angiogram fine vessels can be seen on the surface of the lesion. There is a rim of blocked choroidal fluorescence surrounding this lesion.

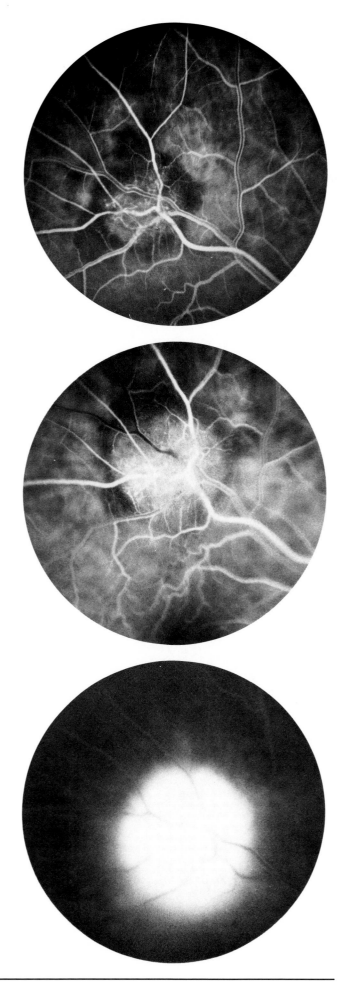

Later in the angiogram there is an obvious retinal branch vein occlusion with the abnormal vessels on the surface of the lesion beginning to leak fluorescein.

The late angiogram shows diffuse leakage of fluorescein from the abnormal vessels and also from the lesion itself. There appears to be late staining of the disc-like subretinal lesion.

AUTHOR'S NOTE

This is a case of probable metastatic fungal chorioretinitis developing during systemic Trichosporon sepsis in a patient with remissions and exacerbations of acute myelogenous leukemia. The increase in size of the lesion occurred during one of the exacerbations of the patient's leukemia with an increase in the manifestations of systemic trichosporosis. *Trichosporon beigelii* has angioinvasive properties, and this could account for the arterial narrowing and eventual branch retinal vein occlusion. There are an increased number of chorioretinic fungal lesions occurring in immunocompromised patients.

Vasculitis—Periphlebitis
(etiology unknown)

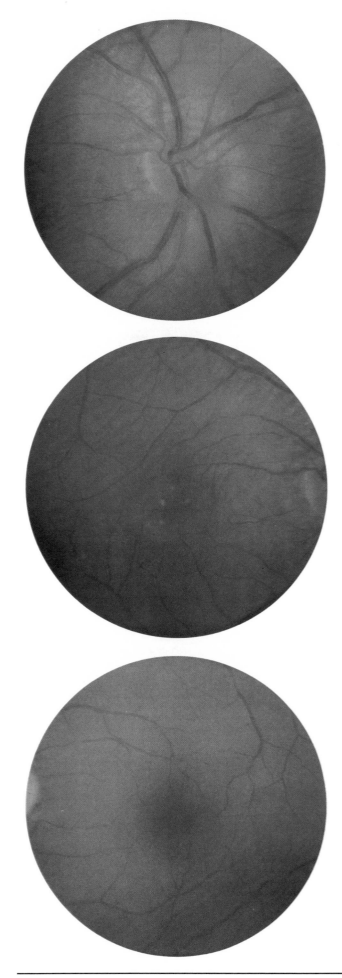

The optic nerve and retinal vasculature appear normal.

In the macular region, there are yellowish deposits within the sensory retina. Whether this is hard exudate or inflammatory material is difficult to distinguish.

The macular region of the left eye appears normal. The distal portion of the inferior temporal vein shows irregularity in its caliber.

During the venous phase of the fluorescein angiogram in the right eye, there is some abnormal hyperfluorescence of the venous walls. This can be seen along the inferior nasal vein and the smaller caliber venules superior to the macula.

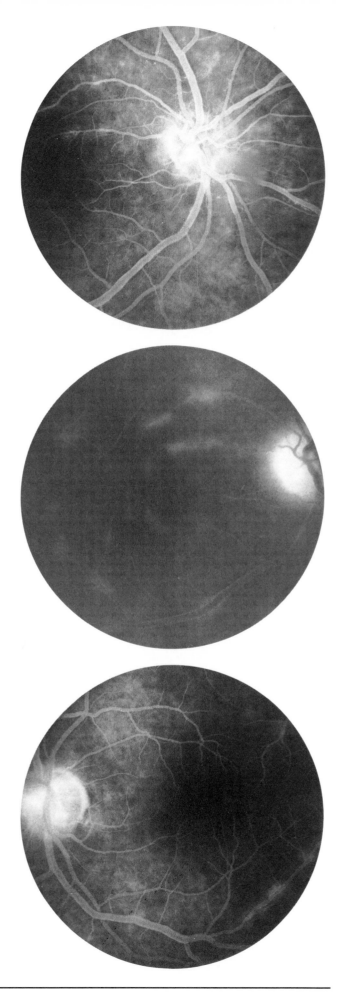

The late angiogram of the right eye shows staining of many of the branch retinal veins, indicating a breakdown in the blood-retinal barrier secondary to inflammation.

In the left posterior pole, there is staining of the inferior temporal retinal vein and also evidence of irregularity in the caliber of the vein.

AUTHOR'S NOTE

This patient was completely worked up for a possible systemic cause for the periphlebitis. However, the work-up was completely negative.

Bibliography

Algvere P: Fluorescein studies of retinal vasculitis in sarcoidosis: Report of a case. *Acta Ophthalmol* 18:1129, 1970.

Allaire J: *Contribution a l'etudes des hemorrhagies de la retine.* Paris, Arnette, 1925.

Archer DB: Neovascularization of the retina—Treacher Collins Prize Essay, 1976. *Trans Ophthalmol Soc UK* 96:471–493, 1976.

Archer DB: Tributary vein obstruction: Pathogenesis and treatment of sequelae. *Doc Ophthalmol* 40:339–360, 1976.

Archer DB, Ernest JT, Newell FW: Classification of branch vein occlusion. *Trans Am Acad Ophthalmol Otolaryngol* 78:148–165, 1974.

Armaly MF, Araki M: Optic nerve circulation and ocular pressure. *Invest Ophthalmol* 14:724–731, 1975.

Ashford TP, Freiman DG: The role of the endothelium in the initial phases of thrombosis: An electron microscopic study. *Am J Pathol* 50:257–273, 1967.

Ashton N: Neovascularization in ocular disease. *Trans Ophthalmol Soc UK* 81:145–161, 1962.

Ashton N: Pathogenesis and aetiology of Eales' disease. In Pandit YK: *XIX Concillium Ophthalmologicum.* Bombay, Times of India Press, 1962, vol 2, p 828.

Ashton N, Cook C: Studies on developing retinal vessels. I. Influence of retinal detachment. *Br J Ophthalmol* 39:449–456, 1955.

Ashton N, Ward B, Serpell G: Effect of oxygen on developing retinal vessels with particular reference to the problem of retrolental fibroplasia. *Br J Ophthalmol* 38:397–432, 1954.

Barton CH, Vaziri ND: Central retinal vein occlusion associated with hemodialysis. *Am J Med Sci* 277:39–47, 1979.

Becker B, Post LT: Retinal vein occlusion: Clinical and experimental observations. *Am J Ophthalmol* 34:677–686, 1951.

Birchall CH, Harris GS, Drance SM, et al: Visual field changes in branch vein occlusion. *Arch Ophthalmol* 94:747–754, 1976.

Blankenship GW, Okun E: Retinal tributary vein occlusion: History and management by photocoagulation. *Arch Ophthalmol* 89:363–368, 1973.

Bonnet P: Le "signe de prethrombose" observe sur les vaisseaux de la retine dans l'hypertension arterielle. Sa valeur semiologique. *Arch Ophthalmol (Paris)* 11:12–34, 1951.

Boyce SW, Platia EV, Green WR: Drusen of the optic nerve head. *Ann Ophthalmol* 10:695–704, 1978.

Brodrick JD: Drusen of the disc and retinal haemorrhages. *Br J Ophthalmol* 57:299–306, 1973.

Campbell CJ, Wise GN: Photocoagulation therapy of branch vein obstructions. *Am J Ophthalmol* 75:28–31, 1978.

Charamis J, Karsourakis N, Mandras G: Etude de la circulation cerebro-retinienne au moyen l'injection intraveineuse de fluorescein. *Bull Soc Fr Ophthalmol* 78:576–587, 1965.

Cleasby GW, Hall DL, Fung WE, et al: Retinal branch vein occlusion: Treatment by photocoagulation. *Mod Probl Ophthalmol* 12(0):254–260, 1974.

Clements DB, Elsby JM, Smith WD: Retinal vein occlusion—A comparative study of factors affecting the prognosis, including a therapeutic trial of atromid S in this condition. *Br J Ophthalmol* 52:111–116, 1968.

Clemett RS: Retinal branch vein occlusion changes at site of obstruction. *Br J Ophthalmol* 58:548–554, 1974.

Clemett RS, Kohner EM, Hamilton AM: The visual prognosis in retinal branch vein occlusion. *Trans Ophthalmol Soc UK* 93:523–535, 1973.

Coats G: A case of thrombosis of the central vein pathologically examined. *Trans Ophthalmol Soc UK* 24:161–173, 1904.

Coats G: Thrombosis of the central vein of the retina. *R Lond Ophthalmol Hosp Rep* 16:62–122, 1904.

Coats G: Der Verschluss der Zentralvene der Retina: Fine ubersicht uber pathologisch-anatomisch untersuchte Falle. *Albrecht von Graefes Arch Ophthalmol* 86:341–393, 1913.

Colyear BH: Retinal vascular lesions treated by photocoagulation. *Am J Ophthalmol* 63:262–270, 1976.

Constantinides G, Francois P, Madelein F: Dechiurures retinennes au decours des thromboses veineuses. *Ann Ocul* 204:1249, 1971.

Cox MS, Whitmore PV, Gutow RF: Treatment of intravitreal and prepapillary neovascularization following branch retinal vein occlusion. *Trans Am Acad Ophthalmol Otolaryngol* 79:387–393, 1975.

Cross AG: Vasculitis retinae. *Trans Ophthalmol Soc UK* 83:133, 1963.

Cross AG: Vasculitis retinae: Prognosis and treatment. *Trans Ophthalmol Soc UK* 85:11, 1965.

Dayton G: The value of photocoagulation in occlusive vascular disease of the retina. *Pacif Med Surg* 76:26–30, 1968.

Dolenek A, Blatnij J, Navratil P: Thrombolyse bei Verschlusz von Netzhautvenen. *Klin Monatsbl Augenheilkd* 153:403–408, 1968.

Dollery CT, Hodge JV, Engel M: Studies of the retinal circulation with fluorescein. *Br Med J* 2:1210–1215, 1962.

Donders PC: Eales's disease. *Doc Ophthalmol* 12:1, 1958.

Dryden RM: Central retinal vein occlusion and chronic simple glaucoma. *Arch Ophthalmol* 73:659–663, 1965.

Duff IF, Falls HF, Linman JW: Anticoagulation therapy in occlusive vascular disease of the retina. *Arch Ophthalmol* 46:601–615, 1951.

Eales H: Cases of retinal haemorrhage associated with epistaxis and constipation. *Birmingham Med Rev* 9:262, 1880.

Elliot AJ: Recurrent intraocular hemorrhage in young adults (Eales's disease): A report of 31 cases. *Trans Am Ophthalmol Soc* 52:811, 1954.

Elliot AJ: Thirty-year observation of patients with Eales's disease. *Am J Ophthalmol* 80:404, 1975.

Elliot AJ, Harris GS: The present status of the diagnosis and treatment of periphlebitis retinae (Eales' disease). *Can J Ophthalmol* 4:117, 1969.

Ellis CJ, Hamer DB, Hunt RW, et al: Medical investigation of retinal vascular occlusion. *Br Med J* 2:1093–1098, 1964.

Elschnig A: Anastomasenbildgen an den Netzhautvenen. *Klin Monatsbl Augenheilkd* 36:55, 1898.

Emery JM, Landis D, Paton D, et al: The lamina cribrosa in normal and glaucomatous human eyes. *Trans Am Acad Ophthalmol Otolaryngol* 78:290–297, 1974.

Ennema MC: *Over Venesluiting in Het Netvlies.* Assen, Dissertatie, Amsterdam, 1940.

Ennema MC, Zeeman WPC: Venous occlusions in the retina. *Ophthalmologica* 126:229–347, 1953.

Everbusch O: Ein Auch in anatomischer Hinsicht bemerenswerter Fall von einseitiger traumatischer Thrombose der Netzhautvenen, verbunden mit Blutug in Centralhanal das Glaskorpers. *Klin Monatsbl Augenheilkd* 37:1, 1899.

Flindall RJ: Photocoagulation in chronic cystoid macular edema secondary to branch vein occlusion. *Can J Ophthalmol* 7:395–404, 1972.

Francois J, Cambie E, deLaez JJ: Argon laser slitlamp photocoagulation: Indications and results. *Ophthalmologica* 169:362–370, 1974.

Freiman DG: Disorders of the circulation: Thrombosis, embolism, infarction. In Brunson JG, Goll EA: *Concepts of Disease: A Textbook of Human Pathology.* New York, MacMillan, 1971, pp 313–314.

Freyler H, Nichorlis S: Lictkoagulation bei retinalen Venenthrombosen. *Klin Monatsbl Augenheilkd* 165:750–755, 1974.

Fujino T, Curtin VT, Norton EWD: Experimental central vein occlusion. *Trans Am Ophthalmol Soc* 66:318–378, 1968.

Fukuchi S: *Photocoagulation in Retinal Vein Symposium: Proceedings of the International Symposium on Fluorescein Angiography.* Tokyo, Igaku Shoin Ltd., 1972.

Gass JDM: A fluorescein angiographic study of macular dysfunction. II. Retinal vein obstruction. *Arch Ophthalmol* 80:550–568, 1968.

Gass JDM: *Stereoscopic Atlas of Macular Diseases: A Funduscopic and Angiographic Presentation.* St Louis, CV Mosby, 1970.

Gitter KA, Cohen G, Baber BW: Photocoagulation in venous occlusive disease. *Am J Ophthalmol* 79:578–581, 1975.

Goldberg MF: The role of ischemia in the production of vascular retinopathies. In Lynn JR, Snyder WB, Vaisen A: *Diabetic Retinopathy*. New York, Grune & Stratton, 1974, pp 47–64.

Green WR, Chan CC, Hutchins GM, et al: Central retinal vein occlusion: A prospective histopathologic study of 29 eyes in 28 cases. *Retina*, 1:27–55, 1981.

Greenwood A: Thrombosis of the central retinal vein and its branches. *JAMA* 82:92, 1924.

Gutman FA, Zegarra H: The natural course of temporal retinal branch vein occlusion. *Trans Am Acad Ophthalmol Otolaryngol* 78:178–192, 1974.

Hamilton AM, Kohner EM, Rosen D, et al: Experimental retinal branch vein occlusion in rhesus monkeys. I. Clinical appearances. *Br J Ophthalmol* 63:377–387, 1979.

Hamilton AM, Marshall J, Kohner EM, et al: Retinal new vessel formation following experimental vein occlusion. *Exp Eye Res* 20:493–497, 1975.

Harms C: Anatomische untersuchungen uber gefaszerkarkungen im Gebiete der Arteria und Vena centralis retinae und ihre Folgen fur die Cirkulation mit besonderer Beruchsichtigung des sogenannten hemorrhageschen Infarktes der netzhaut Graefes. *Arch Ophthalmol (Munchen)* 61:1, 245, 1905.

Hayreh SS: An experimental study of the central retinal vein occlusion. *Trans Ophthalmol Soc UK* 84:586–593, 1964.

Hayreh SS: Occlusion of the central retinal vessels. *Br J Ophthalmol* 49:626–645, 1965.

Hayreh SS: Pathogenesis of occlusion of the central retinal vessels. *Am J Ophthalmol* 72:998–1101, 1971.

Hayreh SS: Optic disc vasculitis. *Br J Ophthalmol* 56:652, 1972.

Hayreh SS, van Heuven WAJ, Hayreh MS: Experimental retinal vascular occlusion. I. Pathogenesis of central retinal vein occlusion. *Arch Ophthalmol* 96:311–323, 1978.

Heydenreich A: Lichtkoagulation bei Erkrankugen der Netzhautmitte. *Klin Monatsbl Augenheilkd* 160:146–154, 1972.

Hill DW: Fluorescein studies in retinal vascular occlusion. *Br J Ophthalmol* 52:1–12, 1968.

Hill DW, Griffiths JD: The prognosis in retinal vein thrombosis. *Trans Ophthalmol Soc UK* 90:309–322, 1970.

Hitchings RA Spaeth GL: Chronic retinal vein occlusion in glaucoma. *Br J Ophthalmol* 60:694–699, 1976.

Holmin N, Ploman KG: Thrombosis of central vein of retina treated with heparin. *Lancet* 1:664–665, 1938.

Hunter CP, Thompson HS: Papillophlebitis. In Blodi FC: *Current Concepts in Ophthalmology*. St Louis, CV Mosby, 1974, vol 4, p 353.

Jensen VA: Clinical studies of tributary thrombosis in the central retinal vein. *Acta Opthalmol Suppl* 10:1–93, 1936.

Joondeph HC, Goldberg MF: Rhegmatogenous retinal detachment after tributary vein occlusion. *Am J Ophthalmol* 80:253–257, 1975.

Kannel WB: Role of blood pressure in cardiovascular morbidity and mortality. *Prog Cardiovasc Dis* 17:5–24, 1974.

Karel I, Votockova J, Peleska M: Fluorescence angiography in unusual forms of idiopathic retinal vasculitis. *Ophthalmologica* 168:446–461, 1974.

Kearns TP, Hollenhorst RW: Venous stasis retinopathy of occlusive disease of the carotid artery. *Proc Mayo Clin* 38:304–312, 1963.

Kelley JS, Patz A, Schatz H: Management of retinal branch vein occlusion: The role of argon laser photocoagulation. *Ann Ophthalmol* 6:1123–1134, 1974.

Kirkham TH, Wrigley PFM, Holt JM: Central retinal vein occlusion complicating iron deficiency anemia. *Br J Ophthalmol* 55:777–781, 1971.

Klien BA: Obstruction of the central retinal vein: A clinicohistopathologic analysis. *Am J Ophthalmol* 27:1339–1354, 1944.

Klien BA: Prevention of retinal venous occlusion. *Am J Ophthalmol* 33:175–184, 1950.

Klien BA: Occlusion of the central retinal vein: Clinical importance of certain histopathologic observations. *Am J Ophthalmol* 36:316–324, 1953.

Klien BA, Olwin JA: A survey of the pathogenesis of retinal venous occlusion. *Arch Ophthalmol* 56:207–247, 1956.

Kloti R, Martenet AC, Speiser P: Zur Pathogenese der sekendarem Netzhautablosungen. *Mod Probl Ophthalmol* 10:236–244, 1972.

Kohner EM, Cappin JM: Do medical conditions have an influence on central retinal vein occlusions? *Proc R Soc Med* 67:20–22, 1974.

Kohner EM, Dollery CT, Shakib M, et al: Experimental retinal branch vein occlusion. *Am J Ophthalmol* 69:778–825, 1970.

Kohner EM, Schilling JS, Clemett RS: Clinical aspects of retinal branch vein occlusion significant for the understanding of its pathogenesis and preventive therapy. *Doc Ophthalmol Proc Series* 5:153–160, 1974.

Kohner EM, Schilling JS, Hamilton AM: The role of avascular retina in new vessel formation. *Metabol Ophthalmol* 1:15–23, 1976.

Kottow M, Metzler P, Hendrickson P: Vision and circulation. In Cant JS: *Proceedings of the Third William Makenzie Memorial Symposium*. London, Kimpton, 1976.

Koyanagi Y: Die Bedeutung der Gafeszkreuzung fur die Entstchung der Astthrombose der retinalen Aentralvene. *Klin Monatsbl Augenheilkd* 81:219–231, 1928.

Koyanagi Y: Die Pathologische Anatomie und Pathogenese de Krusungsphanomens der Netzhautgefasze bei Hochdruck. *Albrecht von Graefes Arch Ophthalmol* 135:526–536, 1936.

Koyanagi Y: Veranderungen an der Netzhaut bei Hocdruk. *Pathol Anat 15 Int Kogr Ophthalmol* 1:143–283, 1937.

Krill AE, Archer DB, Newell FW: Photocoagulation in complications secondary to branch vein occlusion. *Arch Ophthalmol* 85:48–60, 1971.

Kutschera E: Expectation of life in cases of retinal circulatory disturbances. *Wien Klin Wochenschr* 76:773–775, 1964.

Leber T: Die Krankheite der Netzhaut U. des Schnerven. *Handb Ges Ophthalmol Graefe-Saemisch, Leipsig* 5:531, 1877.

Listar A, Zwink FB: The course of thrombosis of the retinal veins. *Trans Ophthalmol Soc UK* 73:55–71, 1953.

Lyle TK, Wybar K: Retinal vasculitis. *Br J Ophthalmol* 45:778, 1961.

Meredith TA, Willerson D, Aaberg TM: Angiomatosis retinae presenting as branch vein occlusion: Report of a case. *Palestra Oftalmol Panamericana* 1:33–38, 1977.

Metzler V, Hohmann R, Kaskel D: Netzhautablosungen bei ver-Schliissen der Zentralvene Oder Ihrer Aste. *Klin Monatsbl Augenheilkd* 164:251–254, 1974.

Meyer-Schwickerath G: *Light Coagulation*. St Louis, CV Mosby, 1960.

Michaelson, IC, Campbell, ACP: Anatomy of the finer retinal vessels. *Trans Ophthamol Soc UK* 60:71–111, 1940.

Michaelson, IC, Herz E, Lewkowitz, E, et al: Effect of increased oxygen on the development of the retinal vessels: An experimental study. *Br J Ophthalmol* 38:577–587, 1954.

Michel, J: Die spontane Thrombose de Vena centralis des Opticus. *Albrecht von Graefes Arch Klin Ophthalmol* 24:37–70, 1878.

Michels RG, Gass JDM: The natural course of retinal branch vein obstruction. *Trans Am Acad Ophthalmol Otolaryngol* 78:166–177, 1974.

Michelson PE, Knox DL, Green WR: Ischemic ocular inflammation. *Arch Ophthalmol* 86:274–280, 1971.

Mierlobenstezn M van, Riaskoff S, Zahn KJ: Fluorescein photography of retinal vein occlusion in relation to photocoagulation and laser treatment. *Doc Ophthalmol Proc Series 3, The Hague, Junk*, 1973.

Moore, RF: Retinal vein thrombosis. *Br J Ophthalmol* 8(Suppl 2):1–90, 1924.

Neubauer H: Kollateralkreislauf der Netzhaut nach Astverschluss der Zentralvene. *Ber Dtsch Opthalmol Ges* 63:498, 1960.

Novotny HR, Alvis DL: A method of photographing fluorescein in circulating blood in the human retina. *Circulation* 24:82, 1961.

Okun E, Collins EM: Histopathology of experimental photocoagulation in the dog eye. Part III. Microaneurysm-like formations following branch vein occlusion. *Am J Ophthalmol* 56:40–45, 1963.

Oosterhuis JA: Fluorescein fundus photography in retinal vein occlusion. In Henkes HE: *Perspectives in Ophthalmology.* Amsterdam, Excerpta Medica, 1968.

Oosterhuis JA, Sedney SC: Photocoagulation in retinal vein thrombosis. *Ophthalmologica* 171:365–379, 1975.

Orth DH: Vascular occlusions. *Int Ophthalmol Clin* 17:97–112, 1977.

Orth DH, Fine BS, Fagman W, et al: Clarification of foveomacular nomenclature and grid for quantitation of macular disorders. *Trans Am Acad Ophthalmol Otolaryngol* 83:506–513, 1977.

Orth DH, Patz A: Retinal branch vein occlusion. *Surv Ophthalmol* 22:357–376, 1978.

Pandolfi M, Hedner N, Nilsson IM: Bilateral occlusion of the retinal veins in a patient with inhibition of fibrinolysis. *Ann Ophthalmol* 2:481–484, 1970.

Paton A, Rubinstein K, Smith VH: Arterial insufficiency in retinal venous occlusion. *Trans Ophthalmol Soc UK* 84:559–595, 1964.

Patz A: A guide to argon photocoagulation. *Surv Ophthalmol* 16:249–257, 1972.

Patz A, Orth DH, Fine SL: Macular edema secondary to branch retinal venous occlusion. In *Symposium on Retinal Diseases.* St Louis, CV Mosby, 1977.

Rabinowicz IM, Litman S, Michaelson IC: Branch venous thrombosis—A pathological report. *Trans Ophthalmol Soc UK* 88:191–210, 1969.

Ramos-Umpierre A, Berrocal JA: Retinal detachment following branch vein occlusion. *Ann Ophthalmol* 9:339–340, 1977.

Ring CP, Pearson TC, Sanders MD, et al: Viscosity and retinal vein thrombosis. *Br J Ophthalmol* 60:397–410, 1976.

Rosengren B, Stenstrom S: 30 Falle nov Venenthrombose der Netzhaut, behandelt mit Heparin. *Acta Ophthalmol* 20:145–152, 1942.

Rossmann H: Die thrombolytische Behandlung von Gefassverschliissen der Netzhaut. *Klin Monatsbl Augenheilkd* 149:874–880, 1966.

Rubinstein K, Jones EB: Retinal vein occlusion: Long-term prospects—10 years' follow-up of 143 patients. *Br J Ophthalmol* 60:148–150, 1976.

Schatz H, Yannuzzi L, Stransky TJ: Retinal detachment secondary to branch vein occlusion. *Ann Ophthalmol* 8:1437–1471, 1976.

Scott TM: Disturbances of body water, electolytes and circulation of blood. In Anderson WAD: *Pathology,* ed 4. St Louis, CV Mosby, 1961, pp 78–115.

Seitz R: Klinik und Pathologie der Netzhautgefasse. *Ferdinand Enke Verlag* 94: 1968.

Seitz R, Kersting G: Die Drusen der Schnervenpapille und des Pigmentepithels. *Klin Monatsbl Augenheilkd* 140:75–88, 1962.

Shimizu K, Tobari I: Treatment of retinal obstruction by photocoagulation. *Jpn J Clin Ophthalmol* 25:25, 1971.

Shoch D, Vail D: Differential diagnosis of retinal vein occlusion: Vascular diseases in ophthalmology. *Bibl Ophthalmol* 76:91–98, 1968.

Snyder WB, Allen L, Frazier O: Fluorescence angiography: An aid in the diagnosis of occluded vessels. *Arch Ophthalmol* 77:168–175, 1976.

Spitznas M, Meyer-Schwickerath G, Stephan B: The clinical picture of Eales' disease. *Albrecht von Graefes Arch Klin Ophthalmol* 194:73–85, 1975.

Spitznas M, Meyer-Schwickerath G, Stephan B: Treatment of Eales' disease with photocoagulation. *Albrecht von Graefes Arch Klin Ophthalmol* 194:193–198, 1975.

Stowe GC III, Zakov AN, Albert DM: Central retinal vascular occlusion associated with oral contraceptives. *Am J Ophthalmol* 86:798–801, 1978.

Theodossiadis G: Fluorescein angiography in Eales' disease. *Am J Ophthalmol* 69:271, 1970.

Theodossiadis G, Charamis J, Velissaropoulos P: Behandlungsergebnisse der Lichtkoagulation bei Ast-und Zentralvenen verschluss. *Klin Monatsbl Augenheilkd* 164:713–721, 1974.

Theodossiadis G, Velissaropoulos P: Choroidal vascular involvement in Eales' disease. *Ophthalmologica* 166:1, 1973.

VanLoon JA: The causes and therapy of thrombosis of the retinal veins. *Ophthalmologica* 141:467–475, 1961.

Vannas S, Orma H: Experience of treating retinal venous occlusion with anticoagulant and antisclerosis therapy. *Arch Ophthalmol* 58:812–828, 1957.

Vannas S, Raitta C: Anticoagulant treatment of retinal venous occlusion. *Am J Ophthalmol* 62:874–884, 1966.

Vannas S, Raitta C: Die Prognose der Zentravenenverschlusse. *Klin Monatsbl Augenheilkd* 153:457, 1968.

Verhoeff RH: Obstruction of central retinal vein. *Arch Ophthalmol* 36:1, 1907.

Von Barseuisch B: Ablatio durch retinale Gefasserkrankungen. *Mod Probl Ophthalmol* 10:294, 1972.

Wessing A: Fluorescenz—Serien-Angiographie am Augenhintergrund. *Dtsch Ophthalmol Ges* 67:132–140, 1965.

Wessing A, Meyer-Schwickerath G: Fluorescein studies in Eales' disease and related lesions of the retina. In *Proceedings of the International Symposium on Fluorescein Angiography.* Basel, Karger, 1971, p 608.

Wise GN: Macular changes after venous obstruction. *Arch Ophthalmol* 58:544–557, 1957.

Wise GN: Arteriosclerosis secondary to retinal vein obstruction. *Trans AM Ophthalmol Soc* 56:361–382, 1958.

Wise GN: Factors influencing retinal new vessel formation. *Am J Ophthalmol* 52:637–650, 1961.

Wise GN, Dollery CT, Henkind P: *Retinal Circulation.* New York, Harper & Row, 1971.

Wise GN, Wangvivat Y: The exaggerated macular response to retinal disease. *Am J Ophthalmol* 61:1359–1363, 1966.

Wolter JR: Retinal pathology after central retinal vein occlusion. *Br J Ophthalmol* 45:683–694, 1961.

Zauberman H: Retinopathy of retinal detachment after major vascular occlusions. *Br J Ophthalmol* 52:117–121, 1968.

Zweng HCH, Fahrenbruch RC, Little HL: Argon laser photocoagulation in the treatment of retinal vein occlusions. *Mod Probl Ophthalmol* 12:261–270, 1974.

CHAPTER 3

Arterial, Venous, and Capillary Insufficiency or Occlusion

Differential Diagnosis

A. DIABETES MELLITUS
B. RADIATION RETINOPATHY
C. SICKLE CELL RETINOPATHY
D. RETROLENTAL FIBROPLASIA

E. SUBACUTE BACTERIAL ENDOCARDITIS
F. OTHER

Diabetic Retinopathy

Diabetic retinopathy is the most commonly encountered retinal vascular disorder. Diabetic retinopathy can be classified clinically into three types: (1) background retinopathy; (2) preproliferative retinopathy; and (3) proliferative retinopathy. Usually, maturity-onset diabetics complain of visual loss from macular edema, whereas juvenile-onset diabetics usually complain of their first episodes of visual loss secondary to vitreous hemorrhage. Fluorescein angiography has been one of the major technological advancements in allowing investigators to understand the hemodynamic changes which occur in diabetic retinopathy. Argon and xenon photocoagulation has been shown to be beneficial in certain stages of proliferative retinopathy. In patients who have advanced to stages of vitreous hemorrhage and tractional retinal detachment, trans-pars plana vitrectomy has been a major surgical breakthrough in restoring useful vision to many patients who previously were without hope.

In background retinopathy, the vascular abnormalities are contained within the sensory retina. The vascular abnormalities in proliferative retinopathy are either on the retinal surface or extend into the vitreous cavity.

In certain selected cases of diabetic macular edema, photocoagulation has appeared to be of some benefit. There are certain favorable prognostic findings and certain nonfavorable prognostic findings which can help the surgeon make a decision as to whether photocoagulation might be of some benefit.

Favorable Prognostic Factors for Macular Edema

1. A circinate ring of hard exudate of short duration extending toward the retinal avascular zone
2. Focal leakage sites causing macular edema can clearly be visualized
3. Very mild or absent cystoid macular edema
4. Good perifoveal capillary perfusion

Nonfavorable Prognostic Factors for Macular Edema

1. Organized, long-standing hard exudate within the fovea
2. Diffuse macular edema throughout the posterior pole
3. Moderate or advanced cystoid macular edema
4. Lamellar or full-thickness macular hole
5. Extensive perifoveal capillary dropout
6. Significant systemic hypertension
7. Renal decompensation

Classification of Diabetic Retinopathy

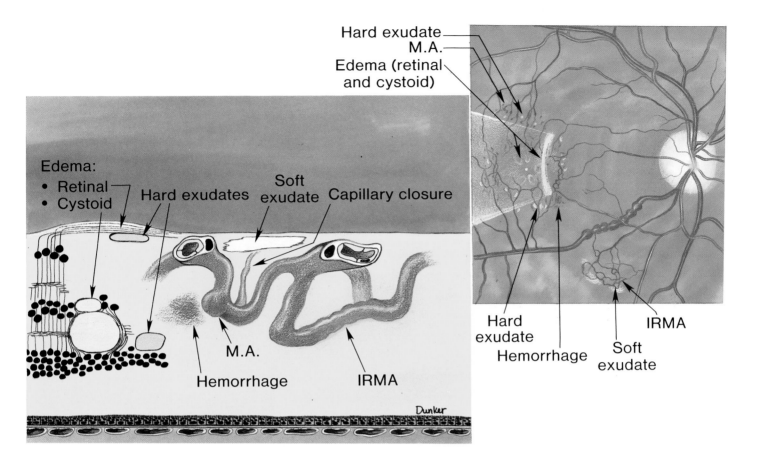

Background Diabetic Retinopathy (BDR)

1. Hemorrhages/microaneurysms
2. Hard exudates
3. Soft exudates
4. Venous abnormalities
   a. Beading
   b. Duplication

5. Arterial abnormalities
6. Intraretinal microvascular abnormalities
7. Arterio-venous nicking
8. Retinal edema

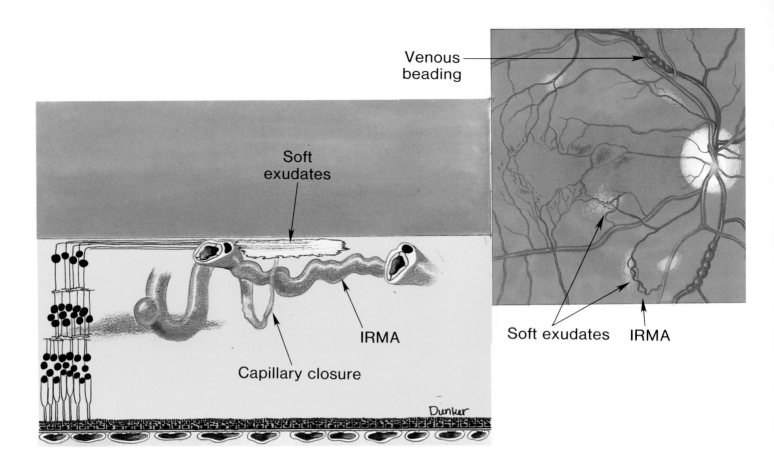

Venous beading

Soft exudates

IRMA

Capillary closure

Soft exudates   IRMA

Dunker

Preproliferative Retinopathy

1. Soft exudates
2. Venous beading
3. IRMA (intraretinal microvascular abnormalities)
4. Moderate to severe retinal hemorrhages and/or microaneurysms

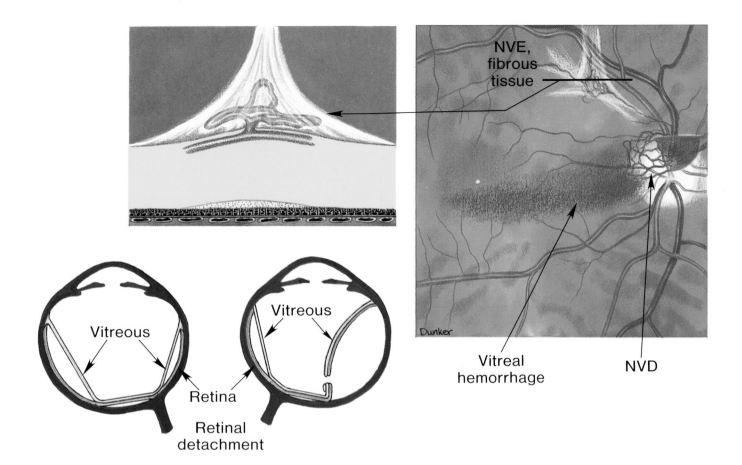

Proliferative (PDR)

1. Progress of vasoproliferation
   (NVD, NVE, fibrous tissue)
2. Preretinal hemorrhage
3. Vitreous hemorrhage
4. Retinal detachment

Reader's Notes

Background Diabetic Retinopathy (a single microaneurysm)

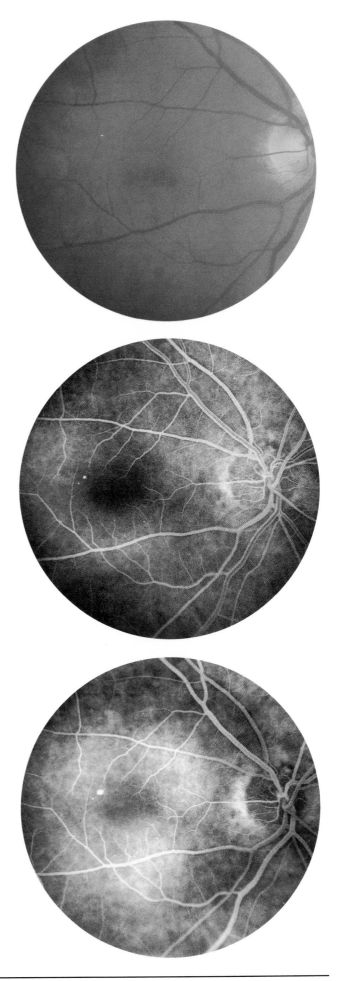

In the posterior pole of the right eye there is a single red dot temporal to the fovea. There is no other evidence of diabetic retinopathy.

During the laminar phase of the angiogram there is an area of increased hyperfluorescence which corresponds to the red dot seen on the color photographs.

This pinpoint area of hyperfluorescence slightly leaks fluorescein in the late phase and is, therefore, characteristic of a microaneurysm.

AUTHOR'S NOTE

This case shows the earliest change of background diabetic retinopathy, which is the formation of microaneurysms. The fluorescein angiogram clearly distinguishes dot hemorrhages from actual microaneurysms. Clinically, these can be difficult to differentiate.

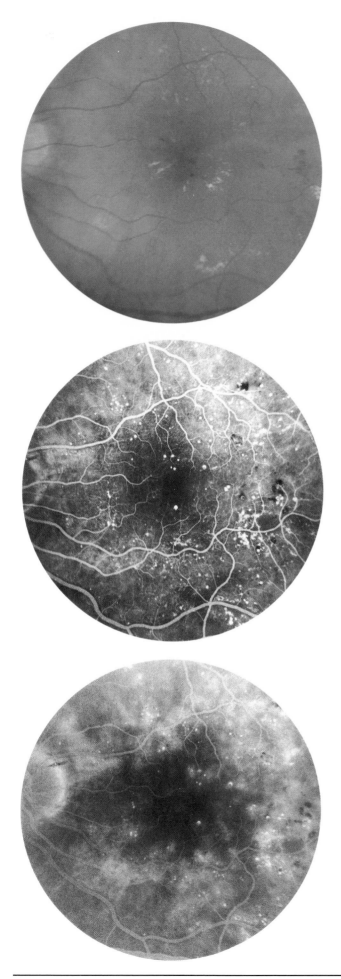

Background Diabetic Retinopathy (microaneurysms and hard exudate)

In the posterior pole of the left eye are scattered dot and blotch hemorrhages, microaneurysms, and deposition of hard exudate.

The fluorescein angiogram shows pinpoint areas of hyperfluorescence which correspond to the microaneurysms. The areas of intraretinal dot and small blotch hemorrhages block the background choroidal fluorescence. The hard exudates do not cause any significant blockage of the background fluorescence or any fluorescein leakage.

Late in the angiogram there is diffuse intraretinal accumulation of fluorescein dye from the leaking microaneurysms, indicating retinal edema. The intraretinal hemorrhage continues to block the background choroidal fluorescence.

Background Diabetic Retinopathy (microaneurysms, hard exudate, soft exudates, and disruption of the perifoveal capillaries)

This aphakic left eye shows scattered dot and blotch hemorrhages, microaneurysms, and deposition of hard exudate. There are several areas of soft exudate superior and inferior to the macula.

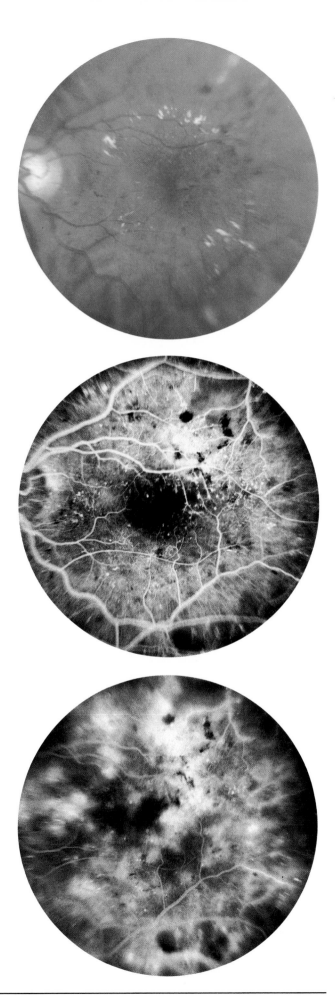

The fluorescein angiogram shows punctate areas of hyperfluorescence corresponding to microaneurysms. The intraretinal hemorrhages block the background choroidal fluorescence. There are several areas of capillary dropout and nonperfusion superior and inferior to the macula, corresponding to the soft exudates seen on the color photographs. There is significant disruption of the perifoveal capillary net.

The late angiogram shows diffuse intraretinal accumulation of fluorescein dye from the leaking microaneurysms and dilated capillaries. This indicates the presence of retinal and a partial cystoid macular edema. The intraretinal hemorrhages continue to block the background choroidal fluorescence late in the angiogram.

AUTHOR'S NOTE

The superior and inferior aspects of the color photograph and angiogram are blurred due to the fact that these photographs were taken of an aphakic eye.

Background Diabetic Retinopathy (cystoid macular edema)

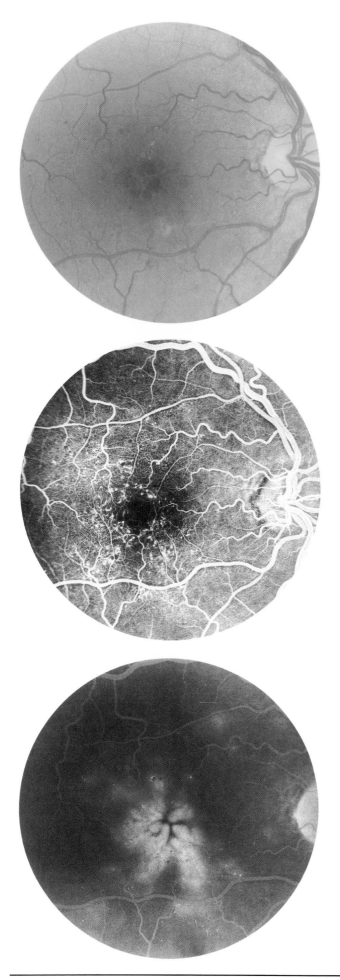

In the posterior pole of the right eye there are a few scattered microaneurysms and dot hemorrhages. There is also some intraretinal hard exudate. In the center of the macula, typical cystoid spaces can be seen.

During the venous phase of the angiogram, punctate areas of hyperfluorescence can be seen, corresponding to the leaking microaneurysms. Some of the microaneurysms have developed on the inner perifoveal capillary ring.

The late angiogram shows diffuse intraretinal accumulation of fluorescein dye from the leaking microaneurysms. In addition, the cystic spaces are also filled with fluorescein dye and give the appearance of a "flower petal."

Background Diabetic Retinopathy (deposition of hard exudate with cystic spaces)

The right posterior pole shows some scattered dot and blotch hemorrhages and microaneurysms. In the perifoveal region there is deposition of hard exudate intraretinally in a "flower petal" type of configuration. There is also an area of soft exudate inferior to the macula.

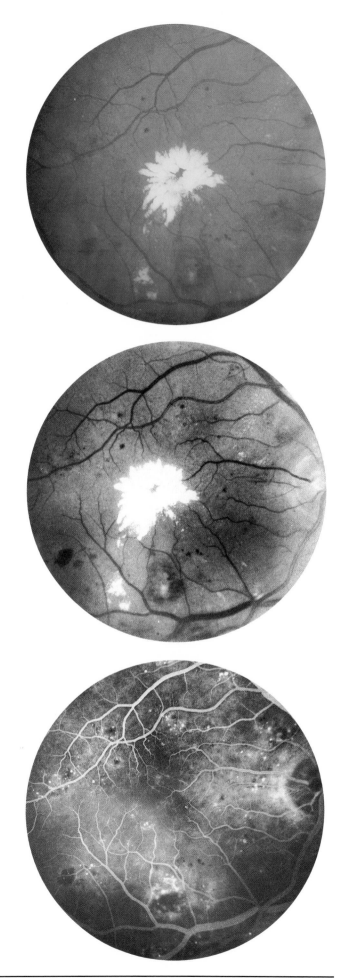

The red-free photograph clearly shows the punctate hemorrhages and microaneurysms in contrast to the deposition of intraretinal hard exudate.

The fluorescein angiogram shows that there is minimal blockage of the background fluorescence by the dense deposition of hard exudate in the macular region. The intraretinal dot and blotch hemorrhages block the background choroidal fluorescence. The intraretinal microaneurysms appear as punctate dots and diffusely leak fluorescein intraretinally.

AUTHOR'S NOTE

Because of the "flower petal" appearance of the deposition of the hard exudate in the perifoveal region, it is assumed that this hard exudate is most likely present within cystic spaces. However, no histopathologic correlation has been obtained in this case. The cystic spaces usually develop in the outer plexiform layer of the sensory retina.

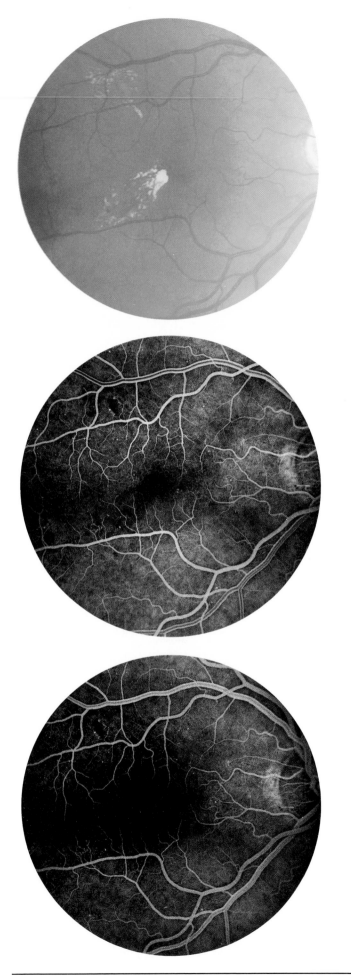

Background Diabetic Retinopathy (with hard exudate encroaching on the fovea—pre- and post-argon laser photocoagulation)

The right eye shows deposition of hard exudate with encroachment of the exudate toward the center of the fovea. A few scattered microaneurysms can also be seen.

During the laminar phase of the angiogram there is evidence of scattered microaneurysms in the vicinity of the intraretinal hard exudate seen on the color photograph.

Later in the angiogram there is slight leakage from these microaneurysms.

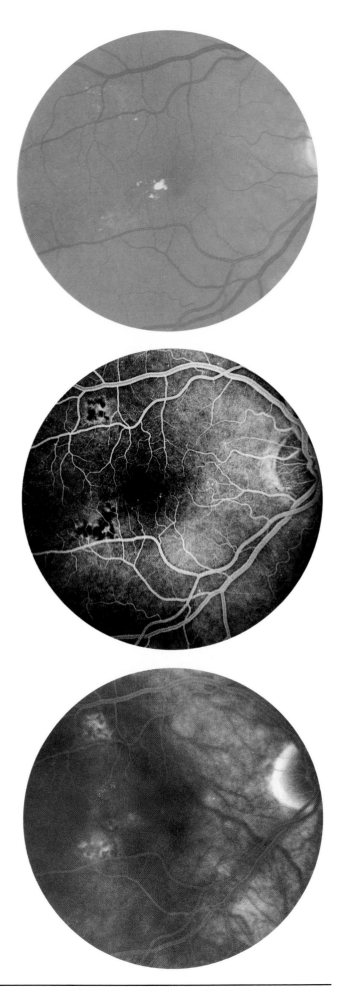

The post-treatment color photograph shows the photocoagulation scars inferior temporal to the fovea. There is still some hard exudate in the proximity of the center of the fovea. However, this exudate appears to be less dense.

During the laminar phase of the post-treatment angiogram the photocoagulation scars can be seen as blocking the background choroidal fluorescence. There is no significant blockage of the background fluorescence by the hard exudate.

The late angiogram shows some very subtle hyperfluorescence around the photocoagulation scars. There does not appear to be any significant intra-retinal accumulation of fluorescein dye.

AUTHOR'S NOTE

Although there was no significant leakage of fluorescein from microaneurysms, the patient's vision was reduced to 20/70 due to the deposition of hard exudate in close proximity to the center of the fovea. After argon laser photocoagulation treatment, the vision improved to 20/30. The only indication for treatment in this case was the concern about an increased amount of organized hard exudate occurring in the center of the macula and causing further reduction of central vision.

Background Diabetic Retinopathy (hard exudate with macular edema—pre- and post-argon laser photocoagulation treatment)

The right posterior pole shows scattered dot and blotch hemorrhages and microaneurysms. There is a considerable amount of intraretinal hard exudate with areas of hard exudate in close proximity to the fovea.

The red-free photograph clearly shows the deposition of hard exudate throughout the posterior pole. The intraretinal dot and blotch hemorrhages and microaneurysms appear as dark areas.

The fluorescein angiogram demonstrates the punctate areas of hyperfluorescence from microaneurysms.

The post-treatment color photograph of the right posterior pole shows a significant decrease in the deposition of hard exudate. The hard exudate in the perifoveal region is less dense than in the pretreatment stage of the retinopathy. The photocoagulation scars appear as light brown areas.

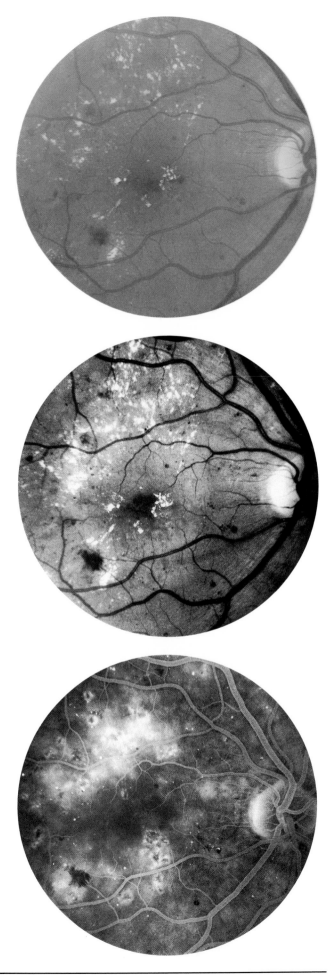

The red-free photograph of the right eye shows much less hard exudate as compared to the pretreatment red-free photograph.

The late fluorescein angiogram shows staining around the photocoagulation scars and some mild leakage of fluorescein from a few remaining scattered microaneurysms.

AUTHOR'S NOTE

This patient's vision was 20/80 pretreatment and improved to 20/30 after treatment. The technique of photocoagulation treatment for diabetic macular edema consists of treating each leaking microaneurysm which appears to be contributing to the macular edema. The areas of hard exudate, per se, are not treated directly with photocoagulation. The microaneurysms merely need to be blanched with the argon laser beam to stop them from leaking intraretinally.

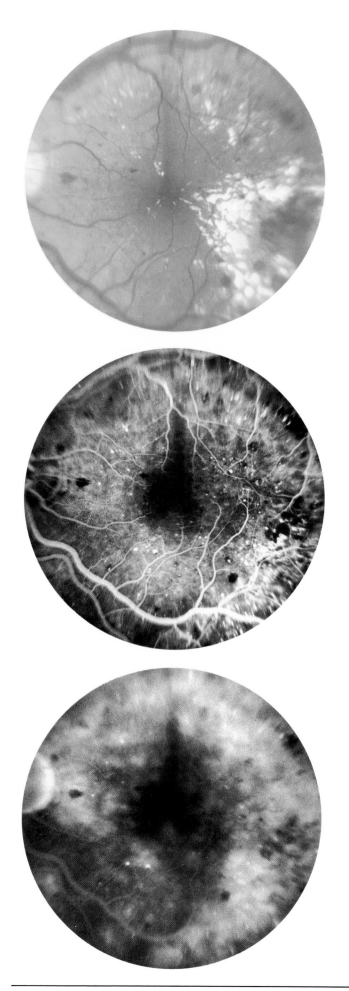

Background Diabetic Retinopathy (circinate ring of hard exudate with encroachment toward the center of the fovea)

The posterior pole of the left eye shows scattered dot and blotch hemorrhages and microaneurysms. There is a circinate ring of hard exudate temporal to the macula with the hard exudate beginning to encroach toward the center of the fovea.

The fluorescein angiogram shows scattered dot and blotch hemorrhages blocking the background choroidal fluorescence. The microaneurysms are present in their greatest density within the center of the ring of hard exudate seen on the color photograph.

The late angiogram shows diffuse intraretinal leakage of fluorescein dye from the microaneurysms, indicating retinal and macular edema.

Six weeks after argon laser photocoagulation, there has been a marked reduction in the amount of intraretinal hard exudate. There are still a few scattered areas of hard exudate and scattered dot and blotch hemorrhages with microaneurysms.

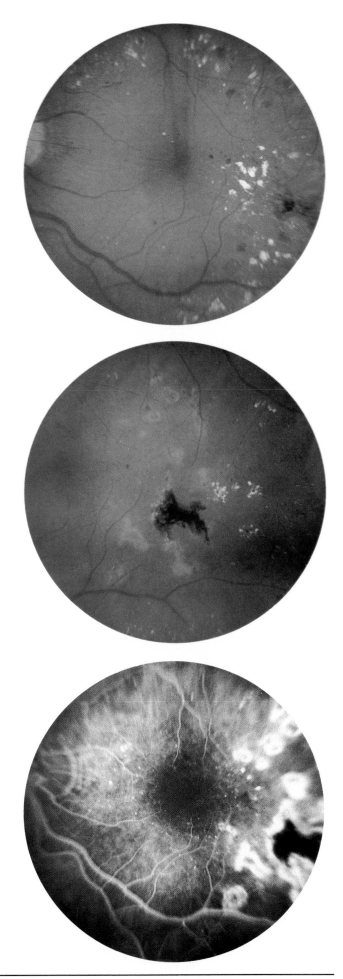

Three months after the initial treatment and some further treatment for the residual microaneurysms, there has been nearly complete disappearance of the hard exudate in the macular region.

The post-treatment fluorescein angiogram shows staining around the heavier photocoagulation scar which was within the center of the circinate ring. There is also staining of the photocoagulation scars outside the circinate ring of hard exudate. A few residual microaneurysms can still be seen. However, there is no significant leakage and, therefore, minimal macular edema.

AUTHOR'S NOTE

This patient's pretreatment vision was 20/50 in the left eye. The patient's right eye had been enucleated because of trauma during childhood. It was felt that this left eye should be treated because the patient was monocular and the hard exudate was beginning to encroach toward the center of the fovea. The post-treatment vision improved to 20/20.

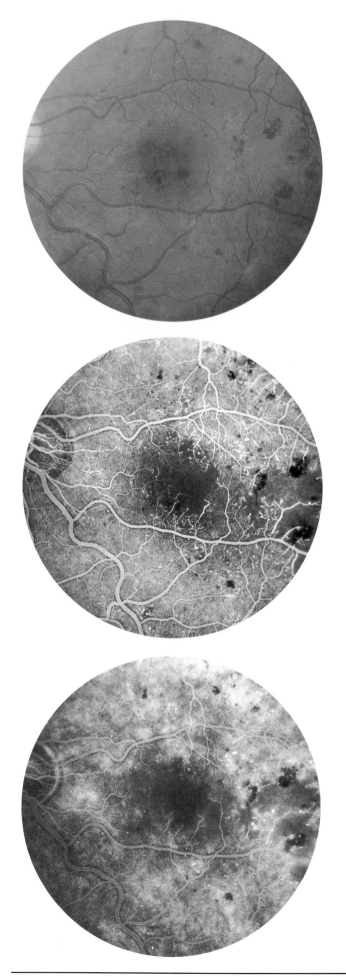

Preproliferative Diabetic Retinopathy (disruption of the perifoveal capillary net and areas of nonperfusion temporal to the macula)

In the left posterior pole there are scattered dot and blotch hemorrhages and scattered microaneurysms.

The fluorescein angiogram shows disruption of the perifoveal capillary net. Scattered microaneurysms with fine intraretinal microvascular abnormalities can be seen. There is an area of capillary dropout and nonperfusion temporal to the macula.

The late angiogram shows intraretinal accumulation of fluorescein dye from the leaking microaneurysms and the fine intraretinal microvascular abnormalities.

The right eye of the patient shows scattered dot and blotch hemorrhages and microaneurysms. A few scattered areas of intraretinal hard exudate can also be seen. Along the inferior temporal arcade is an area of soft exudate.

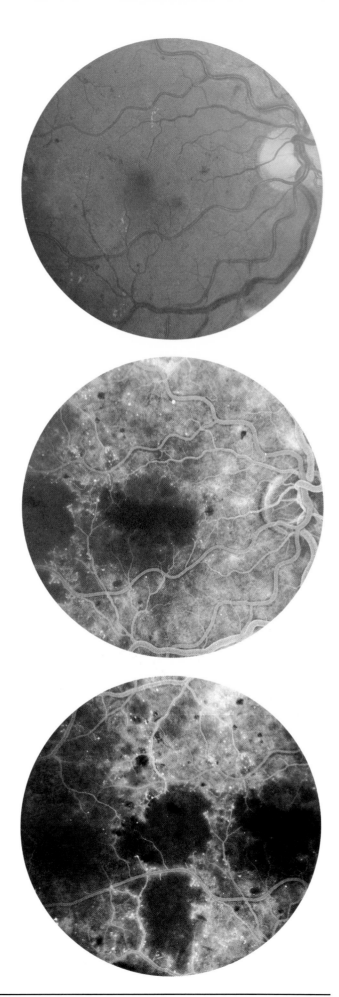

During the venous phase of the angiogram there is evidence of intraretinal fluorescein accumulation from the leaking microaneurysms and intraretinal microvascular abnormalities. There is a large area of capillary dropout and nonperfusion involving the center of the macula.

Temporal to the macula is an additional area of capillary dropout and nonperfusion. This area is surrounded by very fine intraretinal microvascular abnormalities which slightly leak fluorescein. The vessels passing through the areas of nonperfusion and on the border of the nonperfused area also stain with fluorescein dye, indicating a loss of the endothelial cell junction integrity.

AUTHOR'S NOTE

There are frequently fairly large areas of capillary dropout and nonperfusion temporal to the macula in patients with preproliferative retinopathy. These areas are frequently the initial sites for development of neovascularization as part of the proliferative stage.

Preprolifferative Diabetic Retinopathy (IRMA; large areas of nonperfusion)

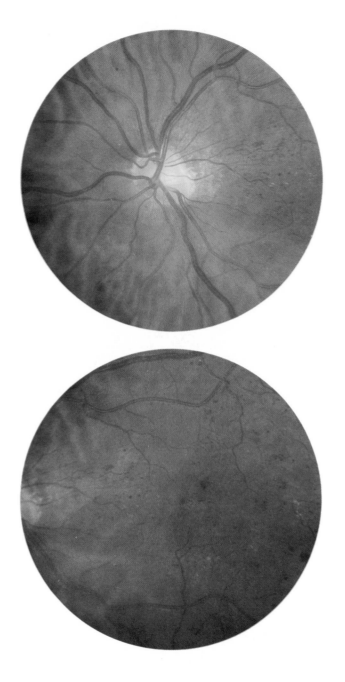

The left optic nerve appears normal. Temporal to the nerve are very fine IRMA. There are also a few scattered dot and blotch hemorrhages and micro-aneurysms.

In the posterior pole of the left eye, scattered dot and blotch hemorrhages and deposition of hard exudate can also be seen. There appears to be a very lacy area of vessels adjacent to the fovea. This could either be a small frond of neovascularization or IRMA.

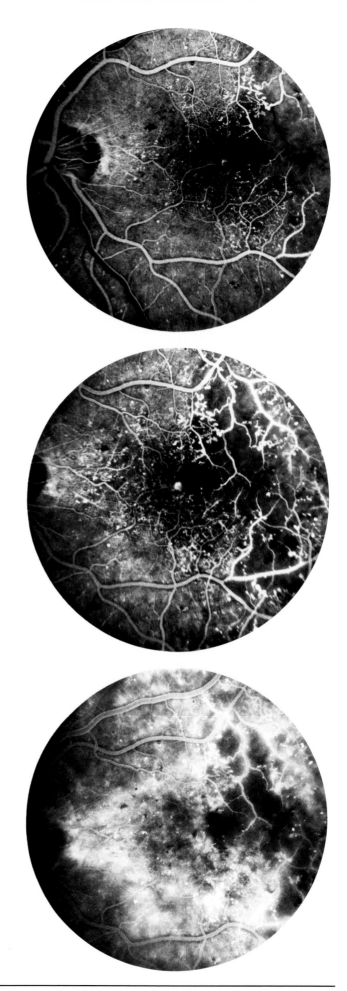

During the early laminar phase of the fluorescein angiogram, these scattered microaneurysms can clearly be seen. IRMA are also visible. At the nasal edge of the retinal avascular zone, i.e. fovea, the lacy network of vessels appears to be hyperfluorescent.

The area of hyperfluorescence at the nasal edge of the fovea shows slight leakage. There is also some slight leakage of fluorescein from the scattered microaneurysms. There are large areas of capillary dropout and nonperfusion involving the temporal macula. The perifoveal capillary net is completely disrupted.

The late angiogram shows diffuse intraretinal accumulation of fluorescein dye from the leaking microaneurysms and slight leakage from IRMA. The areas of capillary dropout and nonperfusion are still evident, with the vessel walls in these nonperfused areas staining with the fluorescein dye.

AUTHOR'S NOTE

Clinically, it was difficult to determine whether this was a small frond of neovascularization involving the fovea, a large microaneurysm, or IRMA. Careful follow-up evaluation of the left eye was recommended without any specific treatment at this stage of the retinopathy.

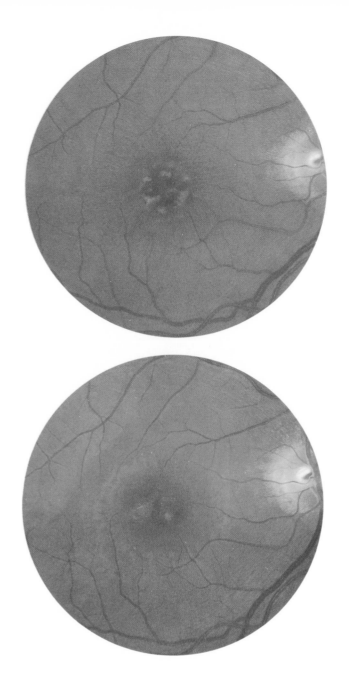

Subacute Bacterial Endocarditis (with macular involvement)—Pre- and Post-treatment

In the posterior pole of the right eye, there is evidence of intraretinal yellowish material. This material involves the center of the fovea. Temporal to the macula, there are very fine intraretinal splinter hemorrhages.

After systemic treatment for subacute bacterial endocarditis, retinal pigment epithelial mottling changes can be seen. There is less intraretinal yellowish material surrounding the macula and fovea. The small intraretinal splinter hemorrhages are no longer present.

AUTHOR'S NOTE

This 23-year-old white male was admitted with intermittent episodes of chills and fever. He was diagnosed as having definite subacute bacterial endocarditis which both the cardiologist and infectious disease specialists felt should be treated with systemic antibiotics. At the time of the initial hospitalization, the patient was complaining of decreased vision in the right eye to the 20/100 level. After aggressive systemic antibiotic treatment, the patient's symptoms improved, as did his vision, to the 20/40 level, with marked clearing of the yellowish material in the macular region. It is hypothesized that the material seen in the macula may have been embolic vegetation related to the subacute bacterial endocarditis. No other source for septic embolization could be found. The changes appear to selectively involve the paramacular capillaries and smaller caliber arterioles.

During the acute phase of subacute bacterial endocarditis, the early fluorescein angiogram shows an abnormal hyperfluorescence in the normally dark foveal region. There appears to be increased blockage of the background choroidal fluorescence in a ring-type configuration around the macula. The perifoveal capillary net is also not well visualized.

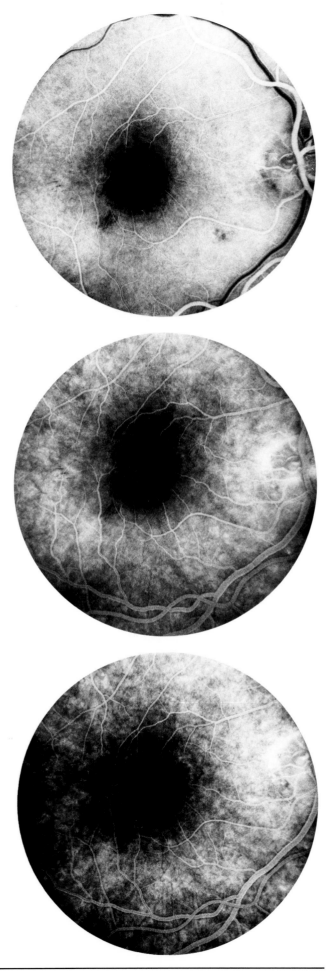

Later in the angiogram, there is persistence of the hyperfluorescence in the center of the macula. There does not appear to be any significant leakage of fluorescein dye. The fine splinter hemorrhages temporal to the macula block the background choroidal fluorescence.

The post-treatment late fluorescein angiogram shows a marked reduction in the hyperfluorescence which was seen during the fulminant stage of subacute bacterial endocarditis. There is also a ring of irregular hyperfluorescence surrounding the macula. This change may indicate some minimal disturbance at the level of the retinal pigment epithelium.

Leukemic Infiltration of the Retina—Bilateral (soft exudates and Roth spots)

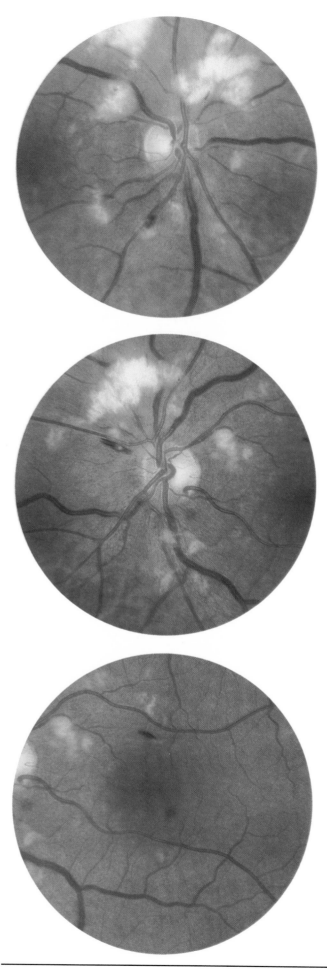

The optic nerve of the right eye appears normal. The retinal veins appear to be slightly engorged. Surrounding the optic nerve are cotton-wool spots or soft exudates, which indicate nerve fiber layer infarcts. A few scattered intraretinal splinter and dot hemorrhages can also be seen.

The left optic nerve appears normal. As in the right eye, surrounding the optic nerve are fluffy cotton-wool spots, or soft exudates, at the level of the nerve fiber layer. Nasal to the optic nerve is an intraretinal splinter hemorrhage with a whitish center, frequently referred to as a "Roth spot." The retinal veins are slightly engorged.

The foveal region appears normal. Superior to the macula is a splinter hemorrhage and a few scattered areas of soft exudate.

During the early laminar phase of the fluorescein angiogram, there appears to be some dilatation of the capillaries on the surface of the optic nerve. The capillary bed around the nerve and along the superior temporal vessels also appears to be abnormally dilated. There are several areas of capillary dropout and nonperfusion corresponding to the soft exudates seen on the color photograph. The splinter hemorrhage nasal to the optic nerve just below one of the nasal branches of the central retinal artery blocks the background choroidal fluorescence. The hemorrhage above the macula also blocks the background choroidal fluorescence.

The late angiogram shows intraretinal leakage of fluorescein from the dilated capillary bed. There is also staining of the optic nerve from leaking surface capillaries. The spot nasal to the optic nerve shows some hyperfluorescence in the center of the splinter hemorrhage, which continues to block the background choroidal fluorescence.

The late angiogram of the right eye shows similar intraretinal leakage of fluorescein from the dilated capillary bed. Much of the fluorescein leakage surrounds areas of capillary dropout and nonperfusion. There is also some staining of the optic nerve tissue from dilated capillaries. Inferior to the optic nerve, the intraretinal hemorrhage continues to block the background fluorescence.

AUTHOR'S NOTE

This patient was diagnosed as having definite acute myelogenous leukemia. In patients with soft exudates which indicate nerve fiber layer infarct, there is frequently fluorescein leakage late in the angiogram surrounding the areas of capillary dropout or nonperfusion. This leakage is usually due to dilatation of the capillary bed, intraretinal microvascular abnormalities, or microaneurysmal changes at the border of the nonperfused areas.

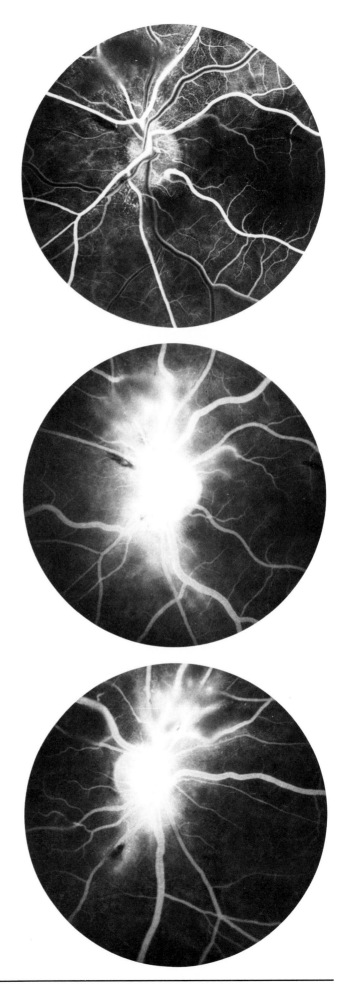

Bilateral Nerve Fiber Layer Infarct (secondary to presumed *Pneumocystis carinii*)

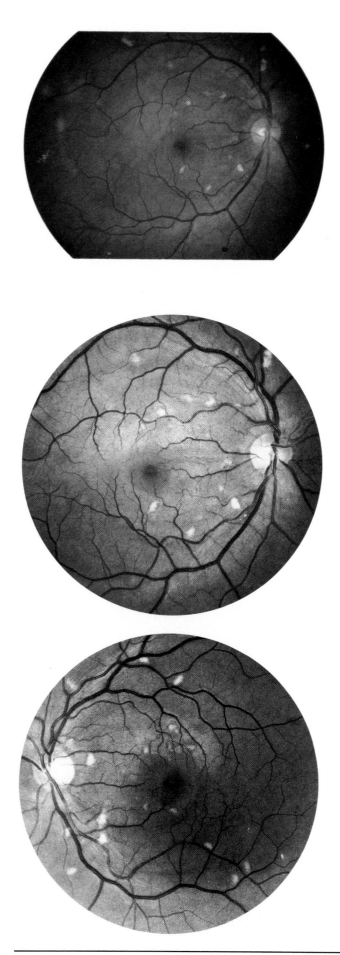

The wide angle color photograph of the right eye reveals multiple small soft exudates in the posterior pole. The retinal vasculature appears to be essentially normal. Below the inferior temporal arcade there is a small intraretinal hemorrhage.

The red-free photograph of the right eye clearly demonstrates the multiple nerve fiber layer infarct as evidenced by the soft exudates.

The red-free photograph of the left eye shows similar small nerve fiber layer infarcts along the arcades and in the posterior pole.

During the laminar phase of the fluorescein angiogram, there are pinpoint areas of hyperfluorescence corresponding to dilated capillaries and, perhaps, small microaneurysms. Subtle areas of capillary dropout corresponding to the soft exudates seen on the color photograph and red-free photograph are also evident.

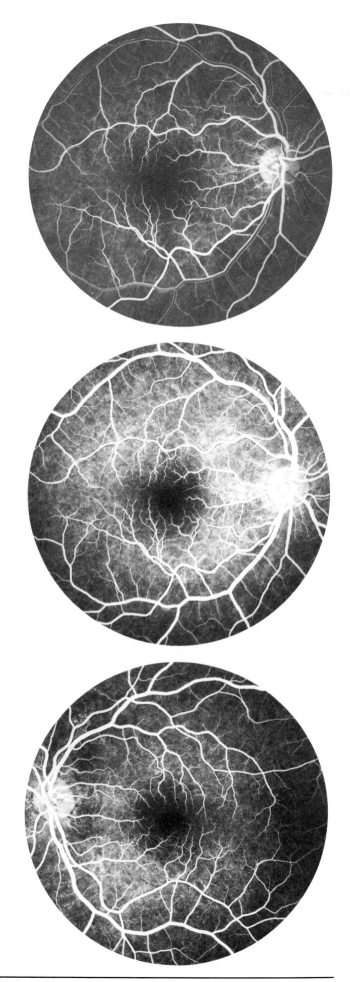

Later, during the venous phase of the fluorescein angiogram, the small pinpoint microaneurysms can be seen superior to the optic nerve and along the superior temporal vein.

During the venous phase of the angiogram in the left eye, similar dilatation of the capillary bed in the posterior pole and what appear to be pinpoint microaneurysms along the superior temporal arcade above the optic nerve can be seen.

AUTHOR'S NOTE

This is a case of a 21-year-old black male who initially presented with blurriness of vision in both eyes. Medical history revealed that the patient was a member of the "gay community." Complete medical work-up revealed *Pneumocystis carinii* on pulmonary biopsy. No other systemic infection was determined in this patient and he was treated for the symptoms of pneumocystosis.

Bibliography

Aaberg TM: Macular holes: A review. *Surv Ophthalmol* 15:139, 1970.

Aaberg TM, Blair CJ, Gass JDM: Macular holes. *Am J Ophthalmol* 69:555, 1970.

Aiello LM: Fluorescein angiographic interpretation of microcirculatory abnormalities of diabetic retinopathy. In L' Esperance FA: *Current Diagnosis and Management of Chorioretinal Diseases.* St Louis, CV Mosby, 1977, p 192.

Amalric P: New considerations concerning the evolution and the treatment of diabetic retinopathy. *Ophthalmologica* 154:151–160, 1967.

Amalric P: Diabetic retinopathy with macular holes and pseudoholes. *Bull Soc Ophthalmol Fr* 79:1021, 1979.

Amemiya T, Yoshida H: Macular hole in diabetic maculopathy. *Ophthalmologica* 177:188, 1978.

Appen RE, Chandra SR, Klein R, et al: Diabetic papillopathy. *Am J Ophthalmol* 90:203–209, 1980.

Awan KJ: Arterial vascular anomalies of the retina. *Arch Ophthalmol* 95:1197, 1977.

Blankenship GW: Diabetic macular edema and argon laser photocoagulation: A prospective randomized study. *Trans Am Acad Ophthalmol Otolaryngol* 86:69, 1979.

Boghen DR, Glaser JS: Ischemic optic neuropathy: The clinical profile and natural history. *Brain* 98:689, 1975.

Bresnick GH: Evaluation and treatment of diabetic retinopathy. *J Cont Educ Ophthalmol* 4:15, 1979.

Bresnick GH, DeVenecia G, Myers FL, et al: Retinal ischemia in diabetic retinopathy. *Arch Ophthalmol* 93:1300–1310, 1974.

Brinkley JR, Ryan SJ: Bruch's membrane and vascular growth. *Invest Ophthalmol* 15:433, 1976.

Brinkley JR, Ryan SJ: Cystoid macular edema, preretinal membrane formation and macular holes. In Yanuzzi LA, Gitter KA, Schatz H: *The Macula. A Comprehensive Text and Atlas.* Baltimore, Williams & Wilkins, 1979, p 265.

Cheng H, Blach RK, Hamilton A, et al: Diabetic maculopathy. *Trans Ophthalmol Soc UK* 92:407, 1972.

Cogan DG, Toussaint D, Kuwabara T: Retinal vascular patterns. IV. Diabetic retinopathy. *Arch Ophthalmol* 66:366, 1961.

Cunha-vaz J, De Abreu F, Campos AJ, et al: Early breakdown of the blood-retinal barrier in diabetes. *Br J Ophthalmol* 59:649, 1975.

David MD, Myers FL, Bresnick GH, et al: Natural evolution. In L'Esperance FA: *Current Diagnosis and Management of Chorioretinal Diseases.* St Louis, CV Mosby, 1977, p 179.

Diddie KR, Ernest JT: The effect of photocoagulation on the choroidal vasculature and retinal oxygen tension. *Am J Ophthalmol* 84:62, 1977.

Ellenberger C, Keltner JL, Burde RM: Acute optic neuropathy in older patients. *Arch Neurol* 28:182, 1973.

Ellenberger C, Messner KH: Papillophlebitis: Benign retinopathy resembling papilledema or papillitis. *Ann Neurol* 3:438, 1978.

Ellis W, Little HL: Leukemic infiltration of the optic nerve head. *Am J Ophthalmol* 75:867, 1973.

Freund M, Carmon A, Cohen AM: Papilledema and papillitis in diabetes: A report of two cases. *Am J Ophthalmol* 60:18, 1965.

Friberg TR: Traumatic retinal pigment epithelial edema. *Am J Ophthalmol* 88:18, 1979.

Gass JDM: A fluorescein angiographic study of dysfunction secondary to retinal vascular disease. IV. Diabetic retinal angiopathy. *Arch Ophthalmol* 80:583, 1968.

Gass JDM: *Stereoscopic Atlas of Macular Diseases. A Funduscopic and Angiographic Presentation.* St Louis, CV Mosby, 1970, p 175.

Gass JDM: Lamellar macular hole: A complication of cystoid macular edema after cataract extraction: A clinicopathologic case report. *Trans Am Ophthalmol Soc* 73:231, 1975.

Gass JDM: *Stereoscopic Atlas of Macular Diseases.* St. Louis, CV Mosby, 1977, pp 334–339.

Henkind P: Histopathologic changes. In L'Esperance FA: *Current Diagnosis and Management of Chorioretinal Diseases.* St Louis, CV Mosby, 1977, p 185.

Hill DW, Dollery CT, Mailer CM, et al: Arterial fluorescein studies in diabetic retinopathy. *Proc R Soc Med* 58:535–537, 1965.

Justice J Jr, Lehmann RP: Cilioretinal arteries: A study based on review of stereo fundus photographs and fluorescein angiographic findings. *Arch Ophthalmol* 94:1355, 1976.

Kaback MB, Tanenbaum HL: The macula in diabetes. *Can J Ophthalmol* 9:202–207, 1974.

Kohner EM: The evolution and natural history of diabetic retinopathy. *Int Ophthalmol Clin* 18:1, 1978.

Kohner EM, Dollery CT: Fluorescein angiography of the fundus in diabetic retinopathy. *Br Med Bull* 26:166–170, 1970.

Kohner EM, Dollery CT, Paterson JW, et al: Arterial fluorescein studies in diabetic retinopathy. *Diabetes* 16:1–11, 1967.

Le Compte PM, Gepts W: The pathology of juvenile diabetes. In Volk BW, Wellman KF: *The Diabetic Pancreas.* New York, Plenum Press, 1977, p 327.

Lonn LI, Hoyt WF: Papillophlebitis: A cause of protracted yet benign optic disc edema. *Eye Ear Nose Throat Mo* 45:62, 1966.

Lubow M, Makley TA: Pseudopapilledema of juvenile diabetes mellitus. *Arch Ophthalmol* 85:417, 1971.

Maumenee AE: Further advances in the study of the macula. *Arch Ophthalmol* 78:151, 1967.

McMeel JW, Trempe CL, Franks EB: Diabetic maculopathy. *Trans Am Acad Ophthalmol Otolaryngol* 83:OP476, 1977.

Merin S, Yanko L, Ivry M: Treatment of diabetic maculopathy by argon laser. *Br J Ophthalmol* 58:85–91, 1974.

Patz A, Fine S: Evaluation and photocoagulation treatment of diabetic maculopathy: In L'Esperance FA: *Current Diagnosis and Management of Chorioretinal Disease.* St Louis, CV Mosby 1977, p 256

Patz A, Fine SL: Observations in diabetic macular edema. *Int Ophthalmol Clin* 18:101, 1978.

Patz A, Schatz H, Berkow J, et al: Macular edema: An overlooked complication of diabetic retinopathy. *Trans Am Acad Ophthalmol Otolaryngol* 77:34, 1973.

Reeser F, Fleischman J, Williams GA, et al: Efficacy of argon laser photocoagulation in the treatment of circinate diabetic retinopathy. *Am J Ophthalmol* 92:762–767, 1981.

Rosenberg MA, Savino PJ, Glaser JS: A clinical analysis of pseudopapilledema. 1. Population, laterality, acuity, refractive error, ophthalmoscopic characteristics, and coincident disease. *Arch Ophthalmol* 97:65, 1979.

Rubinstein K, Myska V: Focal retinal ischemia. *Trans Ophthalmol Soc UK* 91:355, 1971.

Rubinstein K, Myska V: Pathogenesis and treatment of diabetic maculopathy. *Br J Ophthalmol* 58:76, 1974.

Schatz R, Patz A: Cystoid maculopathy in diabetics. *Arch Ophthalmol* 94:761, 1976.

Severin SL: Qualitative photostress testing for the diagnosis of cystoid macular edema. *Am Intra-Ocular Implant Soc J* 6:25, 1980.

Sigelman J: Diabetic macular edema in juvenile- and adult-onset diabetes. *Am J Ophthalmol* 90:287–296, 1980.

Skalka HW: Macular cysts and hole. *J Pediatr Ophthalmol Strabismus* 15:219, 1978.

Spalter HF: Photocoagulation of circinate maculopathy in diabetic retinopathy. *Am J Ophthalmol* 71:242, 1971.

Tattersall R: Diabetic mellitus: Definition, classification, and nosological description of the syndrome. In *Etiology and Pathogenesis of Insulin Dependent Diabetes Mellitus.* Philadelphia, National Institute of Arthritis, Metabolism, and Digestive Disease and Juvenile Diabetes Foundation, 1977, p 3.

The Diabetic Retinopathy Study Research Group: Preliminary report on effects of photocoagulation therapy. *Am J Ophthalmol* 81:383–396, 1976.

Ticho U, Patz A: The role of capillary perfusion in the management of diabetic macular edema. *Am J Ophthalmol* 76:880, 1973.

Walsh FB, Hoyt WF: *Clinical Neuro-ophthalmology.* Baltimore, Williams & Wilkins, 1969, vol 1, pp 600, 614–619.

Welch RB: The treatment of diabetic retinopathy. In Goldberg MF, Fine SL: *Symposium on the Treatment of Diabetic Retinopathy.* Washington DC, Public Health Service Publication No. 1890, 1969, p 563.

CHAPTER 4

Neovascularization (at the Disc and/or Elsewhere)

Differential Diagnosis

A. DIABETES MELLITUS
B. RETROLENTAL FIBROPLASIA
C. SICKLE CELL RETINOPATHY
D. VENOUS OCCLUSION
E. RADIATION RETINOPATHY
F. EALES' DISEASE (IDIOPATHIC PERIPHLEBITIS RETINAE)
G. SARCOIDOSIS
H. SEVERE UVEITIS

I. PARS PLANITIS
J. CHRONIC LEUKEMIA
K. POLYCYTHEMIA
L. CHOROIDAL VITREAL NEOVASCULARIZATION DEVELOPING AFTER PHOTOCOAGULATION FOR RETINAL NEOVASCULARIZATION
M. OTHER

At the present time, most investigators agree that the pathogenesis of the proliferative retinopathies with neovascularization either at the disc or elsewhere in the fundus is secondary to retinal ischemia. Capillary closure causes retinal ischemia which presumably elaborates a soluble polypeptide which stimulates the production of abnormal new blood vessels. These vessels invariably grow at the junction between perfused and nonperfused retina. Due to vitreous traction on these vessels, subsequent vitreous hemorrhage with marked visual impairment results. The current thought regarding the role of photocoagulation in controlling proliferative retinopathy is that extensive photocoagulation converts the retina from a stage of hypoxia, where the vasoproliferative factor is elaborated, to a state of anoxia, where there is no longer a demand for vasoproliferation. The most common etiologic cause for proliferative retinopathy is diabetes mellitus.

Proliferative Diabetic Retinopathy (progression from preproliferative to proliferative retinopathy)

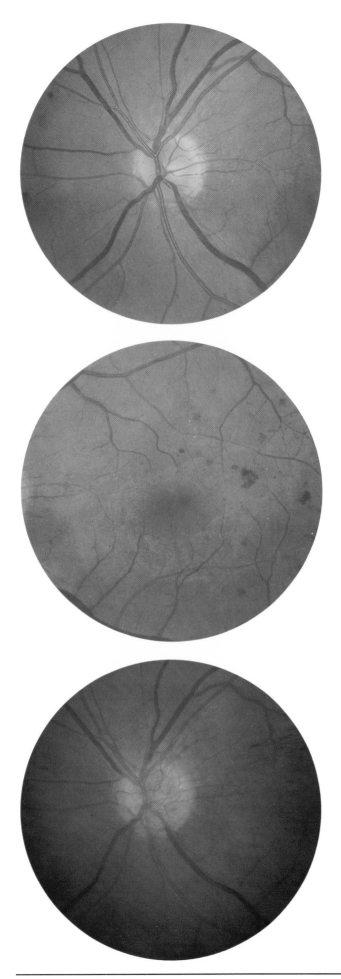

The optic nerve of the left eye appears normal. Scattered around the nerve are multiple dot and blotch hemorrhages.

Scattered throughout the posterior pole are multiple dot and blotch hemorrhages, microaneurysms, and a few scattered areas of hard exudate.

Progression to proliferative retinopathy with disc neovascularization of the left eye is evident.

During the laminar phase of the fluorescein angiogram, there are multiple punctate areas of hyperfluorescence, corresponding to the scattered microaneurysms. The intraretinal dot and blotch hemorrhages block the background choroidal fluorescence.

Along the superior temporal arcade there are venous beading changes. There are multiple areas of capillary dropout and nonperfusion. The intraretinal blotch hemorrhages block the background choroidal fluorescence.

Progression to the stage of proliferative retinopathy shows diffuse leakage of the fluorescein dye into the vitreous from disc neovascularization.

AUTHOR'S NOTE

This is a case of a 26-year-old juvenile-onset diabetic who progressed from a stage of preproliferative diabetic retinopathy within a period of 8 months.

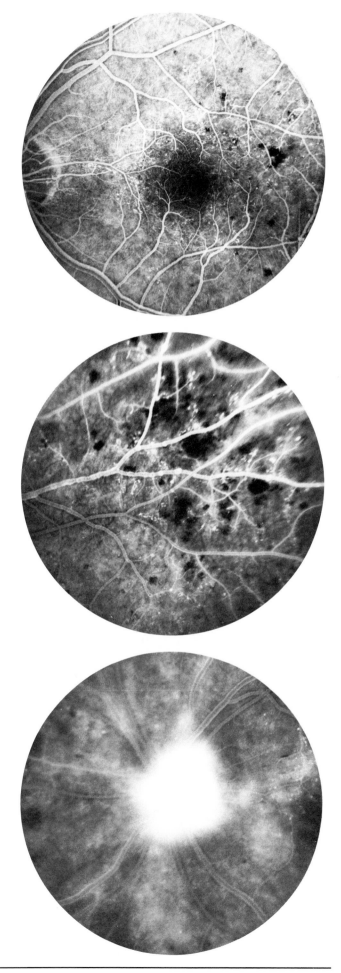

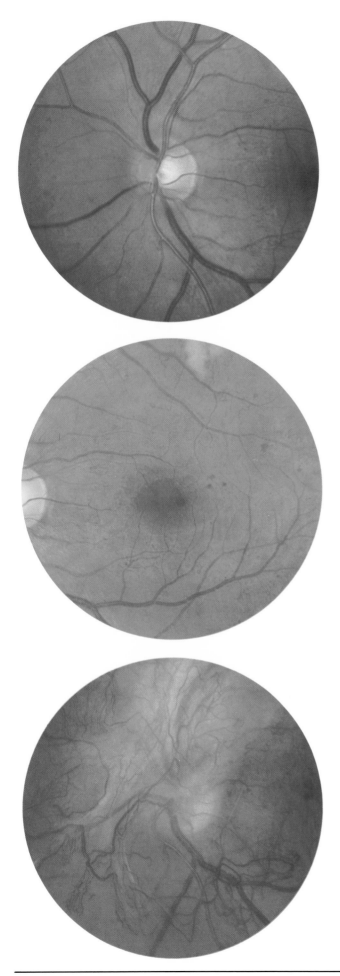

Proliferative Diabetic Retinopathy (progression from preproliferative to severe proliferative retinopathy)

The left optic nerve appears normal. Scattered around the nerve are intraretinal dot hemorrhages and microaneurysms. Fine areas of intraretinal microvascular abnormalities can be seen superior and inferior to the optic nerve.

In the posterior pole are scattered dot and blotch hemorrhages and microaneurysms. Superior to the macula is an area of soft exudate surrounded by intraretinal microvascular abnormalities (IRMA).

There is progression to severe proliferative diabetic retinopathy with extensive fibrovascular proliferation on the surface of the nerve and extending along the arcades.

During the arterial phase of the fluorescein angiogram, the disc neovascularization in the left eye can be seen filling with the fluorescein dye.

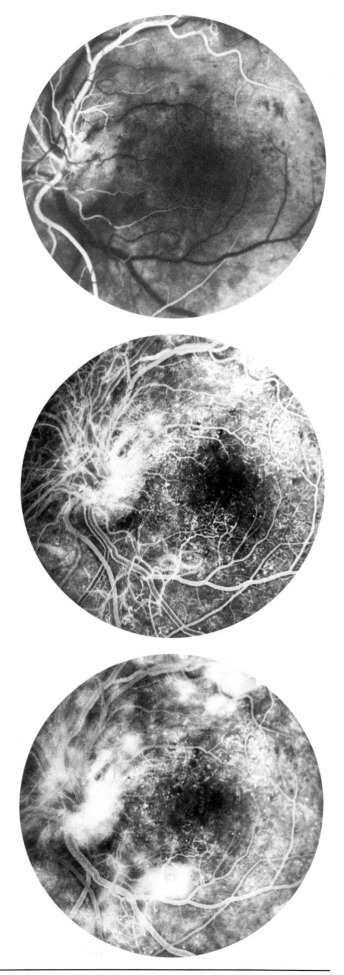

During the laminar phase of the angiogram, the extensive disc neovascularization and fronds of neovascularization overlying the inferior temporal arcade are hyperfluorescing. Multiple microaneurysms and dilatation of the capillary bed with IRMA can be seen throughout the posterior pole.

Late in the angiogram there is leakage of the fluorescein dye into the vitreous from the fronds of neovascularization. There is intraretinal accumulation of fluorescein dye from the leaking microaneurysms and IRMA.

AUTHOR'S NOTE

This 27-year-old juvenile-onset diabetic progressed from a stage of very early preproliferative retinopathy to severe proliferative disease within a period of 16 months. It appears that this rapid progression of preproliferative to proliferative retinopathy occurs more frequently in the juvenile-onset diabetic than in the maturity-onset diabetic population.

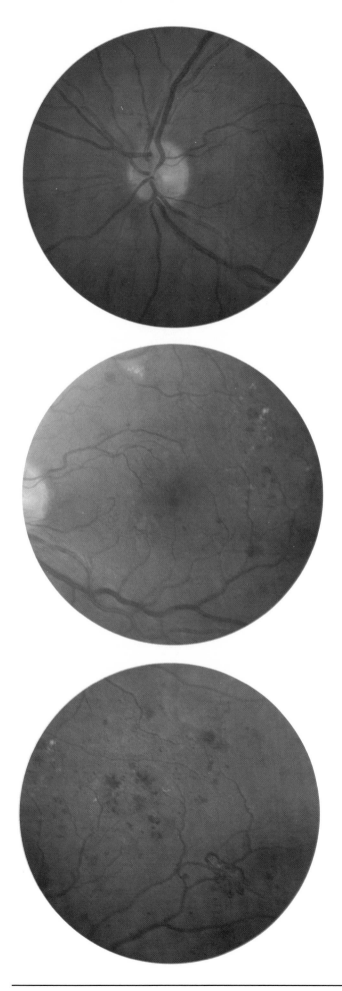

Early Proliferative Diabetic Retinopathy (small fronds of neovascularization away from the disc)

The left optic nerve appears normal. Around the nerve are a few scattered dot and blotch hemorrhages.

In the posterior pole there are scattered dot and blotch hemorrhages, microaneurysms, and some deposition of hard exudate. Superior to the macula is a small area of soft exudate surrounded by fine IRMA.

Temporal to the macula, additional dot and blotch hemorrhages and microaneurysms can be seen. There is a small frond of slightly elevated neovascularization.

During the early laminar phase of the left eye there is hyperfluorescence from the microaneurysms. The intraretinal dot and blotch hemorrhages block the background choroidal fluorescence. Superior to the macula is a triangle-shaped area of nonperfusion, corresponding to the yellow soft exudate seen clinically.

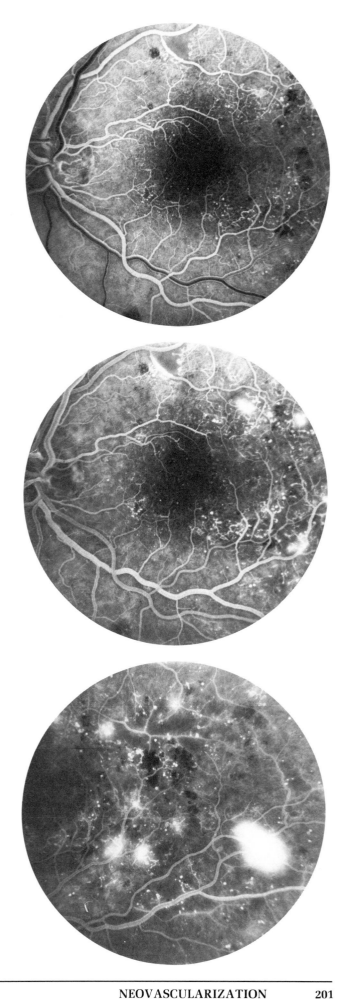

Later in the angiogram there is intraretinal leakage of fluorescein from the scattered microaneurysms and fine areas of intraretinal microvascular abnormalities. The vessel bordering the area of nonperfusion superior to the macula stains with fluorescein dye, indicating a breakdown in the blood-retinal barrier.

Temporal to the macula, the small fronds of neovascularization in association with the larger frond diffusely leak fluorescein into the vitreous. The intraretinal blotch hemorrhages block the background choroidal fluorescence.

AUTHOR'S NOTE

It is the impression of the author that very early proliferative disease with small fronds of neovascularization frequently develops temporal to the macula. These areas appear to be more susceptible to capillary dropout and nonperfusion early in the stages of preproliferative and proliferative retinopathy. It is useful to look for fine areas of neovascularization with red-free illumination.

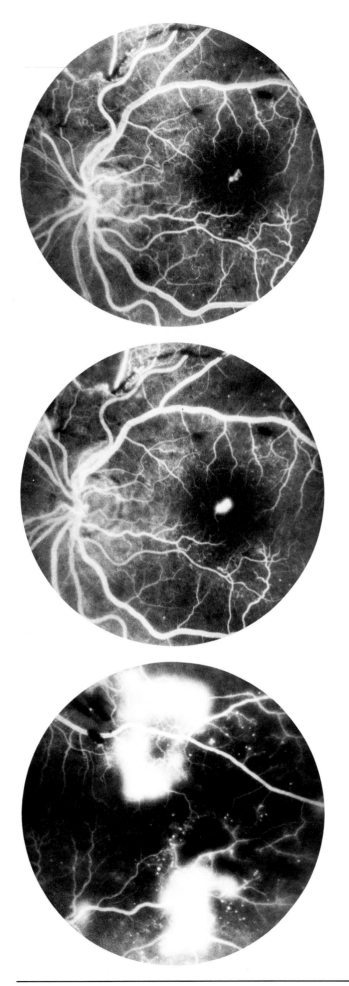

Proliferative Diabetic Retinopathy (with neovascularization in the fovea and elsewhere)

The late laminar phase of the left eye shows a small frond of neovascularization within the retinal avascular zone, i.e. fovea. Intraretinal blotch hemorrhages below the superior temporal vein block the background choroidal fluorescence. There are multiple areas of IRMA superior to the optic nerve.

Later in the angiogram there is leakage of fluorescein from the small proliferative frond in the center of the macula. Scattered microaneurysms can be seen. The intraretinal and linear preretinal hemorrhages superiorly block the background choroidal fluorescence. Superior to the optic nerve are several areas of capillary dropout and nonperfusion.

Temporal to the macula there is diffuse leakage of fluorescein from neovascularization. There are multiple leaking microaneurysms and areas of nonperfusion.

AUTHOR'S NOTE

Neovascularization directly in the center of the macula, i.e. fovea, is quite unusual. Direct focal treatment of the neovascularization in this location would certainly be contraindicated.

Reader's Notes

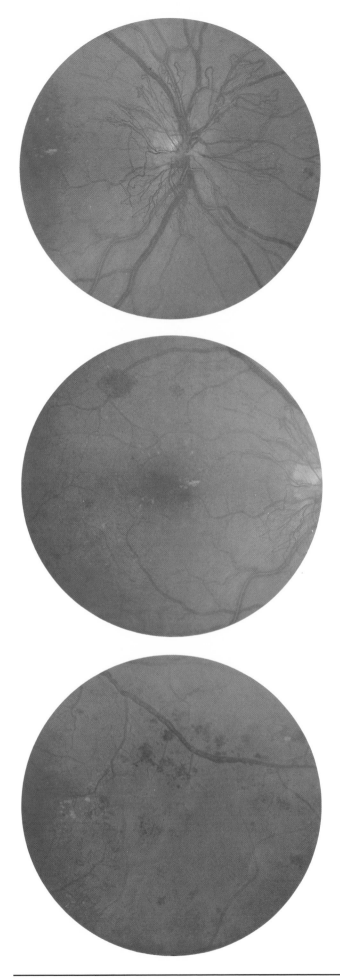

Proliferative Diabetic Retinopathy (disc neovascularization; large areas of capillary dropout and nonperfusion; IRMA; venous changes)

The right eye shows extensive neovascularization 360° around the optic nerve.

In the posterior pole there are scattered dot and blotch hemorrhages, microaneurysms, and deposition of hard exudate. Superior to the macula is a small frond of neovascularization.

In the inferior nasal quadrant, there is marked irregularity in the caliber of the inferior nasal vein. Multiple dot and blotch hemorrhages and microaneurysms can be seen. IRMA and deposition of hard exudate are also present.

The early laminar phase of the fluorescein angiogram shows the disc neovascularization filled with the fluorescein dye. There are multiple punctate microaneurysms throughout the posterior pole. There is also some dilatation of the capillary bed.

Later in the angiogram there is diffuse leakage of fluorescein into the vitreous from the disc neovascularization. There is intraretinal leakage of fluorescein from the scattered microaneurysms in the posterior pole. The small frond of neovascularization superior to the macula slightly leaks fluorescein.

The inferior nasal quadrant shows marked irregularity and "sausaging" of the retinal vein. There is some slight staining of the walls of the vein. There is a sharp demarcation between an area of capillary dropout and nonperfusion and perfused retina. At the junction of these two areas there is slight leakage from IRMA.

AUTHOR'S NOTE

It is the author's clinical impression that treating large areas of capillary dropout and nonperfusion will frequently result in marked regression of disc neovascularization.

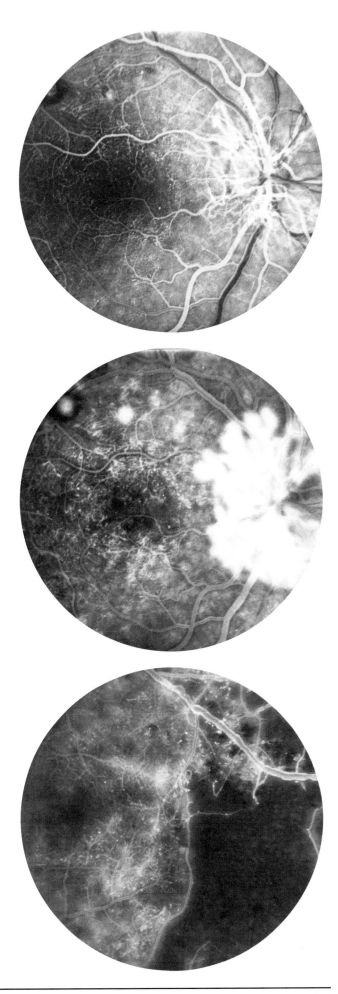

Proliferative Diabetic Retinopathy (with disc neovascularization and cystoid macular edema)

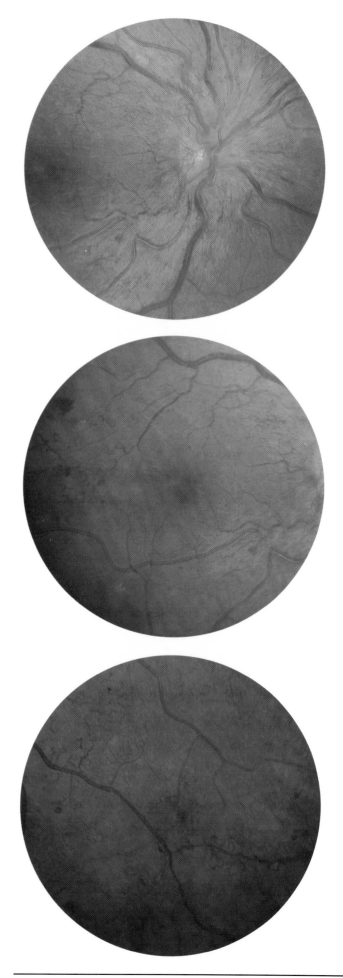

The right eye shows fine disc neovascularization. There are also areas of IRMA nasal and inferior temporal to the optic nerve.

Small cystic spaces can be seen in the perifoveal region. There are scattered dot and blotch hemorrhages and microaneurysms. Temporal to the macula, areas of IRMA can be seen.

In the inferior nasal quadrant there are scattered areas of neovascularization and IRMA. The retinal veins show "sausaging" changes. Scattered dot and blotch hemorrhages and microaneurysms are also present.

During the laminar phase of the fluorescein angiogram, there is hyperfluorescence from the disc neovascularization, IRMA, scattered microaneurysms, and dilatation of the capillary bed.

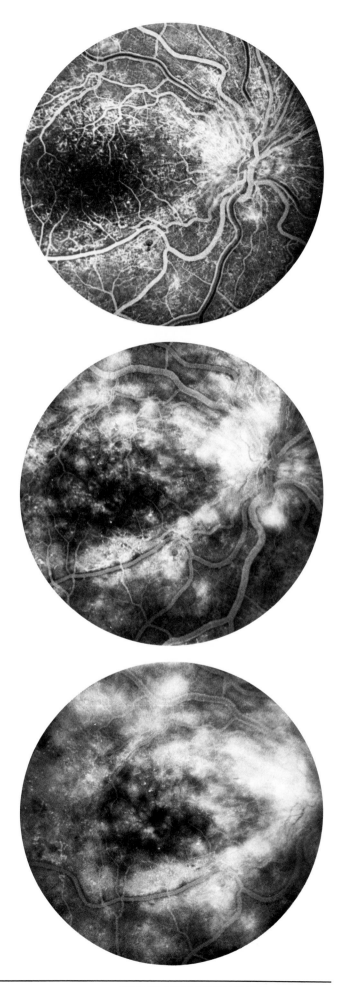

Later in the angiogram there is leakage of fluorescein into the vitreous from the disc neovascularization. There is intraretinal leakage of fluorescein from scattered microaneurysms and IRMA. Perifoveal leakage of the fluorescein dye is also evident.

The late angiogram shows definite perifoveal cystoid macular edema. There is diffuse hyperfluorescence intraretinally secondary to leakage from IRMA and microaneurysms. There is late leakage into the vitreous from the disc neovascularization.

AUTHOR'S NOTE

Frequently, extensive panretinal photocoagulation can compromise macular vision by causing an increase in the amount of macular edema when there is significant edema present prior to treatment.

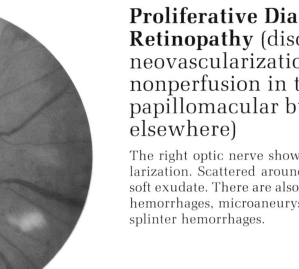

Proliferative Diabetic Retinopathy (disc neovascularization and nonperfusion in the papillomacular bundle and elsewhere)

The right optic nerve shows evidence of neovascularization. Scattered around the nerve are areas of soft exudate. There are also scattered dot and blotch hemorrhages, microaneurysms, and a few scattered splinter hemorrhages.

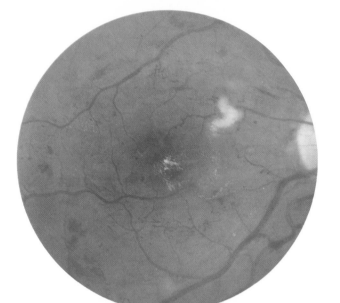

In the posterior pole, scattered dot and blotch hemorrhages, microaneurysms, and deposition of hard exudate in the vicinity of the fovea can be seen. There are multiple areas of IRMA. An area of soft exudate can be seen in the papillomacular bundle.

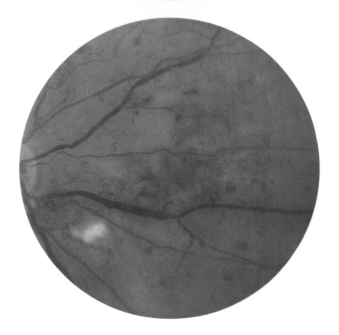

Nasal to the right optic nerve, there are areas of soft exudate. The retinal vein shows marked irregularity and "sausaging" changes. Scattered dot hemorrhages, microaneurysms, and IRMA are also present.

During the laminar phase of the fluorescein angiogram, a large area of capillary dropout and nonperfusion can be seen in the papillomacular bundle. Microaneurysmal changes at the superior aspect of the nonperfused area are also visible. There are scattered microaneurysms and IRMA throughout the posterior pole. Increased hyperfluorescence from leakage of fluorescein can be seen on the surface of the right optic nerve.

Later in the angiogram, there is leakage of fluorescein dye into the vitreous from disc neovascularization. The area of nonperfusion in the papillomacular bundle remains hypofluorescent. There is a small preretinal hemorrhage inferior to the optic nerve which blocks the background choroidal fluorescence. There is extensive intraretinal accumulation of fluorescein dye secondary to leaking microaneurysms and IRMA.

The late angiogram shows staining of the retinal vessel as it passes through the inferior aspect of the nonperfused area in the papillomacular bundle. There is diffuse hyperfluorescence intraretinally throughout the posterior pole from the leaking microvascular abnormalities and microaneurysms. The intraretinal blotch and dot hemorrhages in the posterior pole continue to block the background choroidal fluorescence.

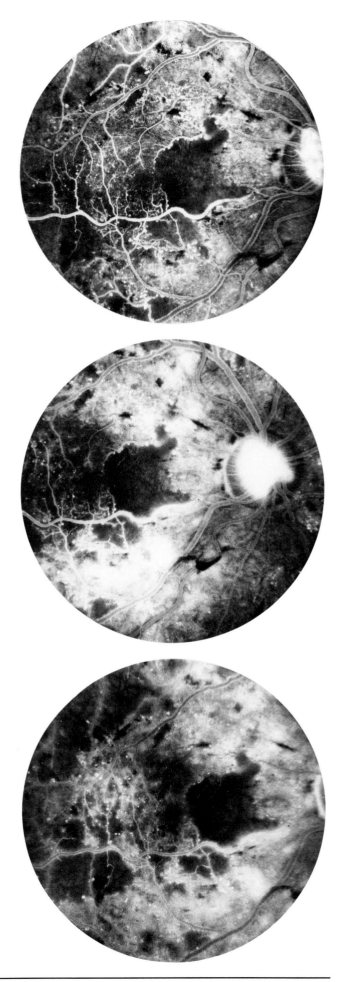

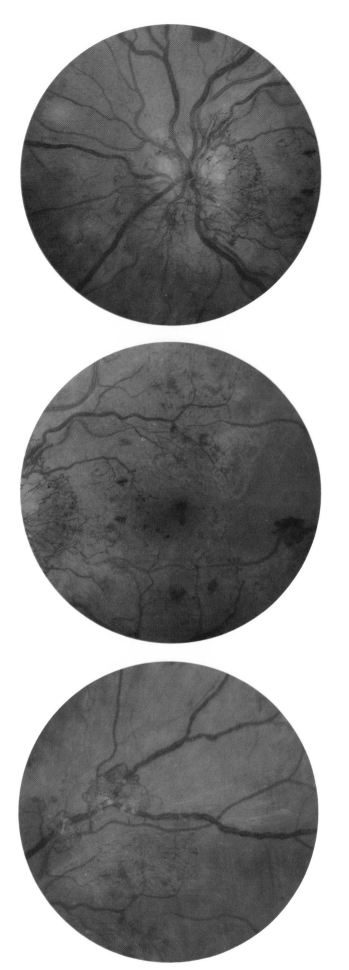

Proliferative Diabetic Retinopathy (with disc neovascularization; neovascularization elsewhere; venous caliber changes and nonperfusion)

The left eye shows extensive neovascularization 360° around the optic nerve. Nasal to the optic nerve is an area of soft exudate. Superior to the optic nerve is a blotch intraretinal hemorrhage.

In the posterior pole of the left eye there are scattered dot and blotch hemorrhages and microaneurysms. Temporal to the fovea there is an area of retinal ischemia, as evidenced by the nonperfused branches which appear as fine, white cords.

Along the superior temporal arcade are fronds of neovascularization. These fronds overlie the superior temporal vein, which shows marked "sausaging" changes.

During the choroidal phase of the fluorescein angiogram, there is filling of the major branches of the disc neovascularization.

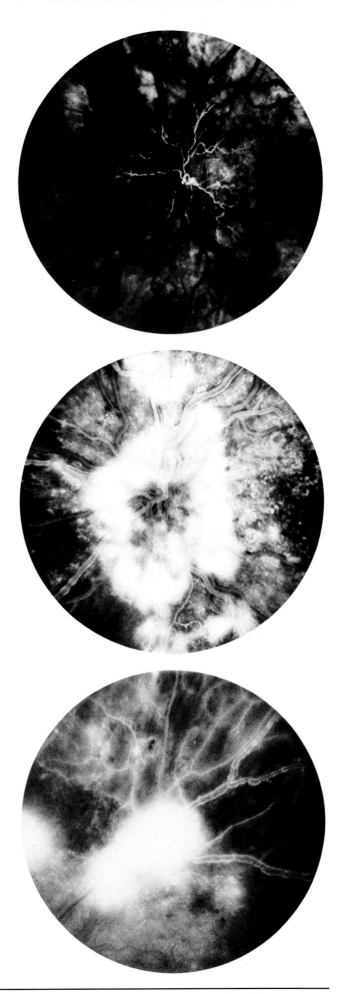

Later in the angiogram there is diffuse leakage of fluorescein into the vitreous from the extensive disc neovascularization. There are scattered areas of intraretinal leakage from scattered microaneurysms and microvascular abnormalities.

Along the superior temporal arcade there is leakage of fluorescein from the neovascularization. The marked irregularities in the branches of the superior temporal vein are evident as these branches course through areas of capillary dropout and nonperfusion.

AUTHOR'S NOTE
Careful focal treatment must be done of these neovascular tufts over major branch veins for fear of causing a major vein occlusion. Hopefully, there will be regression of the disc neovascularization by extensive panretinal photocoagulation treatment specifically to the large areas of nonperfusion.

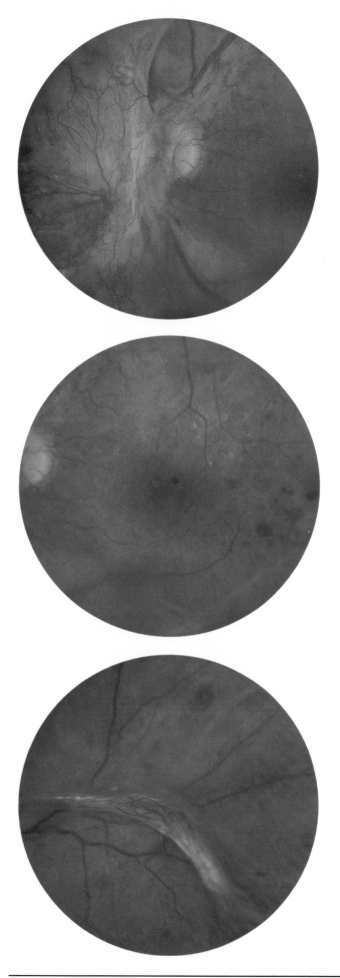

Proliferative Diabetic Retinopathy (with extensive fibrovascular proliferation over the disc and traction along the superior temporal arcades)

There is extensive fibrovascular proliferation overlying the surface of the optic nerve. This proliferative tissue extends nasally and along the superior temporal vessels.

In the posterior pole there are scattered dot and blotch hemorrhages, microaneurysms, and deposition of hard exudate.

Along the superior temporal arcade there is an area of fibrovascular proliferation with slight traction on the sensory retina. Intraretinal dot and blotch hemorrhages and microaneurysms are also present.

During the very early laminar phase of the angiogram, the disc neovascularization can be seen filling with the fluorescein dye. There is some blockage of the background choroidal fluorescence by the intraretinal dot and blotch hemorrhages in the posterior pole.

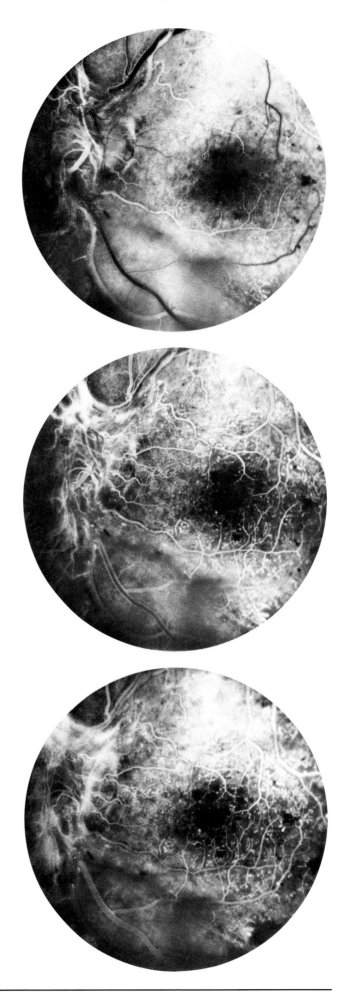

Later in the laminar phase, there is further filling of the disc neovascularization and slight leakage of fluorescein into the vitreous. Multiple microaneurysms can be seen in the macular region.

The late angiogram shows subtle leakage of fluorescein into the vitreous from the disc neovascularization. There is intraretinal accumulation of fluorescein in the macula and superior to the macular region. There is some blockage of the background choroidal fluorescence along the inferior temporal arcade due to a faint vitreous hemorrhage.

AUTHOR'S NOTE

When argon panretinal photocoagulation is considered in these patients, one must be aware of the possible increase in traction on the sensory retina secondary to heating up of the vitreous and pulling on the already present fibrous component to the proliferative tissue.

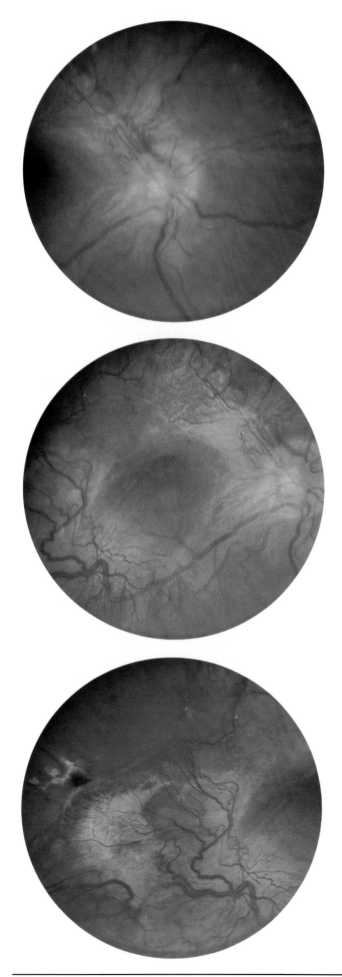

Proliferative Diabetic Retinopathy (with fibrovascular proliferation extending over the posterior pole)

Extending from the surface of the optic nerve is fibrovascular proliferation. This tissue extends along the superior and inferior temporal arcades.

The posterior pole is covered by the fibrovascular proliferative tissue with traction on the center of the macula toward the inferior temporal arcades. A frond of neovascularization can be seen overlying the inferior temporal vessels.

Further temporally, there is extensive fibrovascular proliferation with traction on the sensory retina.

During the venous phase of the angiogram, there is hyperfluorescence within the extensive proliferative tissue overlying the optic nerve and extending along the superior and inferior temporal arcades. The retinal avascular zone is irregular in configuration, indicating tractional changes on the posterior pole.

Later in the angiogram, there is leakage of fluorescein into the vitreous from the fibrovascular proliferative tissue.

The late angiogram shows extensive leakage into the vitreous from the proliferative tissue overlying the optic nerve and along the temporal arcades.

AUTHOR'S NOTE

This patient developed a total tractional detachment of the posterior pole 10 days after argon panretinal photocoagulation treatment. It is certainly conceivable that the photocoagulation treatment caused further tractional change on the posterior pole. It is the author's clinical impression that the krypton red photocoagulation is safer in patients with severe traction.

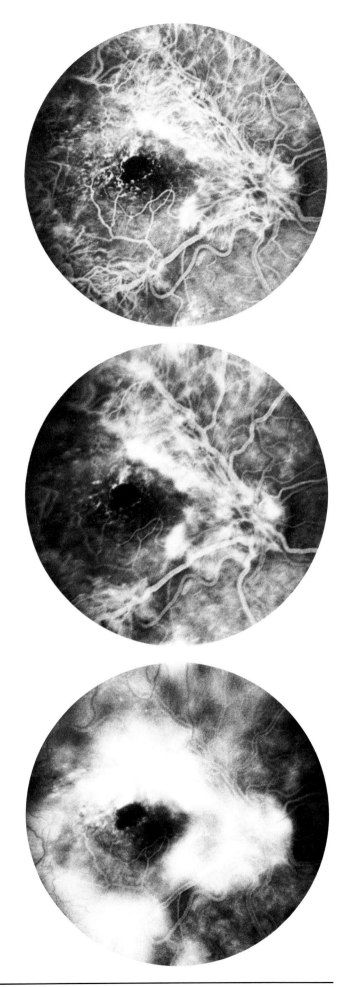

Proliferative Diabetic Retinopathy (with neovascularization elsewhere and preretinal hemorrhage)

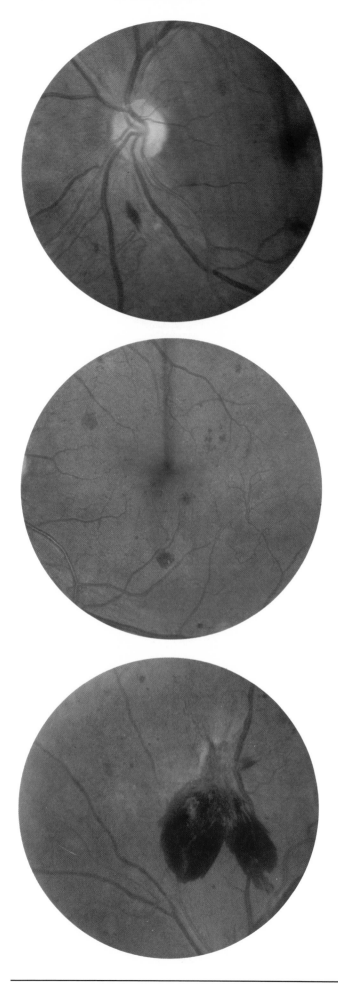

The left optic nerve appears normal. Inferior to the nerve there is a frond of neovascularization overlying one of the major branch veins.

In the posterior pole there are scattered dot and blotch hemorrhages, microaneurysms, and areas of intraretinal microvascular abnormalities (IRMA).

Superior to the optic nerve is an area of preretinal hemorrhage. There appears to be a frond of neovascularization just superior to the hemorrhage.

During the laminar phase of the angiogram, the left posterior pole shows multiple microaneurysms, IRMA, and dilatation of the capillary bed. The small dot and blotch hemorrhages block the background choroidal fluorescence. There is some disruption of the perifoveal capillary net.

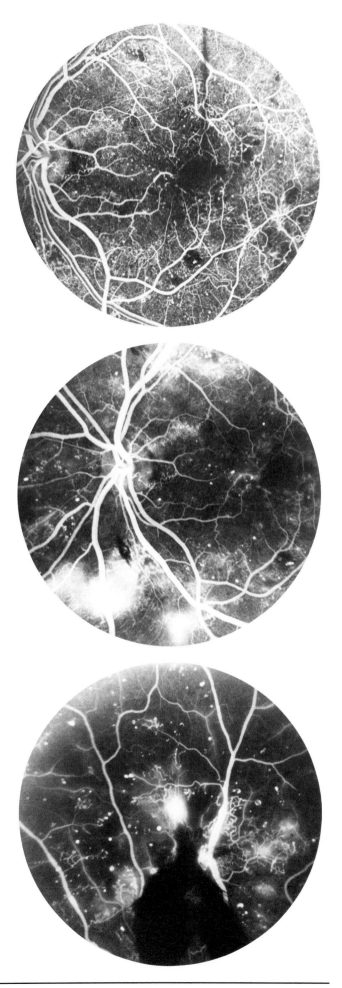

The venous phase of the angiogram shows leakage of fluorescein into the vitreous from the multiple fronds of neovascularization inferior to the optic nerve. The microaneurysms in the posterior pole and surrounding the nerve leak fluorescein intra-retinally.

Superior to the optic nerve there is blockage of the background choroidal fluorescence by the preretinal hemorrhage. A frond of neovascularization can be seen above the hemorrhage leaking fluorescein into the vitreous. The superior quadrant shows extensive areas of capillary dropout and nonperfusion.

Proliferative Diabetic Retinopathy (with subhyaloid hemorrhage)

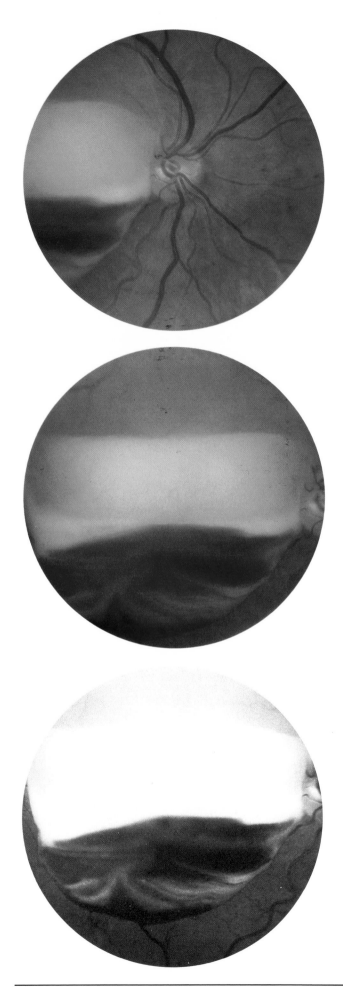

The optic nerve appears normal. Nasal to the nerve are a few scattered dot hemorrhages and microaneurysms.

In the posterior pole, there is a layering out of a subhyaloid hemorrhage. The fovea is obscured by the hemorrhage.

Red-free photograph clearly shows the layering out of the hemorrhage in the posterior pole.

During the venous phase of the angiogram, small fronds of neovascularization nasal to the optic nerve are leaking fluorescein into the vitreous. Scattered microaneurysms can also be seen.

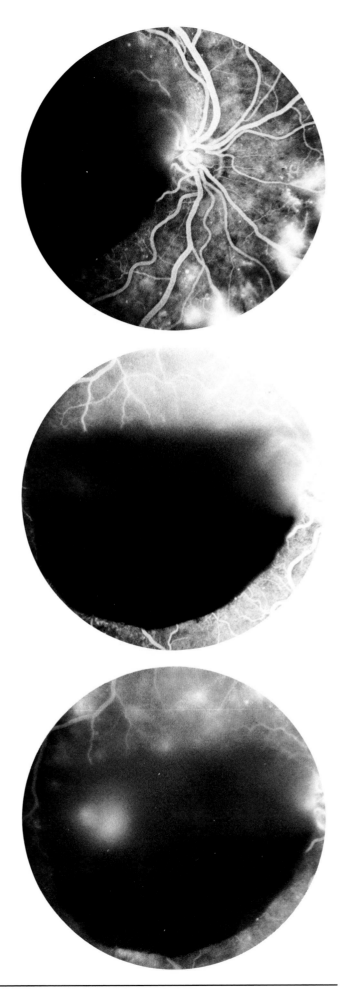

There is blockage of the background choroidal fluorescence by the boat-shaped hemorrhage overlying the posterior pole. Blockage is more intense inferiorly due to the difference in the density of the hemorrhage.

The late angiogram shows sustained blockage of the background fluorescence by the preretinal hemorrhage. There appears to be an area of increased hyperfluorescence and leakage above the more dense hemorrhage temporal to the macula. This area is suspicious for neovascularization.

AUTHOR'S NOTE

Clinically, the hemorrhage overlying the posterior pole appeared to be in the subhyaloid space. Because proliferative retinopathy occurs on the surface of the retina, it was not felt that this hemorrhage was beneath the internal limiting membrane. After clearing of the hemorrhage, there was a definite frond of neovascularization seen temporal to the macula.

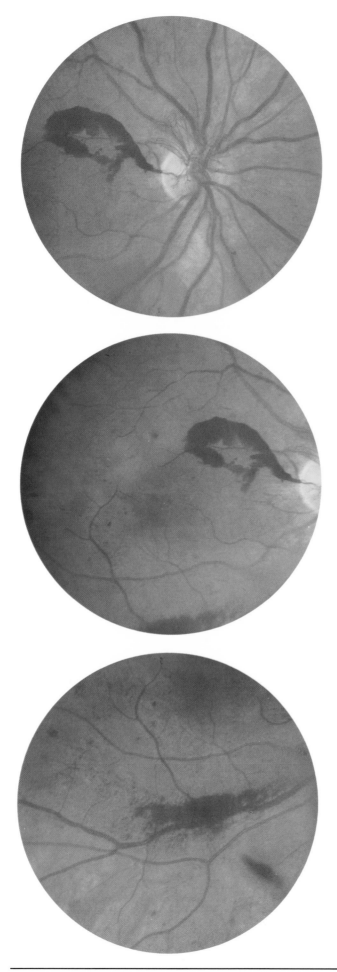

Proliferative Diabetic Retinopathy (with disc neovascularization and preretinal hemorrhage)

The optic nerve shows evidence of neovascularization. Extending temporally from the neovascularization on the surface of the nerve is some preretinal hemorrhage.

In the posterior pole there are scattered dot and blotch hemorrhages and microaneurysms. There appears to be a small area of ischemic retinal whitening above the fovea. The preretinal hemorrhage overlies the papillomacular bundle. There is also some hemorrhage along the inferior temporal arcade.

Along the inferior temporal vein of the right eye, there is evidence of preretinal hemorrhage. In this inferior temporal quadrant, there are scattered dot and blotch hemorrhages and microaneurysms. The branches of the inferior temporal veins show marked caliber irregularities.

During the laminar phase of the angiogram, the disc neovascularization is clearly evident. The preretinal hemorrhage temporal to the optic nerve blocks the background choroidal fluorescence. There are multiple areas of pinpoint hyperfluorescence corresponding to microaneurysms.

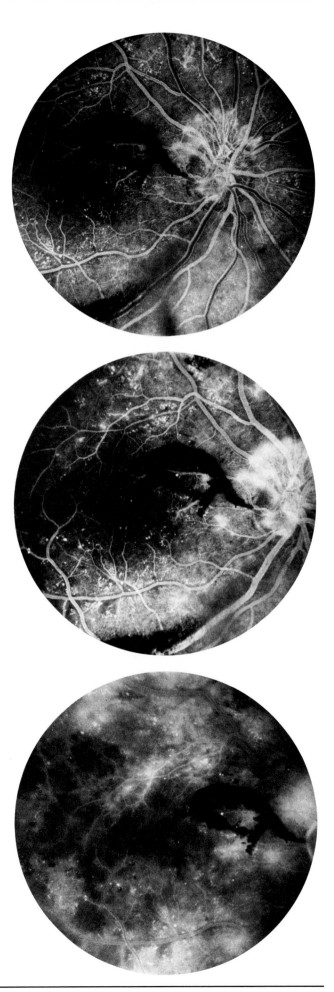

Later in the angiogram, there is leakage of fluorescein into the vitreous from the disc neovascularization. The preretinal hemorrhage temporal to the optic nerve and along the inferior temporal vein blocks the background fluorescence. There is disruption of the perifoveal capillary net. The microaneurysms and IRMA continue to leak fluorescein.

The late angiogram shows continlued blockage of the background fluorescence by the preretinal hemorrhage. There is diffuse intraretinal leakage of fluorescein dye, indicating retinal edema. Areas of nonperfusion continue to persist around the fovea and temporal to the macula.

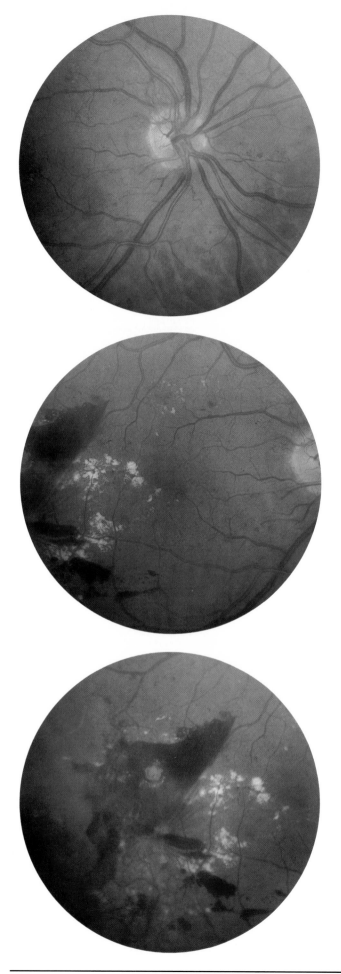

Proliferative Diabetic Retinopathy (with disc neovascularization, neovascularization elsewhere with preretinal hemorrhage)

The optic nerve shows evidence of fine neovascularization. Nasal to the nerve are scattered dot and blotch hemorrhages and microaneurysms.

In the posterior pole there are scattered dot and blotch hemorrhages, microaneurysms, and deposition of hard exudate temporal to the fovea. Temporal to the macula is some preretinal hemorrhage.

Inferior to the preretinal hemorrhage is a frond of neovascularization. Temporal to the hemorrhage is an area of retinal ischemia as evidenced by the loss of the normal sensory retinal sheen and the presence of a nonperfused vessel.

The late angiogram shows leakage of fluorescein into the vitreous from the disc neovascularization. In the posterior pole there is intraretinal accumulation of the fluorescein dye from leaking microaneurysms.

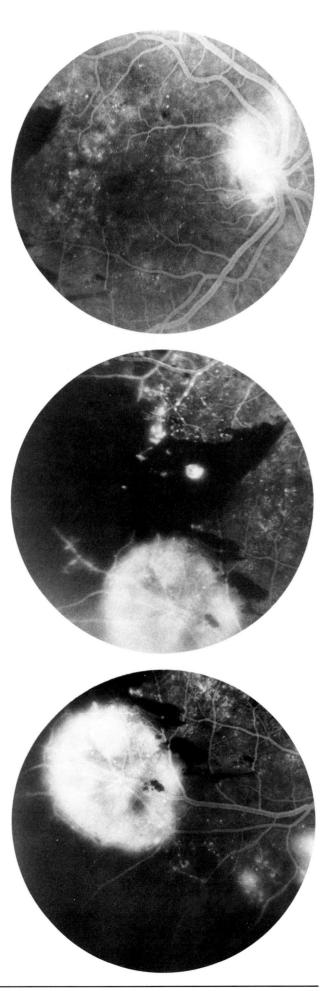

Temporal to the macula there is blockage of the background choroidal fluorescence by the preretinal hemorrhage. Just temporal to the hemorrhage is a large area of capillary dropout and nonperfusion. Inferior to the hemorrhage is leakage of fluorescein from a fairly large frond of neovascularization.

There is diffuse leakage of fluorescein from the neovascularization along the inferior temporal arcade which was also the cause of the preretinal hemorrhage. Inferior to the neovascularization is a large zone of retinal nonperfusion.

AUTHOR'S NOTE

Frequently. fronds of neovascularization away from the disc can be seen at a junction between perfused and nonperfused retina.

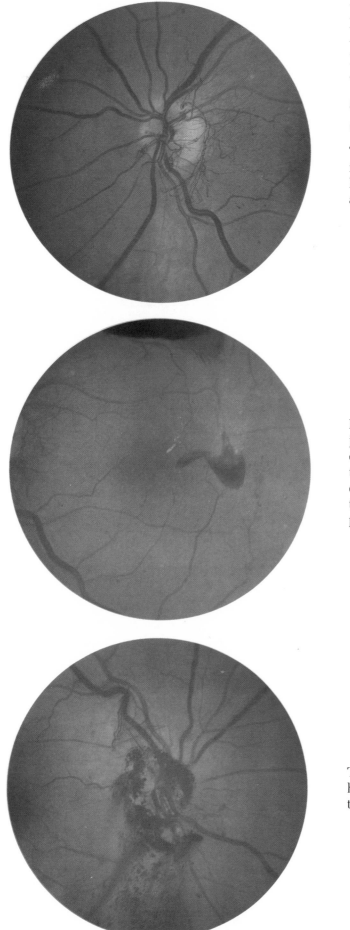

Proliferative Diabetic Retinopathy (disc neovascularization with vitreous hemorrhage; preretinal and vitreous hemorrhage elsewhere)

The left optic nerve shows evidence of neovascularization. Neovascularization extends into the papillomacular bundle and along the superior temporal arcade.

In the posterior pole there is preretinal hemorrhage just temporal to the fovea. There are a few scattered dot and blotch hemorrhages and microaneurysms in the posterior pole. A few scattered areas of hard exudate can be seen in the perifoveal region. Along the superior temporal arcade there is evidence of a preretinal hemorrhage.

The fellow right eye shows preretinal and vitreous hemorrhage emanating from disc neovascularization.

During the laminar phase of the angiogram of the left eye there is blockage of the background choroidal fluorescence by the preretinal hemorrhage temporal to the fovea and the hemorrhage along the superior temporal arcade. There are multiple microaneurysmal changes with dilatation of the capillary bed. The perifoveal capillary net is intact and well visualized. Temporal to the macula are areas of capillary dropout and nonperfusion.

There is diffuse leakage of fluorescein into the vitreous from the disc neovascularization. There is intraretinal accumulation of fluorescein dye from the leaking microaneurysms. The hemorrhage temporal to the fovea and along the superior temporal arcade continues to block the background fluorescence.

Late angiography of the fellow eye shows diffuse leakage into the vitreous from neovascularization of the disc. The preretinal and vitreous hemorrhage overlying the nerve blocks the background fluorescence. Scattered microaneurysms leak fluorescein intraretinally. There is some irregularity in the caliber of the retinal veins, with staining of the venous walls.

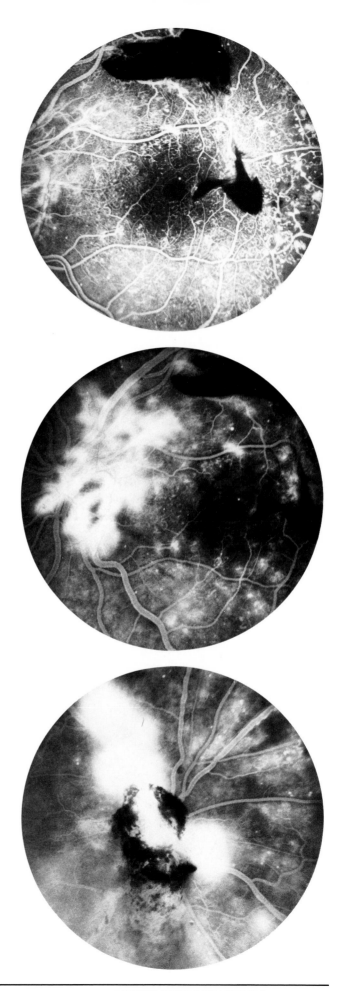

Proliferative Diabetic Retinopathy (with progression of traction in the posterior pole)

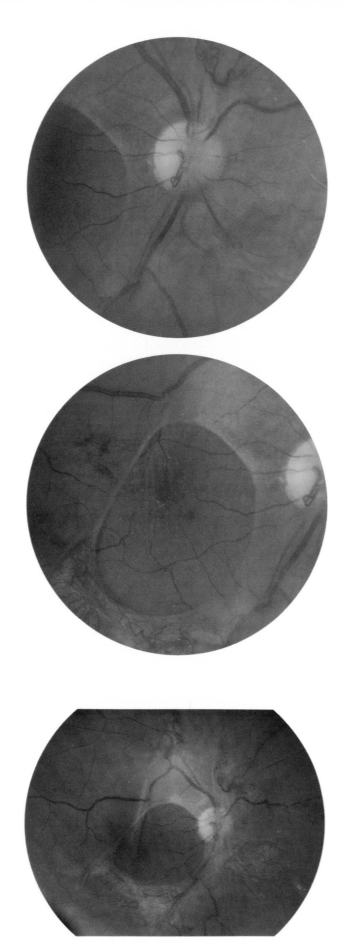

Superior and inferior nasal to the optic nerve there is definite evidence of neovascularization. There is a sheet of fibrovascular proliferation extending over the optic nerve and temporally.

In the posterior pole there is a ring of fibrovascular proliferation causing traction. Vertical striae can be seen extending from the superior temporal vein as it is pulled into the traction. Extensive neovascularization is present along the inferior temporal arcade, intermixed with the fibrous tissue.

Sixty degree photograph of the right eye shows progression of the tractional changes within a period of 2 weeks. The extensive fibrovascular proliferation around the posterior pole is clearly evident. There is now a very prominent retinal fold extending vertically from the superior arcades to the temporal aspect of the macula.

The red-free photograph clearly shows the ring of traction around the macular region with the prominent vascular component along the inferior temporal arcade.

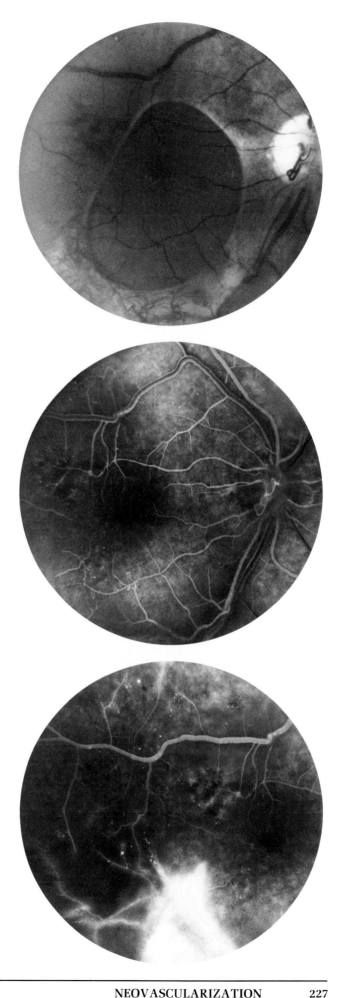

During the laminar phase of the angiogram, there are some scattered microaneurysms. Some slight traction can be seen along the superior temporal vein.

Temporal to the macula is a large area of capillary dropout and nonperfusion. There is leakage into the vitreous from the fibrovascular proliferation along the inferior temporal arcade.

AUTHOR'S NOTE

Extreme caution must be taken if panretinal photocoagulation is considered in this type of case. The heating up of the vitreous could cause rapid contraction of the posterior hyaloid with an increase in tractional changes throughout the posterior pole. The risks of photocoagulation must be weighed against the possibility of doing a vitrectomy if there is a sudden drop of vision from a spontaneous increase in the tractional changes.

Proliferative Diabetic Retinopathy (tractional elevation of the posterior pole with distortion of the fovea)

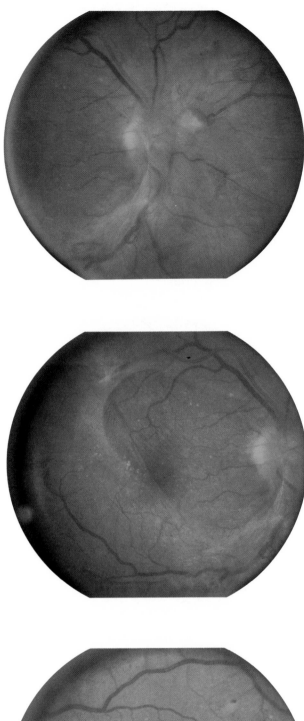

Extensive fibrovascular proliferation can be seen over the optic nerve and extending nasal to the nerve and along the inferior temporal arcade. Neovascularization is present superior nasal to the nerve.

Tractional elevation is present in the macular region with striae extending from an epiretinal center of proliferation along the superior temporal arcade.

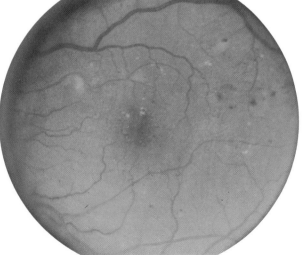

The fellow (left) eye shows scattered dot and blotch hemorrhages, microaneurysms, and areas of soft exudate. There are a few scattered areas of intraretinal hard exudate.

During the venous phase of the fluorescein angiogram, the disc neovascularization slightly leaks fluorescein. Scattered microaneurysms can also be seen in the posterior pole. There is distortion of the normally round perifoveal capillary net due to the traction extending from the superior temporal arcade.

The late angiogram shows diffuse intravitreal leakage of fluorescein dye from the extensive fibrovascular proliferation on the optic nerve, along the inferior temporal arcades, and nasal retina.

The fellow (left) eye shows intraretinal leakage of fluorescein from scattered microaneurysms and intraretinal microvascular abnormalities.

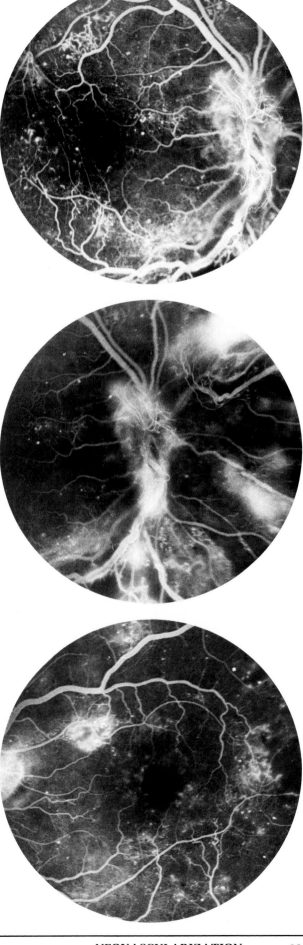

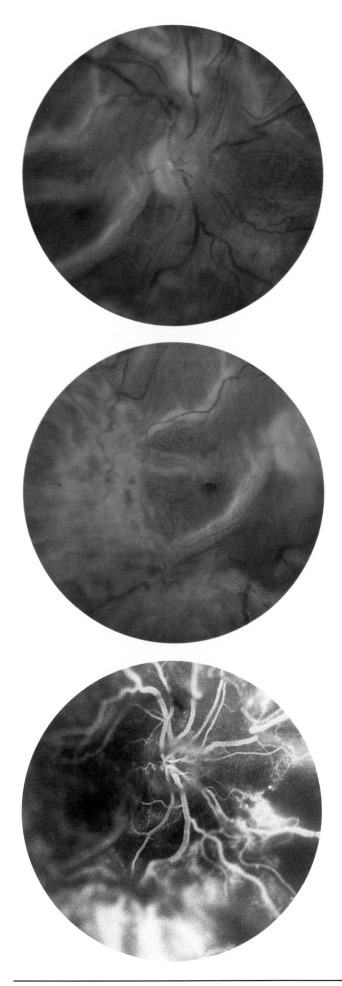

Proliferative Diabetic Retinopathy (extensive tractional and rhegmatogenous detachment)

Overlying the right optic nerve and extending along all the arcades is extensive fibrovascular proliferation. The retina has multiple fixed folds, and there is evidence of subretinal fibrosis.

In the posterior pole, there is evidence of both a tractional and rhegmatogenous retinal detachment. The extensive fibrovascular proliferation can be seen just temporal to the macula. There is also a full-thickness foveal hole.

Fluorescein angiography of the right eye shows extensive leakage of fluorescein into the vitreous from the fibrovascular proliferation. There is blockage of the background choroidal fluorescence by the extensive subretinal fluid from both the tractional and combined rhegmatogenous retinal detachment.

AUTHOR'S NOTE

This patient had both a tractional and rhegmatogenous retinal detachment. The rhegmatogenous component of the detachment was secondary to approximately 15 to 20 atrophic holes along all the arcades and temporal to the macula. The presence of subretinal fibrosis and fixed folds also makes the prognosis for any type of visual improvement poor, and it was decided that this eye should not have surgery.

Reader's Notes

Panretinal Photocoagulation for Proliferative Retinopathy

In most cases, panretinal photocoagulation for proliferative retinopathy can be divided into three separate sessions. When there is significant neovascularization of the optic nerve, photocoagulation is brought up to the edge of the optic nerve along the superior, nasal and inferior borders.

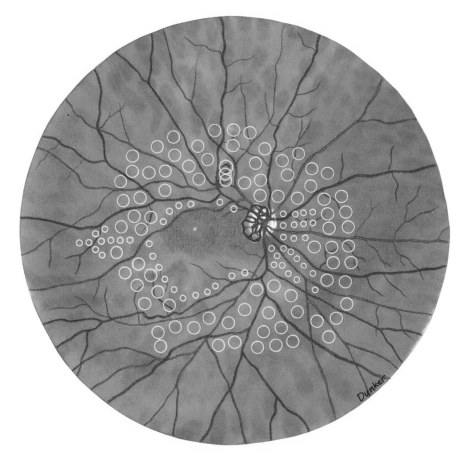

During session one, the initial area is treated with 200-μ spots. The innermost row of photocoagulation temporal to the macula is usually 1½ to 2 disc diameters temporal to the center of the fovea. An arrow pointing toward the far temporal periphery or some other landmark is usually placed so that when the 3-mirror contact lens is used for treatment of the temporal periphery, this landmark or arrow will direct the photocoagulator away from the posterior pole. The photocoagulation burns immediately around the optic nerve and surrounding the posterior pole are usually 200-μ in size. The remainder of the first session can be carried out using 500-μ spot sizes.

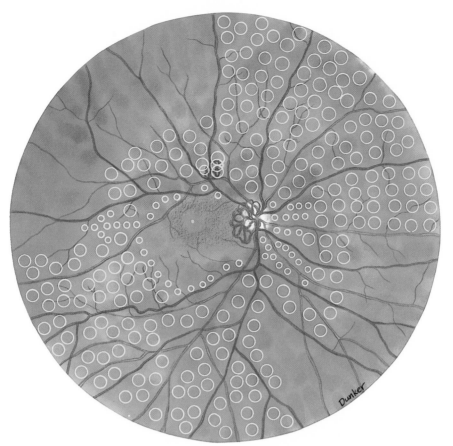

The second session consists of additional 500-μ spot sizes treating the superior nasal and inferior temporal peripheral quadrants.

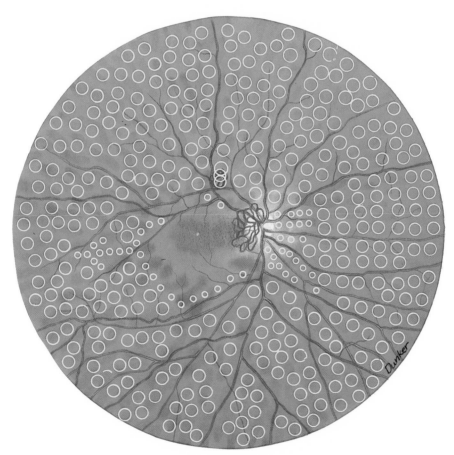

The third and final session consists of treating the superior temporal and inferior nasal quadrants.

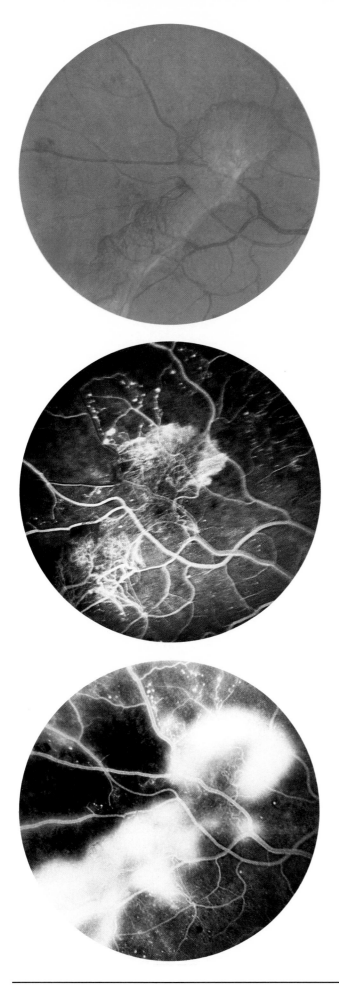

Proliferative Diabetic Retinopathy (with extensive neovascularization elsewhere—pre- and post-treatment)

Temporal to the macula, there is a large area of neovascularization intermixed with fibrous tissue. Scattered areas of intraretinal dot and blotch hemorrhages are also seen.

During the venous phase of the fluorescein angiogram, the neovascularization hyperfluoresces, as do the scattered microaneurysms.

Later in the angiogram, there is diffuse leakage of fluorescein into the vitreous from the extensive neovascularization. This large fibrovascular frond is located at a junction of perfused and nonperfused retina.

Eight weeks after panretinal photocoagulation, there is significant regression of the vascular component of the fibrovascular proliferative tissue. The argon laser photocoagulation scars can be seen temporal and superior to the frond.

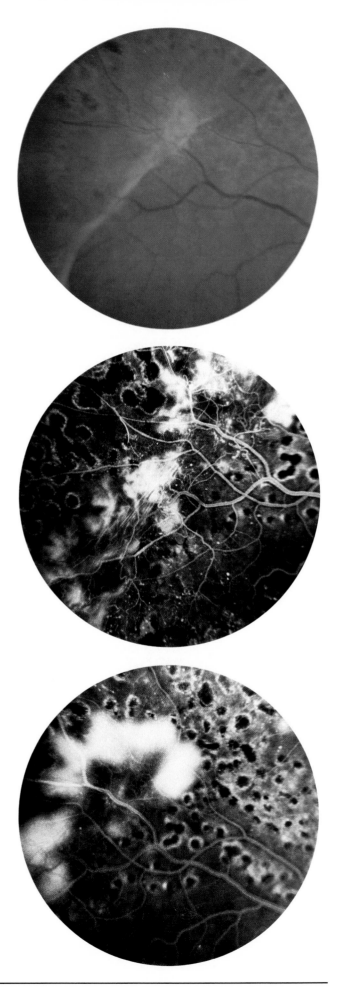

Angiography reveals subtle leakage of fluorescein into the vitreous from residual neovascularization. The photocoagulation scars stain in a typical fashion.

The very late angiogram shows leakage into the vitreous from the residual neovascularization. However, the leakage is much less than prior to treatment.

AUTHOR'S NOTE

Due to the extensive size of the proliferative tissue and the significant fibrotic component, it was decided that focal treatment to the frond should not be done, and extensive panretinal photocoagulation was carried out with particular attention being paid to completely obliterating the nonperfused areas temporal to the neovascularization. This treatment resulted in a dramatic response with marked regression of the vascular component of the fibrovascular tissue. The patient has done well, without any significant hemorrhages, for 3 years since her treatment.

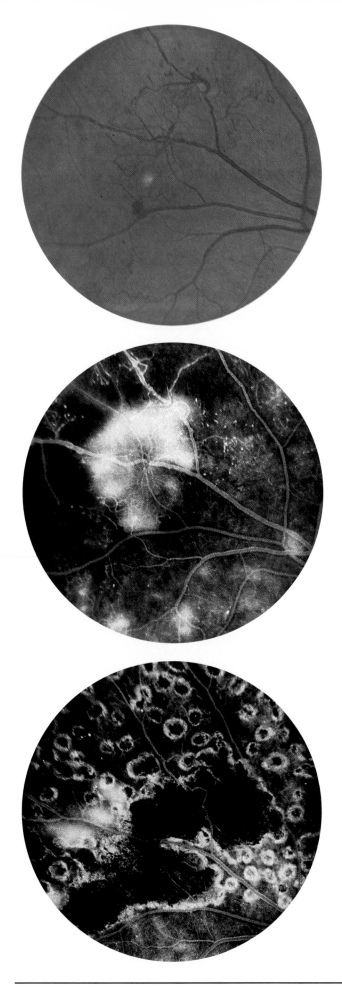

Proliferative Diabetic Retinopathy
(neovascularization elsewhere—pre- and post-treatment)

In the superior temporal quadrant of the right eye, there is evidence of neovascularization. There is a small venous loop at the origin of the neovascular frond. Scattered intraretinal dot and blotch hemorrhages are also present.

There is leakage of the fluorescein dye into the vitreous from the surface neovascularization along the superior temporal arcade. There is a large area of capillary dropout and nonperfusion peripheral to and around the neovascularization. There is marked irregularity in the caliber of the retinal veins. Intraretinal leakage of fluorescein can be seen from the microaneurysms.

There is complete obliteration of the neovascularization by focal argon laser photocoagulation. In addition, panretinal photocoagulation scars can be seen.

AUTHOR'S NOTE

The neovascularization was treated focally in this patient, in addition to extensive panretinal photocoagulation. It was decided that focal treatment could be carried out due to the small caliber of the neovascularization, the fact that it was relatively flat on the surface of the retina, and that there was no significant fibrous component with traction.

Proliferative Diabetic Retinopathy (disc neovascularization—pre- and post-treatment)

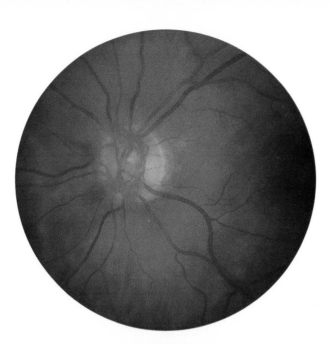

Overlying the surface of the left optic nerve is neo-vascularization.

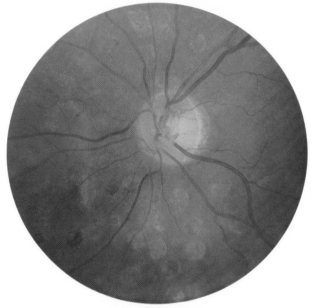

Eight weeks post-photocoagulation treatment, there is marked regression of the neovascularization overlying the surface of the nerve.

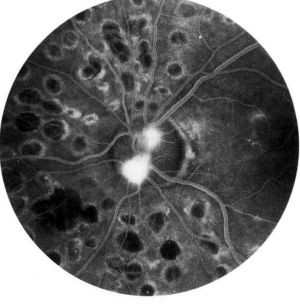

The late angiogram of the left eye shows some very subtle leakage of fluorescein into the vitreous from residual neovascularization. The panretinal photocoagulation scars can be seen staining in a typical fashion.

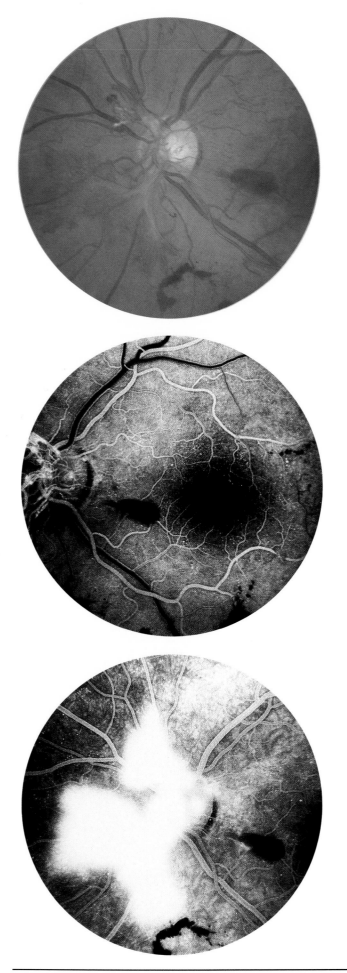

Proliferative Diabetic Retinopathy (extensive disc neovascularization with hemorrhage—pre- and post-treatment)

The left optic nerve shows extensive neovascularization with some fibrous tissue. Preretinal and vitreous hemorrhage can be seen temporal and inferior to the nerve.

Fluorescein angiography during the laminar phase shows early filling of the disc neovascularization. The hemorrhage temporal to the optic nerve blocks the background choroidal fluorescence. Scattered intraretinal microaneurysms can also be seen.

The late angiogram shows diffuse leakage of fluorescein into the vitreous from the extensive disc neovascularization. The hemorrhage temporal and inferior to the nerve continues to block background fluorescence.

Ten weeks after panretinal photocoagulation treatment, there is marked regression in the vascular component of the proliferative tissue emanating from the surface of the optic nerve. The panretinal photocoagulation scars around the nerve are clearly visible.

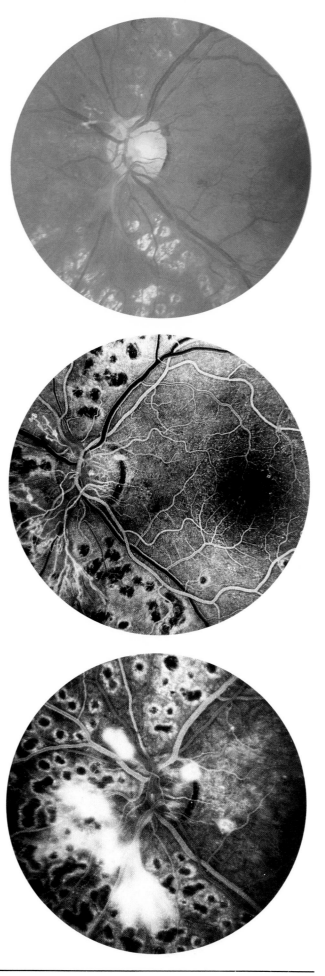

During the laminar phase of the angiogram, there is some minimal filling of the residual disc neovascularization. The pinpoint areas of hyperfluorescence in the macular region correspond to the microaneurysms.

The late angiogram shows leakage of fluorescein into the vitreous from the residual disc neovascularization. However, there is a significant reduction in the amount of proliferative tissue and fluorescein leakage as compared to the pretreatment angiogram.

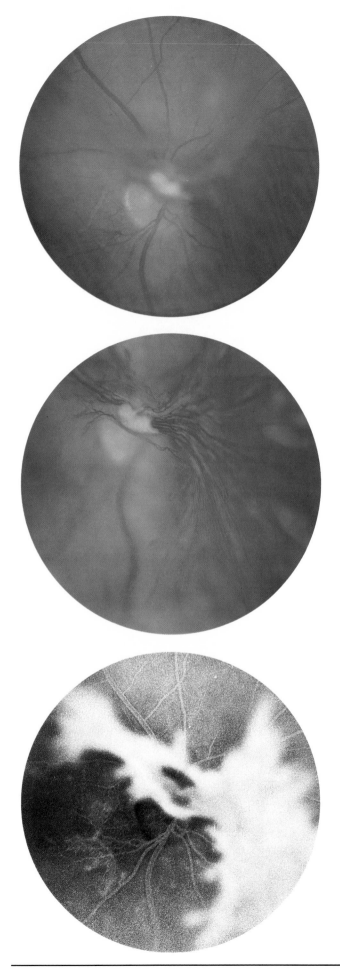

Proliferative Diabetic Retinopathy (extensive elevated disc neovascularization—pre- and post-treatment)

There is some blurriness of the superior disc margin and nasal retina due to the extensive elevated disc neovascularization.

The camera is focused on the elevated fibrovascular frond emanating from the surface of the nerve. This frond extended into the anterior one-third of the vitreous gel. The optic nerve and retinal vessels are out of focus due to the anterior focusing of the camera on the proliferative tissue.

Fluorescein angiography shows extensive leakage of the dye into the vitreous from the disc neovascularization.

Three months post-photocoagulation treatment, there is marked regression of the fibrovascular proliferation with essentially no vascular component to the tissue. The photocoagulation scars can be seen superior and inferior to the optic nerve.

The posterior pole of the right eye is attached. There is a small frond of neovascularization just temporal to the macula.

Fluorescein angiography shows some slight blockage of the background fluorescence by the fibrous tissue, which remains after photocoagulation treatment. There is no leakage of fluorescein into the vitreous, indicating complete regression of the vascular component to the disc proliferation. The photocoagulation scars stain in a typical fashion.

AUTHOR'S NOTE

This patient had a dramatic response to panretinal photocoagulation. There was no focal treatment to any of the disc neovascularization. The patient is now 6 years post-treatment and has had no hemorrhage in the right eye. Vision remains at 20/25. The small frond of neovascularization temporal to the macula has not progressed and has undergone some fibrous change with less of a vascular component.

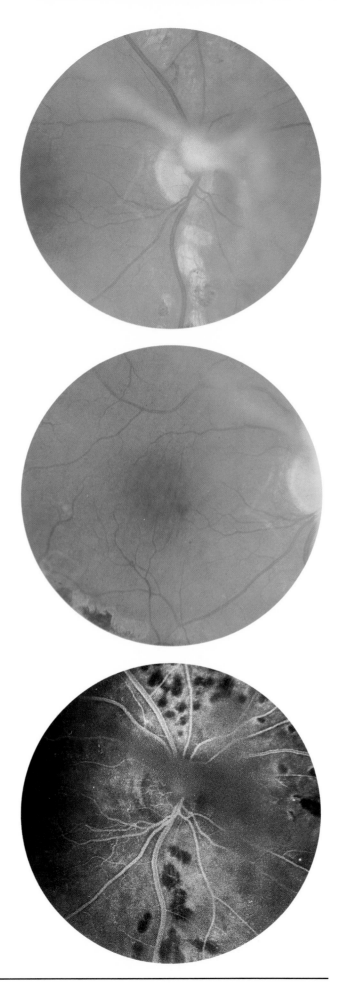

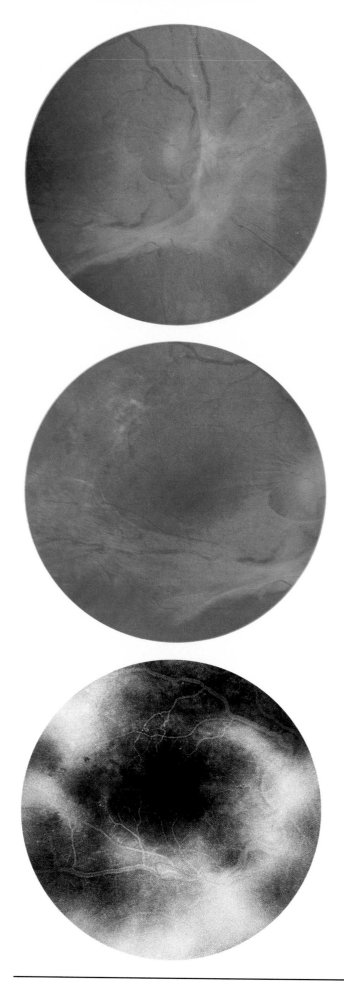

Proliferative Diabetic Retinopathy (severe proliferative retinopathy with traction—pre- and postvitrectomy)

There is extensive fibrovascular proliferation on the surface of the optic nerve. There is traction nasally and along the inferior temporal arcade.

Striae are present through the center of the macula. There is extensive fibrous tissue with neovascularization temporal to the macula.

The late fluorescein angiogram shows diffuse leakage of the dye into the vitreous from the extensive fibrovascular proliferation.

Postvitrectomy, there are multiple epicenters of fibrous tissue. These areas appear on the surface of the optic nerve along the inferior temporal vein and superior nasal to the nerve. The traction between these epiretinal centers was severed during vitrectomy surgery as was the anterior-posterior traction.

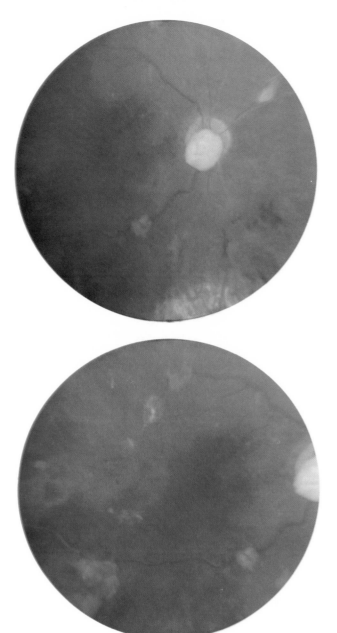

Additional epiretinal centers of proliferation can be seen superior temporal and inferior temporal to the macula. There has been complete relaxation of the sensory retina in the posterior pole with no evidence of striae.

AUTHOR'S NOTE

This 32-year-old white male had finger-counting vision in his right eye. A trans-pars plana lensectomy, vitrectomy and xenon endophotocoagulation were done. The patient's vision has been stable at the level of 20/25 wearing an aphakic contact lens.

Retrolental Fibroplasia

Retrolental fibroplasia (RLF) in the 1950s was one of the major causes of blindness in children throughout the world. Oxygen has been incriminated as the cause of RLF. In the mid and late 1970s there seems to have been a resurgence of cases of both active and cicatritial RLF.

The following is a classification of active stages and cicatritial stages of RLF.

Active Stages of RLF

Stage Ia   Pre-RLF
Stage Ib   Early peripheral vasoproliferative stage
Stage II   Peripheral proliferative and posterior vascular changes
Stage III Further proliferation; vitreoretinal traction

Stage IV   Advanced proliferation and moderate retinal detachment
Stage V   Advanced retinal detachment and proliferation

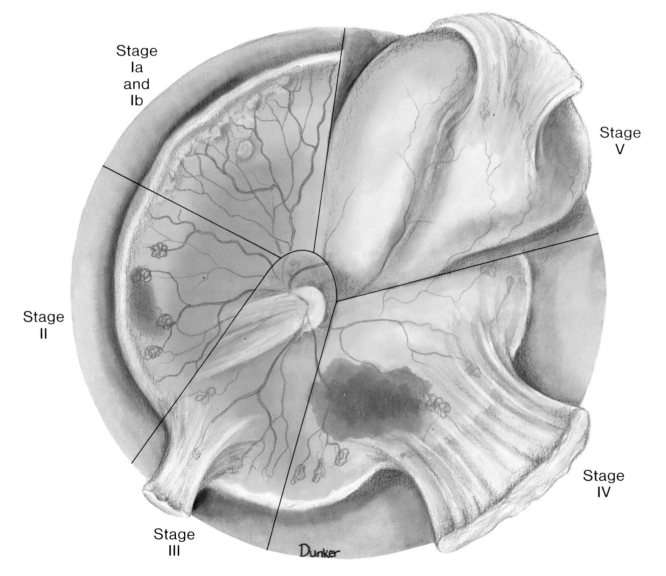

Stage Ia and Ib

Stage V

Stage II

Stage IV

Stage III

Dunker

Cicatritial RLF

Grade I   Minor changes
Grade II   Disc distortion and dragging of the retina temporally

Grade III Retinal folds
Grade IV Incomplete retrolental mass
Grade V Complete retrolental mass

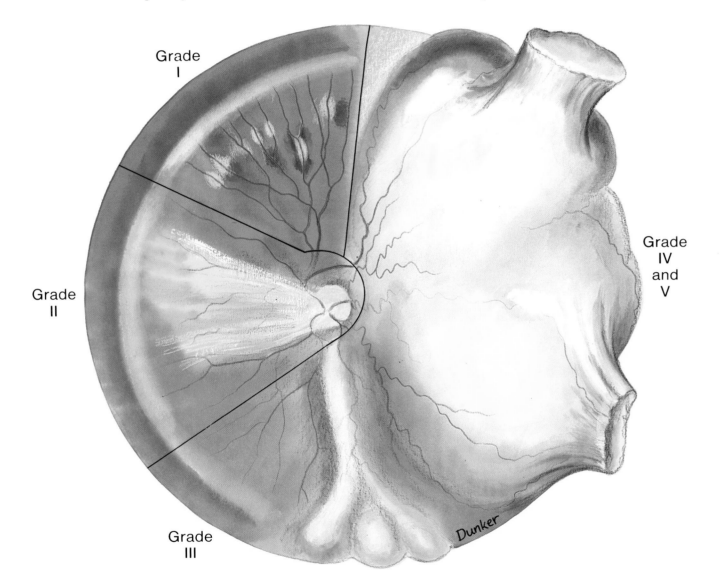

Grade
I

Grade
II

Grade
III

Grade
IV
and
V

Dunker

AUTHOR'S NOTE

These classifications are based on those presented in *Sights and Sounds in Ophthalmology*, vol 2: *Retinal Vascular Disorders*, by Stuart L. Fine, M.D., Arnall Patz, M.D., and David H. Orth, M.D. St. Louis, C.V. Mosby, 1977.

Retrolental Fibroplasia
(peripheral vascular tufts)

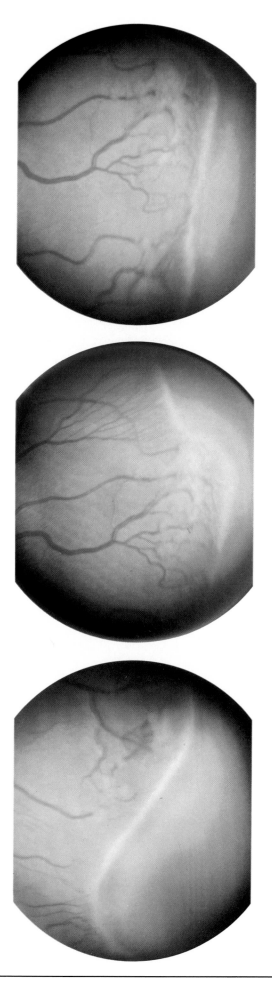

The superior temporal periphery of the left eye demonstrates vascular tufts just posterior to an area of arterio-venous shunting.

Adjacent to the vascular tufts there is a sharp demarcation between perfused and nonperfused peripheral temporal retina.

The inferior temporal periphery showed a larger area of nonperfused retina. There is a sharp, slightly elevated border between perfused and nonperfused retina. Just posterior to this border are additional pinkish-brown elevated vascular tufts.

The early venous phase of the angiogram demonstrates the normal retinal vessels coursing toward the periphery and entering into an area of arterio-venous shunting with the vascular tufts being hyperfluorescent.

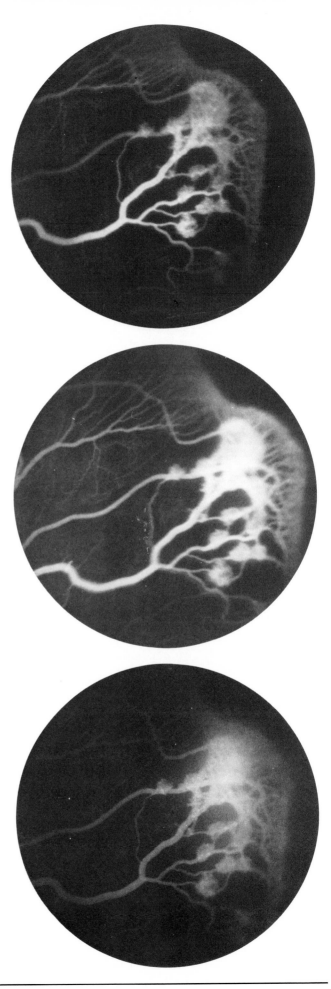

Later in the angiogram the tufts are more hyperfluorescent, and the neovascular tissue at the junction of perfused and nonperfused retina is clearly visible.

The very late venous phase of the angiogram shows the neovascular tissue at the junction of perfused and nonperfused retina to slightly leak fluorescein dye into the vitreous. The round vascular tufts show no leakage of the fluorescein dye.

AUTHOR'S NOTE

This is an unusual presentation of a patient with peripheral vascular tufts in association with arterio-venous shunting and fine neovascularization. The patient was a 950 gm, 28-week-old premature infant. The infant had perinatal asphyxia, respiratory distress syndrome, and a patent ductus arteriosus. The patient required oxygen therapy up to concentrations of 50%, which was finally discontinued after 43 days.

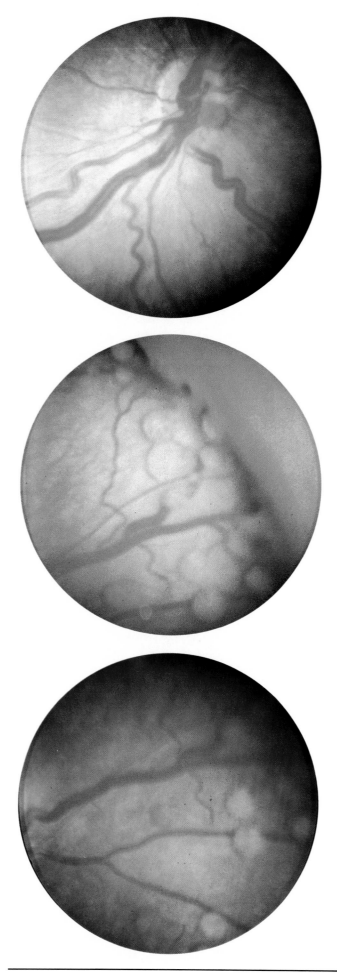

Retrolental Fibroplasia
(vascular tufts over the disc, posterior retina, and peripheral retina)

Overlying the nasal aspect of the optic nerve is a reddish-pink vascular tuft. The retinal veins appear to be slightly engorged.

The superior nasal region of the right eye demonstrates multiple vascular tufts posterior to an elevated border between vascular and avascular retina.

Posterior pole of the right eye demonstrates multiple vascular tufts overlying the major vessels and also present between branches of the retinal vessels.

During the very early phase of the fluorescein angiogram in the right eye, the multiple tufts can be seen. These tufts are not significantly leaking fluorescein dye. A large arterio-venous shunt can also be noted. There is leakage of fluorescein into the vitreous from neovascular tissue peripheral to the tufts and at the junction of vascular and avascular retina.

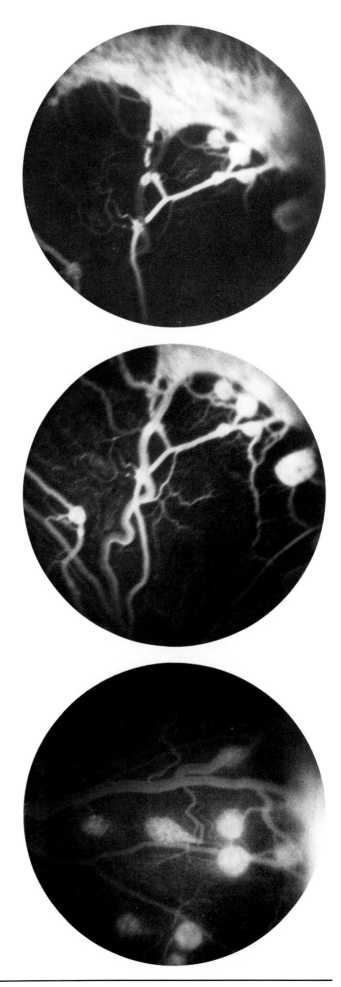

Later in the venous phase of the angiogram, these tufts continue to show no leakage of fluorescein dye. The hyperfluorescent border just peripheral to the tufts is clearly visible.

The late venous phase of the angiogram shows multiple, nonleaking vascular tufts posterior to an area of leaking arterio-venous shunting.

AUTHOR'S NOTE

The arterio-venous shunting tissue just peripheral to the vascular tufts does leak fluorescein dye and can, therefore, be considered neovascular tissue with poor tight junctions between endothelial cells. This is a patient who was born at 26 weeks' gestation and weighed 740 gm. The patient initially received intubation with 100% oxygen for 24 hours. Over a period of 6 days the oxygen therapy varied between 29% and 50%.

Retrolental Fibroplasia
(arrested)

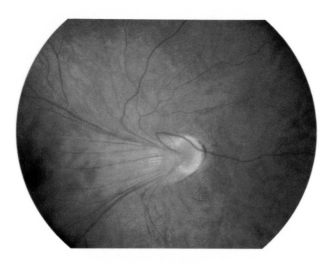

The right optic nerve appears to be oval in shape. The retinal vessels on the temporal portion of the nerve are under stretch and pulled temporally.

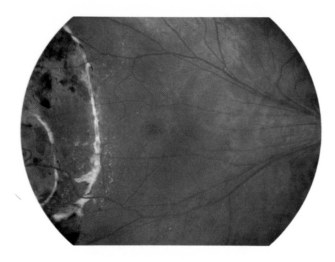

The sensory retina, along with the vessels in the posterior pole, is pulled temporally toward elevated fibrous tissue. Two prominent ridges of fibrous tissue can be seen temporal to the macula.

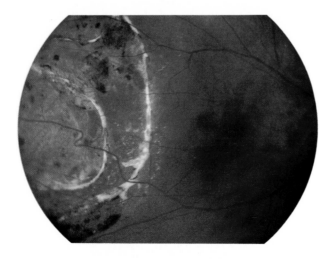

The temporal peripheral retina is markedly atrophic. Diffuse hypo- and hyperpigmentary changes at the level of the retinal pigment epithelium can also be seen.

During the laminar phase of the fluorescein angiogram, there is evidence of the retinal vessels in the posterior pole being pulled temporally. There is increased hyperfluorescence at the level of the retinal pigment epithelium in the macular region and temporal to the macula.

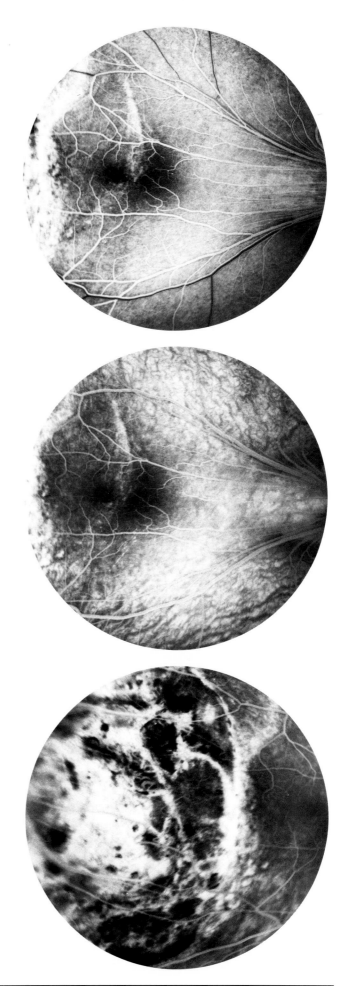

During the venous phase of the angiogram there is persistence of the hyperfluorescence, indicating atrophy of the pigment epithelium. The remainder of the posterior pole appears normal. There is no abnormal leakage of fluorescein from the vessels which are under stretch.

The far temporal periphery shows extensive hypo- and hyperfluorescent change due to atrophy and hyperpigmentation at the level of the retinal pigment epithelium. The retinal vessels coursing through the atrophic elevated retina can also be seen. The vertical ridges of fibrous tissue stain brilliantly with fluorescein dye.

AUTHOR'S NOTE

This 25-year-old white male was born prematurely and was administered oxygen during the first few weeks of life. The right eye shows arrested retrolental fibroplasia, and the left eye has a total retinal detachment secondary to severe complications from retrolental fibroplasia.

Sickle Cell Retinopathy

Sickle cell retinopathy consists of both nonproliferative and proliferative stages in patients who inherit sickle cell hemoglobin. Sickle cell hemoglobin differs from hemoglobin A in that a single gene mutation results in the substitution of amino acid valine for glutamic acid in hemoglobin S. In hemoglobin C, the substitution of lysine for glutamic acid takes place. A genetic defect in the rate of synthesis of the entire protein chain creates another type of hemoglobin protein, causing the disease known as thalassemia. If sickle cell hemoglobin only is inherited from both parents, the resulting disease is called sickle cell anemia, or SS disease. If hemoglobin S is inherited from one parent and hemoglobin C from the other, the offspring has sickle cell C disease, or SC disease. If hemoglobin S is inherited from one parent and hemoglobin A from the other, the offspring has sickle cell traits, or AS hemoglobin. The SS disease, or sickle cell anemia, results in the worst types of systemic problems. These patients have periods of hemolysis, chronic anemia, and painful crises due to hypoxia and in some cases actual infarction. SC and S thal produce milder types of anemia with less severe systemic symptoms. Sickle cell trait (AS hemoglobin) is the mildest of all the sickle cell hemoglobinopathies. Unlike the systemic complications, the most severe ocular complications occur in SC and S thal types of the disease.

Nonproliferative Stages

The funduscopic findings in the nonproliferative stage of sickle retinopathy consist of (1) venous tortuosity; (2) black sunbursts which are probably due to small arteriolar occlusion which causes a small, preretinal, intraretinal, or subretinal hemorrhage. The organization of the hemorrhage in the retina produces a combination of melanin and hemosiderin, resulting in the observable black circumscribed fundus lesion resembling a chorioretinal scar. (A) Salmon patch. (B) Black sunburst. (C) Iridescent spots.

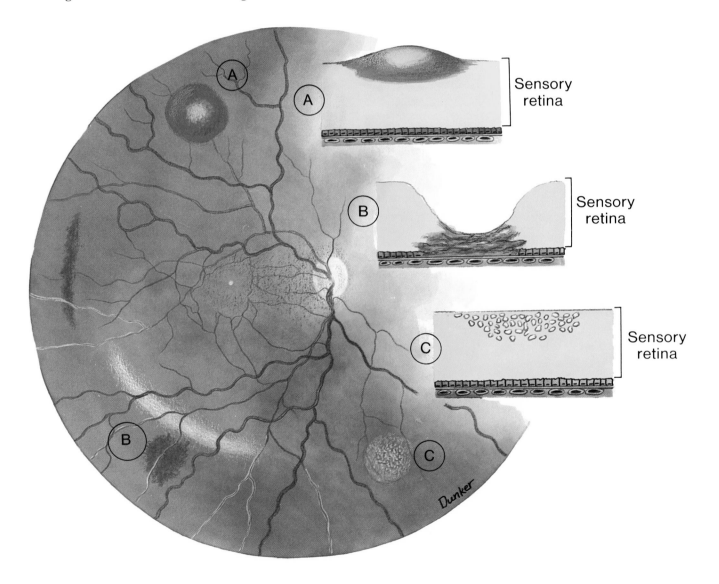

Proliferative Stages

The following classification has been devised for proliferative sickle retinopathy based on funduscopic findings:

Stage I Peripheral arteriolar occlusions

Stage II Peripheral arteriolar anastomoses
Stage III Peripheral neovascularization
Stage IV Vitreous hemorrhage
Stage V Retinal detachment

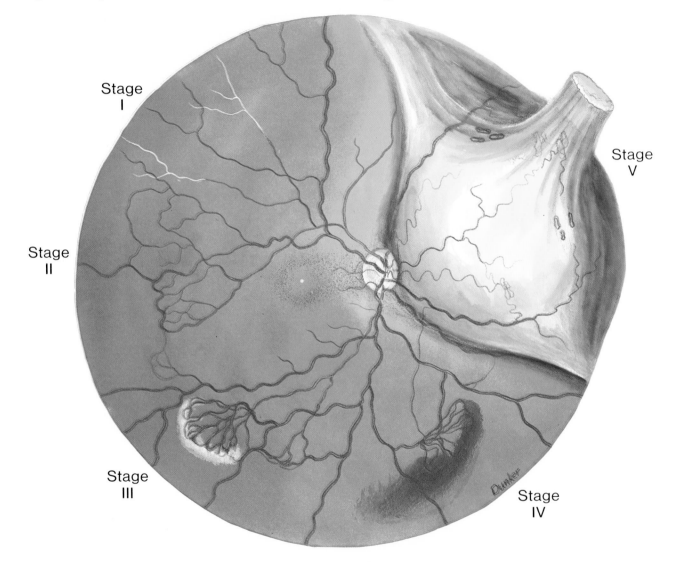

Sickle Cell Retinopathy
("salmon patch" with peripheral retinal nonperfusion)

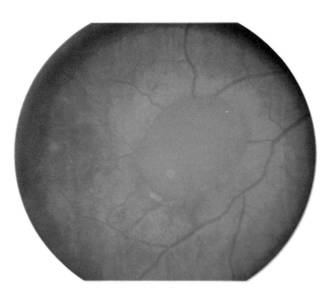

Color photograph of the right eye shows a sharp preretinal hemorrhage which has been termed a "salmon patch."

Fluorescein angiography shows blockage of the background choroidal fluorescence by the round, preretinal hemorrhage.

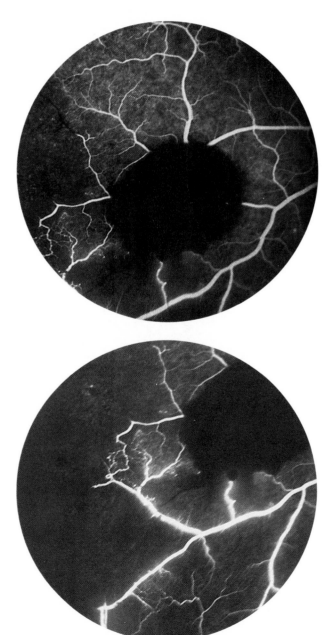

Temporal and inferior to the hemorrhage are areas of retinal avascularity secondary to peripheral arteriolar occlusion. In addition, peripheral arteriolar anastomoses are also present.

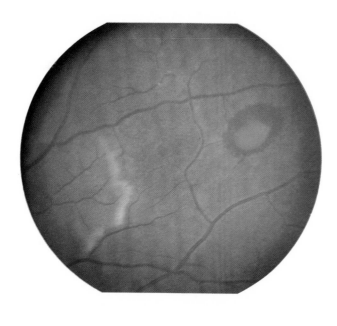

Sickle Cell Retinopathy
(arteriolar occlusion; "salmon patch"; "black sunburst"; neovascularization)

In the temporal periphery of the left eye there is a zone of ischemic retinal whitening. Further temporal, there is a small, round, preretinal hemorrhage.

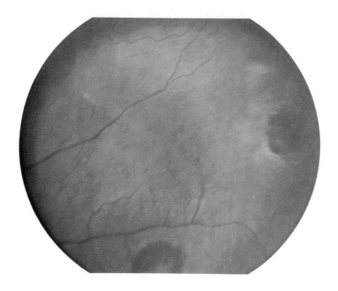

Superior temporal to the preretinal hemorrhage is a small frond of neovascularization, beyond which is an area of hyperpigmentation known as a "black sunburst."

The fluorescein angiogram shows an area of nonperfusion secondary to arteriolar obstruction. Areas of arteriolar anastomoses are present.

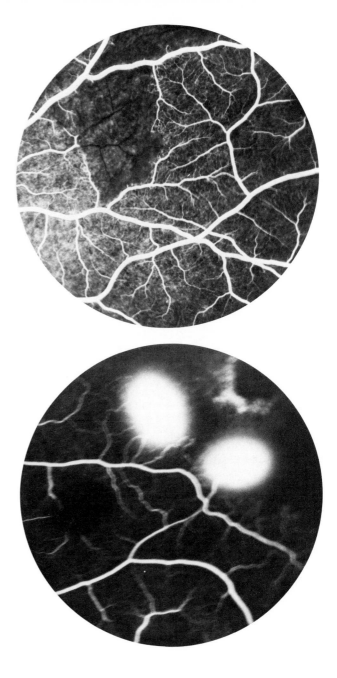

Fluorescein angiography shows blockage of the background choroidal fluorescence by the small, round, preretinal hemorrhage. The neovascular fronds at the junction of perfused and nonperfused retina diffusely leak fluorescein into the vitreous. Beyond the leaking frond is another area of blocked fluorescence secondary to the hyperpigmentation in association with the "black sunburst."

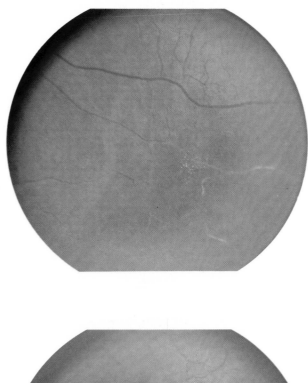

Sickle Cell Retinopathy
(progression to
neovascularization)

In the temporal periphery of the left eye there is occlusion of the peripheral arterioles which appear as silver wires.

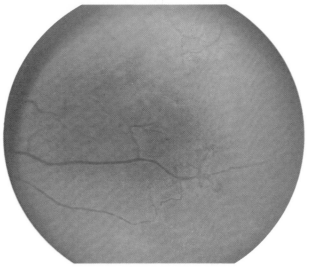

After approximately 1 year, the development of small fronds of neovascularization can be seen.

Fluorescein angiography shows the avascular retina secondary to arteriolar occlusion and the formation of anastomotic channels.

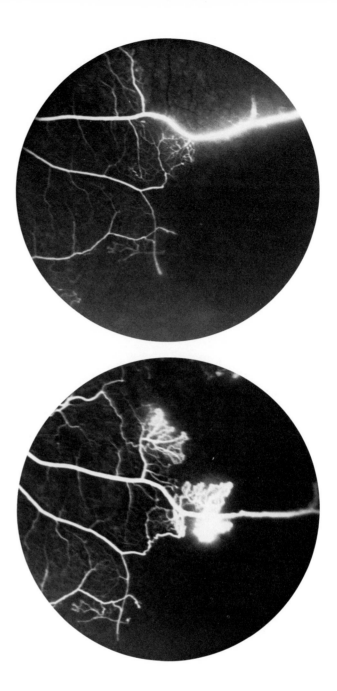

At the junction of perfused and nonperfused retina, the lacy preretinal neovascular fronds hyperfluoresce and leak fluorescein into the vitreous.

Sickle Cell Retinopathy (with progression in size of peripheral neovascularization)

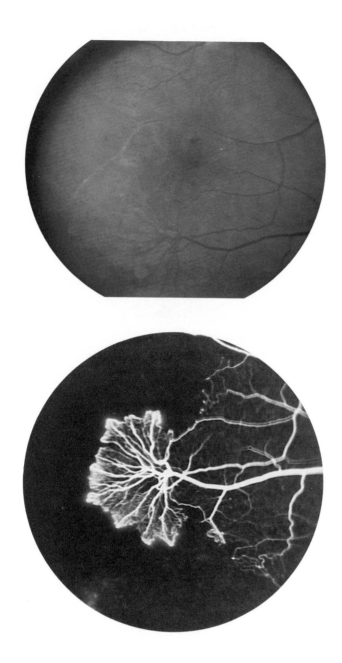

The peripheral retina of the right eye demonstrates areas of arteriolar occlusion which appear as silver wires. Below the whitish occluded vessel is a frond of neovascularization, better known as a "sea fan."

Fluorescein angiography clearly shows the "sea fan" configuration of the neovascularization at the junction of the vascular and avascular retina.

Within a period of 3 months there was marked progression in size of the "sea fan." The feeding vessels to the "sea fan" can be seen as well as the draining vessel, which lacks the fluorescein dye.

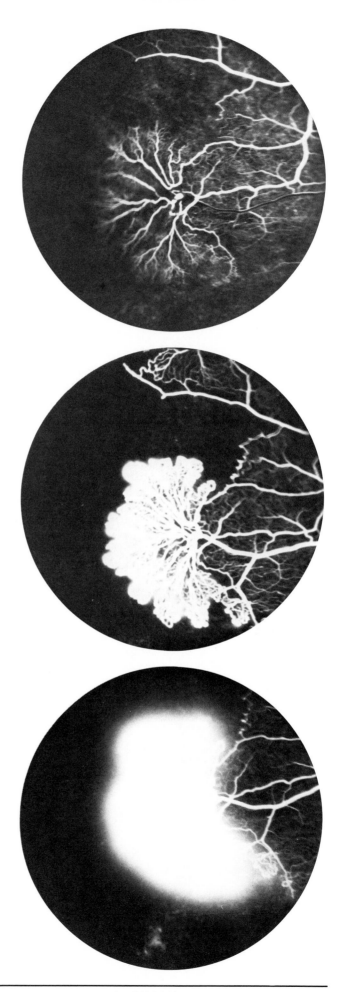

Later in the angiogram, there is increased hyperfluorescence of the "sea fan" with the fluorescein dye beginning to accumulate at the peripheral tufts of the neovascular frond. The "sea fan" extends into the avascular retina.

The late angiogram shows diffuse leakage of fluorescein into the vitreous from the peripheral "sea fan."

AUTHOR'S NOTE

I extend my deepest gratitude and appreciation to Lee Jampol, M.D., and Morton F. Goldberg, M.D. for permitting me to present this series of cases dealing with sickle cell retinopathy.

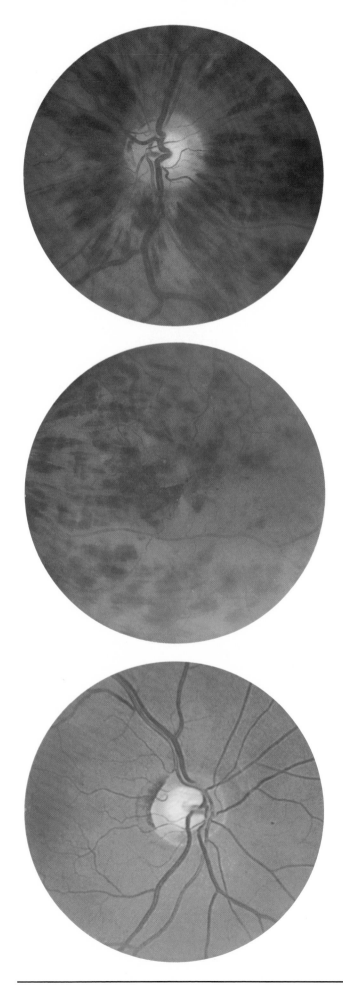

Central Retinal Vein Occlusion
(progression to proliferative retinopathy)

Overlying the temporal aspect of the left optic nerve are a few punctate hemorrhages; 360° around the nerve are multiple intraretinal blotch hemorrhages. The retinal veins appear to be slightly engorged.

In the posterior pole there are extensive intraretinal hemorrhages and thickening of the sensory retina compatible with retinal edema.

The right optic nerve and major branches of the retinal vasculature appear normal. There is a small intraretinal hemorrhage nasal to the optic nerve.

During the laminar phase of the angiogram, there is dilatation of the capillaries on the surface of the optic nerve. Blockage of the background choroidal fluorescence can be seen secondary to the intra-retinal hemorrhages.

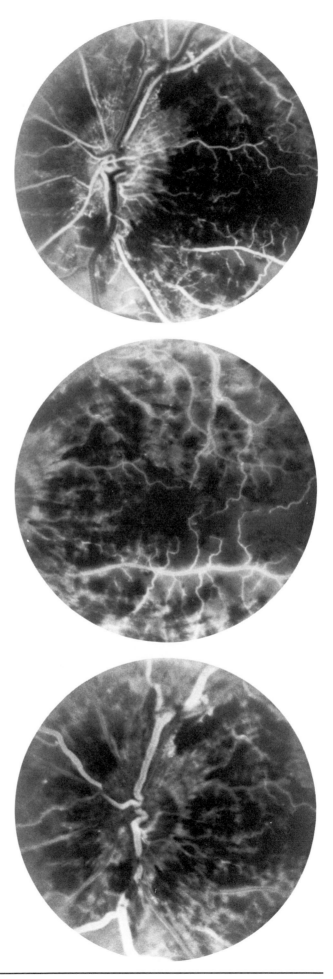

Later in the angiogram, there is further blockage of the background choroidal fluorescence by the intra-retinal hemorrhage. There appear to be areas of nonperfusion in the perifoveal region and temporal to the macula. There is some slight staining of the retinal venous walls with the fluorescein dye, indicating breakdown in the blood-retinal barrier.

The late angiogram shows subtle leakage of fluorescein from the dilated capillaries on the surface of the nerve and surrounding the nerve. The retinal veins appear to be engorged. The intraretinal hemorrhages surrounding the optic nerve and extending toward the macula continue to block the background fluorescence.

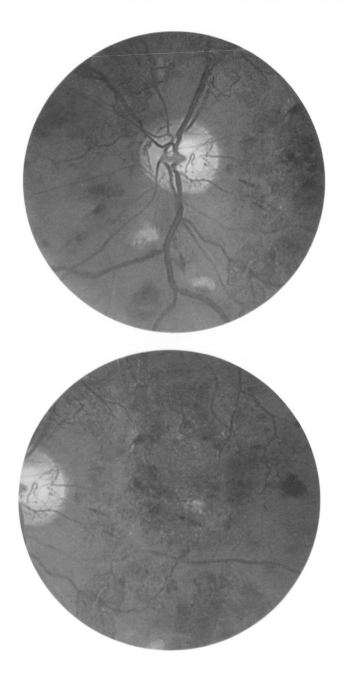

The left optic nerve shows definite evidence of neovascularization. Neovascular fronds can be seen superior temporal and inferior temporal to the optic nerve. Scattered around the optic nerve are intraretinal blotch hemorrhages and areas of soft exudate.

In the posterior pole of the left eye, multiple intraretinal dot and blotch hemorrhages can be seen. There is increased sheen off the internal limiting membrane in the macular region, giving this area a cellophane-like appearance.

AUTHOR'S NOTE

This patient shows progression from a central retinal vein occlusion to proliferative retinopathy with extensive neovascularization of the disc and elsewhere. It is obvious that the extensive amount of avascularity and nonperfusion in the posterior pole must be considered as the possible source for the development of the neovascularization. Disc neovascularization developed approximately 3 months after the onset of the patient's central retinal vein occlusion. This patient underwent extensive panretinal photocoagulation in the hope of reducing the risks of a severe vitreous hemorrhage in the future.

During the very early laminar phase of the fluorescein angiogram of the left eye, the fronds of neovascularization on the surface of the nerve and inferior temporal to the nerve can be seen. A large area of capillary dropout and nonperfusion is present throughout the posterior pole.

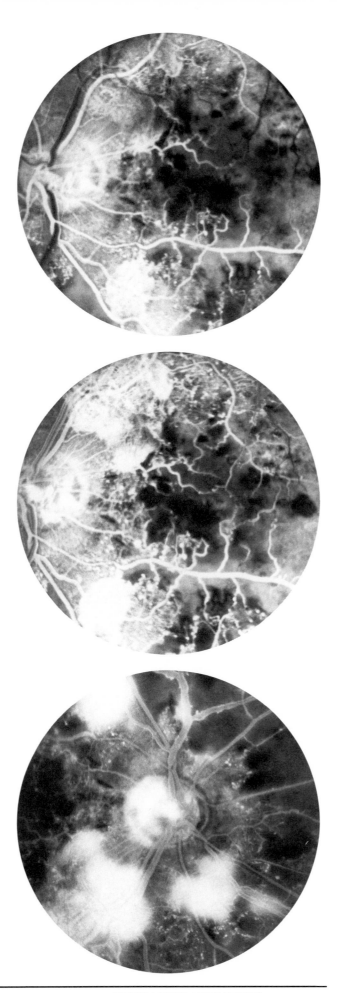

Later in the laminar phase of the angiogram, there is leakage of fluorescein into the vitreous from the neovascular fronds. The extensive areas of capillary dropout and nonperfusion throughout the posterior pole are evident. There is complete loss of the perifoveal capillary ring. A few scattered intraretinal hemorrhages continue to block the background fluorescence.

Very late in the angiogram, there is diffuse leakage of fluorescein from the disc neovascularization and the three fronds of neovascularization elsewhere, two inferior to the disc and one superior to the nerve. The branches of the superior temporal vein stain with fluorescein and show irregularity in their caliber.

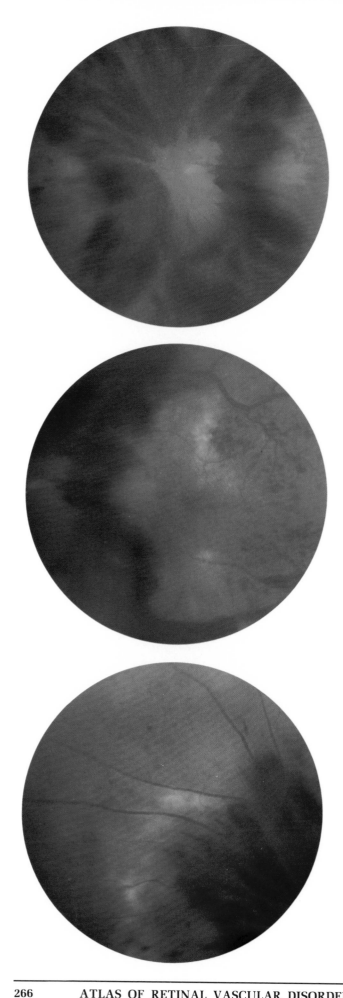

Central Retinal Vein Occlusion
(disc neovascularization)

Extensive intraretinal hemorrhage can be seen surrounding the left optic nerve secondary to a central retinal vein occlusion. Very fine disc neovascularization can be seen.

In the posterior pole of the left eye there is extensive intraretinal dot and blotch hemorrhage and hard exudate.

The intraretinal hemorrhage extends superior nasally. There are intraretinal dot and blotch hemorrhages 360° around the mid-periphery.

During the arterial phase of the fluorescein angiogram, the disc neovascularization fills with the fluorescein dye.

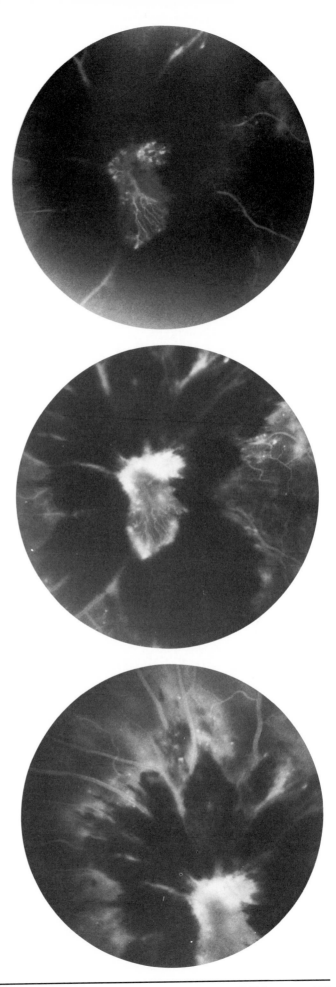

Later in the angiogram, there is leakage of fluorescein into the vitreous from disc neovascularization. The extensive intraretinal hemorrhage around the nerve blocks the background choroidal fluorescence.

Superior to the optic nerve there is further blockage of the background fluorescence by the intraretinal hemorrhage. The retinal veins stain with fluorescein dye, indicating a breakdown in the blood-retinal barrier.

AUTHOR'S NOTE
This patient developed disc neovascularization approximately 6 weeks after the onset of symptoms secondary to her central retinal vein occlusion.

Branch Retinal Vein Occlusion
(with neovascularization)

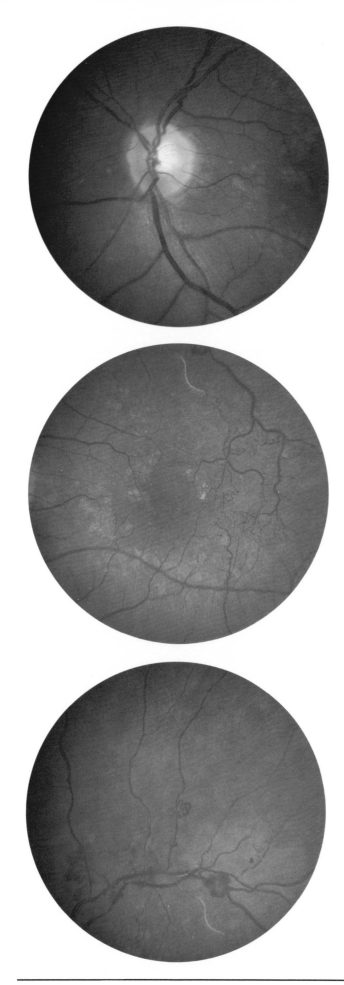

The left eye shows the location where the superior temporal artery crosses the superior temporal vein for the first time.

In the posterior pole, collaterals can be seen temporal to the macula across the horizontal raphe. Intraretinal microvascular abnormalities and microaneurysms are also visible. There is mottling of the retinal pigment epithelium.

Along the superior temporal arcade there are multiple fronds of neovascularization. The branches of the superior temporal vein are irregular. The superior temporal artery shows marked attenuation. One of the branches of the superior temporal artery appears to be completely sclerosed.

Fluorescein angiography of the left posterior pole shows the multiple collaterals being filled with the fluorescein dye. There is no significant leakage from these collaterals. The microaneurysms appear to be hyperfluorescent. Nasal to the fovea there are hyperfluorescent changes due to window defects from atrophy of the pigment epithelium. Above the macula and temporal to the macula are several areas of capillary nonperfusion.

Along the superior temporal arcade there is diffuse leakage of fluorescein from the multiple neovascular fronds. Areas of intraretinal microvascular abnormalities can also be seen.

The late angiogram shows diffuse leakage of fluorescein into the vitreous from the multiple small fronds of neovascularization secondary to the major superior temporal branch vein occlusion.

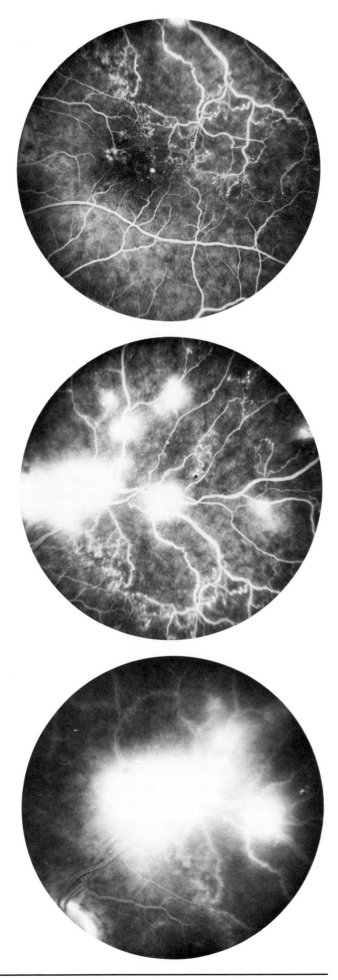

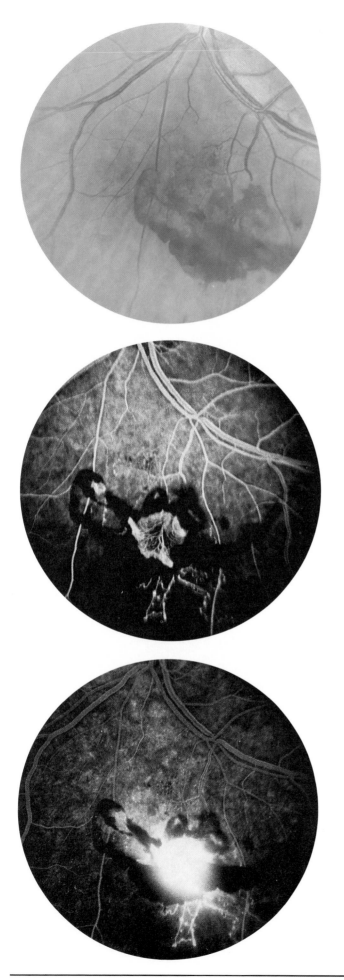

Branch Retinal Vein Occlusion
(with neovascularization and preretinal hemorrhage—pre- and post-treatment)

There is a preretinal hemorrhage in association with surface neovascularization below the inferior temporal arcade. The occlusion site is where the inferior temporal artery crosses one of the branches of the inferior temporal vein as it extends into the inferior temporal quadrant.

The fluorescein angiogram reveals a lacy frond of surface neovascularization. The preretinal hemorrhage around the frond blocks the background choroidal fluorescence. Peripheral to the neovascularization is an area of capillary dropout and nonperfusion.

The late angiogram shows leakage of fluorescein into the vitreous from the surface neovascularization secondary to the branch vein occlusion. The preretinal hemorrhage continues to block the background choroidal fluorescence.

Photocoagulation scars can be seen. There was focal treatment of the surface neovascularization and also photocoagulation treatment in the quadrant involved in the occlusion.

The fluorescein angiogram shows complete destruction of the surface neovascularization by argon laser photocoagulation.

The photocoagulation treatment extended into the area of capillary dropout and nonperfusion. There is no evidence of fluorescein leakage, indicating complete destruction of the surface neovascularization.

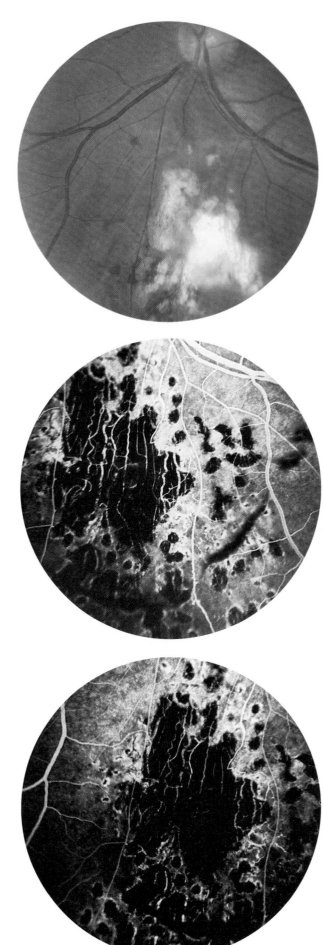

Branch Retinal Vein Occlusion
(with disc neovascularization)

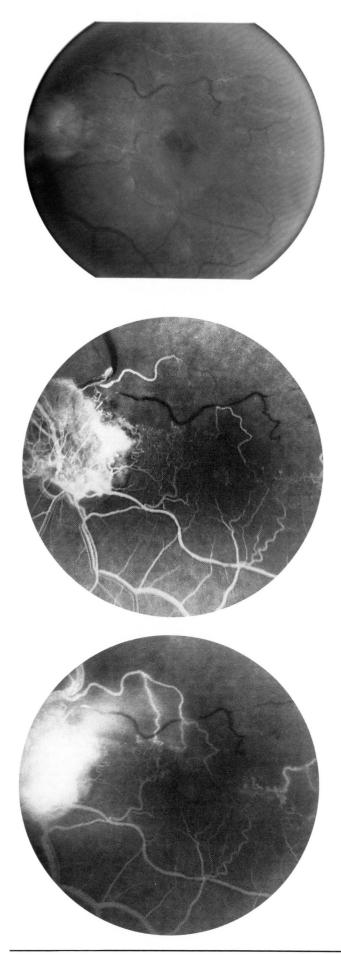

The optic nerve shows fairly extensive disc neovascularization. The retinal arteries show sclerotic changes. This is particularly evident in the superior branches of the central retinal artery. The superior temporal retinal vein shows a marked irregularity in its caliber. In the macular region, large cystic spaces can be seen. Collateralization temporal to the macula is also evident. The retinal vessels superior to the macula are extremely narrowed, and many of them appear to be occluded.

During the laminar phase of the angiogram there is hyperfluorescence of the neovascularization on the surface of the nerve. There is nonperfusion extending from the center of the macula into the superior temporal quadrant and peripherally. The branch retinal veins and artery are void of fluorescein. Collaterals can be seen extending across the horizontal raphe temporal to the macula. The perifoveal capillary net has been completely disrupted.

Later in the angiogram there is diffuse leakage of fluorescein from the disc neovascularization. Collaterals can be seen nasal to the macula. The branch retinal artery running above the macula still shows a lack of filling with the fluorescein dye.

Branch Retinal Vein Occlusion
(with neovascularization)

The right eye shows an old inferior temporal branch vein occlusion. Several of the branched vessels appear as white cords due to complete occlusion. Along the inferior temporal arcade there is a slightly elevated frond of neovascularization. Scattered areas of microaneurysms and intraretinal microvascular abnormalities can be seen superior to the neovascularization.

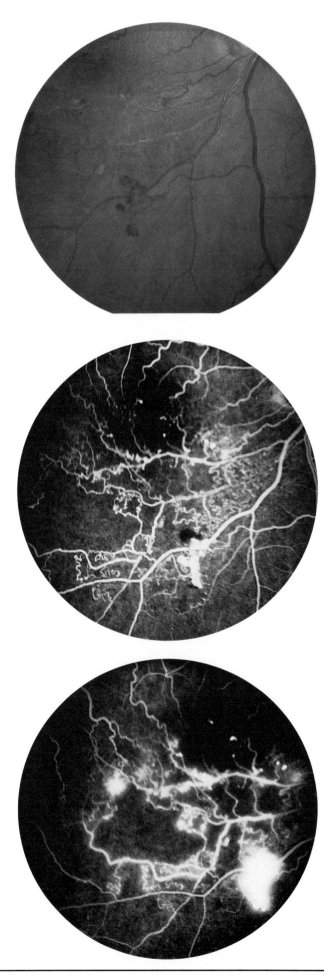

During the laminar phase of the angiogram there are multiple areas of collateralization along the inferior temporal arcades and inferior to the macula. The perifoveal capillary net appears to be completely disrupted. There are several large areas of capillary dropout and nonperfusion. Scattered areas of intraretinal microvascular abnormalities and microaneurysms can also be seen. Along the inferior temporal arcade there is an area of neovascularization.

The late angiogram shows diffuse leakage of fluorescein from the neovascular frond. There is some slight intraretinal leakage of fluorescein from the intraretinal microvascular abnormalities and microaneurysms. The larger collaterals temporal to the macula show no significant leakage. There is some staining of the walls of the larger caliber vessels, indicating a lack of endothelial integrity.

Branch Retinal Vein Occlusion
(with disc neovascularization and vitreous hemorrhage)

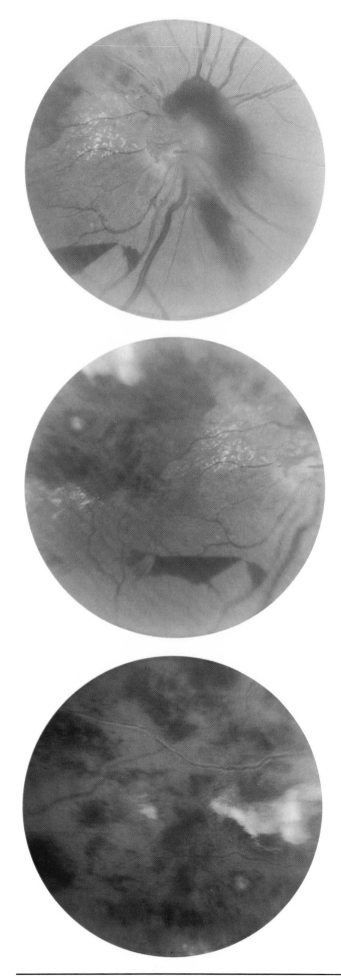

There is disc neovascularization in the right eye. Preretinal and vitreous hemorrhage surrounds the nerve.

In the posterior pole, there are scattered intraretinal blotch hemorrhages. The hemorrhage extends into the center of the macula. There is an area of pre-retinal hemorrhage inferior to the macula. Intra-retinal hard exudate can be seen in the papillomacular bundle.

Along the superior temporal arcade there is extensive blotch hemorrhage secondary to the major superior temporal branch vein occlusion. There are also areas of soft exudate.

During the laminar phase of the angiogram there is hyperfluorescence from the disc neovascularization. The hemorrhage superior to the nerve and inferior to the macula blocks the background choroidal fluorescence. There is also some blockage of the background fluorescence by the intraretinal blotch hemorrhage in the macular region.

Later in the angiogram there is diffuse leakage of fluorescein into the vitreous from the disc neovascularization. The preretinal hemorrhage continues to block the background choroidal fluorescence.

Along the superior temporal arcade there is extensive blockage of the background fluorescence by the extensive blotch hemorrhages. An area of nonperfusion can be seen which corresponds to the soft exudate seen clinically. The walls of the retinal veins stain with fluorescein dye, indicating a loss of endothelial junction integrity and a breakdown in the blood-retinal barrier.

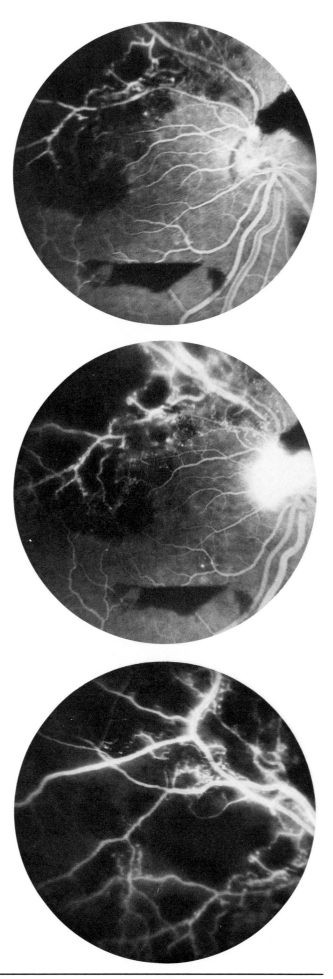

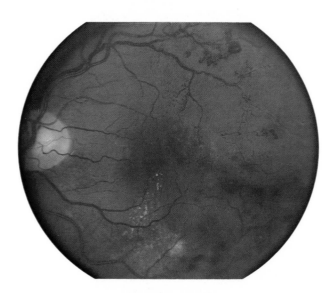

Double Branch Retinal Vein Occlusion (with neovascularization)

Along the inferior temporal arcade and extending into the center of the macula are scattered dot and blotch hemorrhages and deposition of hard exudate. There is some thickening of the sensory retina in the macular region compatible with macular edema. Along the superior temporal arcade surface neovascularization is evident.

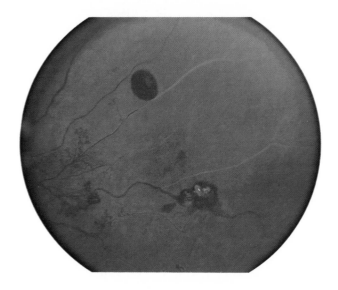

Beyond the neovascularization, extending into the superior temporal quadrant, are several occluded vessels. This area of the retina is ischemic. An area of intraretinal blotch hemorrhage can also be seen. These changes are secondary to a major superior temporal branch vein occlusion.

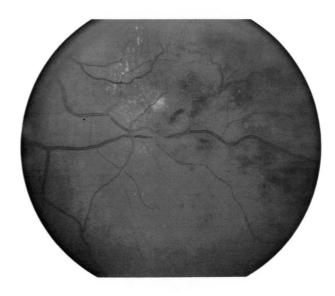

A more recent inferior temporal branch vein occlusion can be seen. The area of the occlusion, where the artery crosses the vein, is clearly evident. There is significant intraretinal dot and blotch hemorrhage with hard exudate along the inferior temporal vessels extending into the inferior temporal quadrant.

The fluorescein angiogram of the left eye shows dilatation of the capillary bed, microaneurysmal change, and intraretinal microvascular abnormalities above and below the horizontal raphe in the vicinity of the macula. There is a definite area of capillary nonperfusion and ischemia temporal to the macula. There is a delay of filling of the superior temporal branch vein distal to the occlusion site.

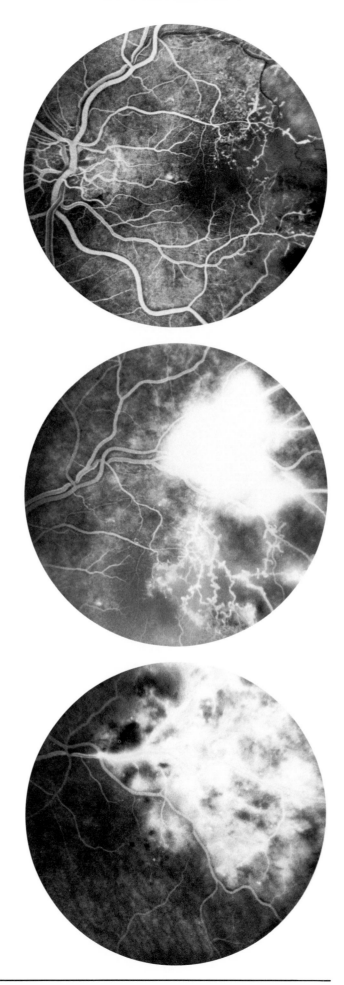

There is diffuse leakage of fluorescein into the vitreous from the surface neovascularization along the superior temporal arcade. The neovascularization is located at the junction between perfused and nonperfused retina.

Along the inferior temporal arcade there is intraretinal leakage of fluorescein from microaneurysms, the dilated capillary bed, intraretinal microvascular abnormalities, and the branch vein involved in the occlusion. There is also some staining of the retinal venous walls, indicating a loss of the endothelial cell tight junctions.

AUTHOR'S NOTE

After the initial superior temporal branch vein occlusion, this patient did not complain of any visual impairment. However, after the second occlusion occurred, involving the inferior temporal quadrant with edema extending into the macula, it became apparent to the patient that there was some visual problem with the left eye. Frequently, a major branch vein occlusion, which spares the macula, will not be noticed by the patient.

Photocoagulation Treatment of Branch Vein Occlusion

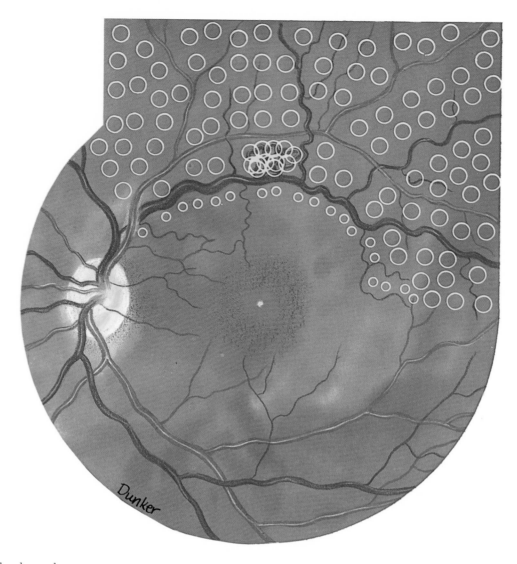

Two hundred- and 500-μ spot sizes are used to treat the quadrant involved in the major retinal branch vein occlusion. Focal overlapping photocoagulation scars are placed over any surface neovascularization.

In treating retinal branch vein occlusion, an attempt is made to treat all the areas of capillary dropout and nonperfusion seen on the angiogram in addition to focally treating the neovascularization.

One should not treat over intraretinal hemorrhage in order to avoid treating the nerve fiber layer and also to prevent increased retinal fibrosis, which can cause traction on the posterior pole. It does not appear necessary to completely fragment the neovascularization. In fact, in some cases, the neovascularization has purposely been avoided, with treatment only to the nonperfused areas, and there has been complete regression of the proliferative tissue.

Reader's Notes

Double Retinal Branch Vein Occlusion (with disc neovascularization, pre- and post-photocoagulation treatment)

There is evidence of disc neovascularization which extends inferior to the optic nerve.

Along the superior temporal arcade, the acute branch vein occlusion can be seen with extensive intraretinal dot and blotch hemorrhages which extend into the superior temporal quadrant and into the macula.

The old branch vein occlusion extends along the inferior temporal arcade where the vessels are completely occluded. There is still some residual intraretinal blotch hemorrhage.

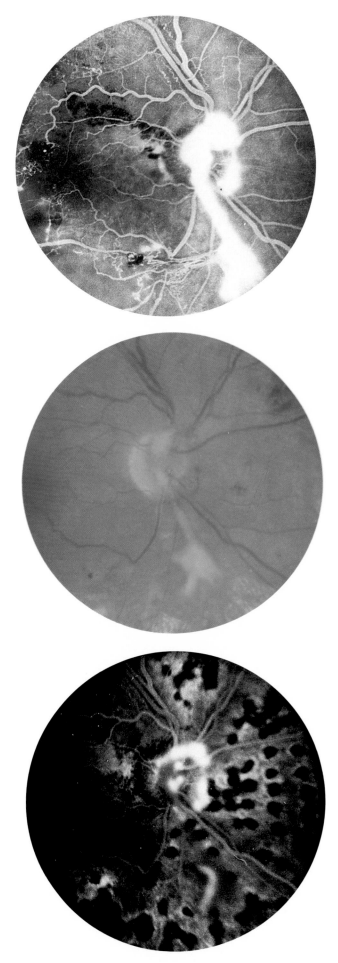

There is diffuse leakage of fluorescein into the vitreous from the elevated disc neovascularization. The double branch vein occlusion involving the superior temporal macular region and inferior temporal region can be seen.

After extensive photocoagulation treatment there is marked regression of the vascular component of the fibrovascular proliferation on the surface of the nerve and extending inferiorly.

Two months after photocoagulation treatment there has been nearly complete regression of the disc neovascularization.

AUTHOR'S NOTE

Branch vein occlusions with disc neovascularization respond very nicely to treatment of the involved quadrant or quadrants which have significant capillary dropout and nonperfusion. There is no need for focal treatment of the disc neovascularization.

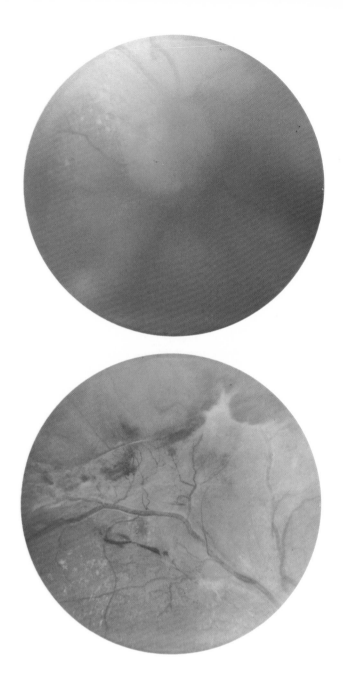

Branch Retinal Vein Occlusion
(with vitreous hemorrhage and tractional retinal elevation— pre- and post-treatment)

The posterior pole of the right eye is obscured due to the presence of vitreous hemorrhage. The optic nerve can be seen. There also appears to be some deposition of intraretinal hard exudate as seen through the diffuse hemorrhage.

Along the superior temporal arcade there is extensive fibrovascular proliferation with tractional elevation of the sensory retina. This proliferative change is secondary to a major superior temporal branch vein occlusion.

Fluorescein angiography shows the superior temporal major branch vein occlusion. The loose vitreous hemorrhage blocks some of the background choroidal fluorescence. Microaneurysms, intraretinal microvascular abnormalities, and capillary dilatation can be seen in the superior macular region.

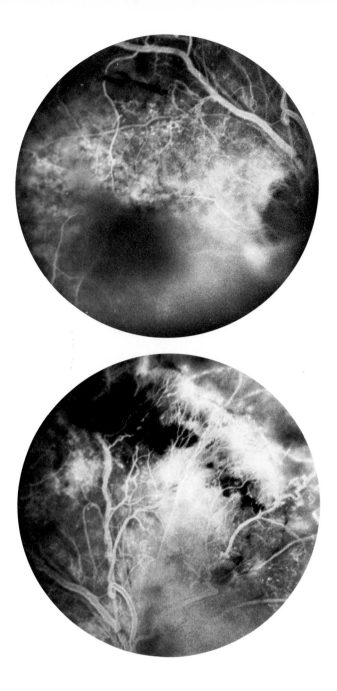

Extending into the superior quadrants there is extensive fibrovascular proliferation with diffuse leakage of fluorescein into the vitreous. The irregularity of the superior temporal vessel, secondary to the branch vein occlusion, can also be seen. The preretinal hemorrhage, in association with the proliferative tissue, blocks the background fluorescence.

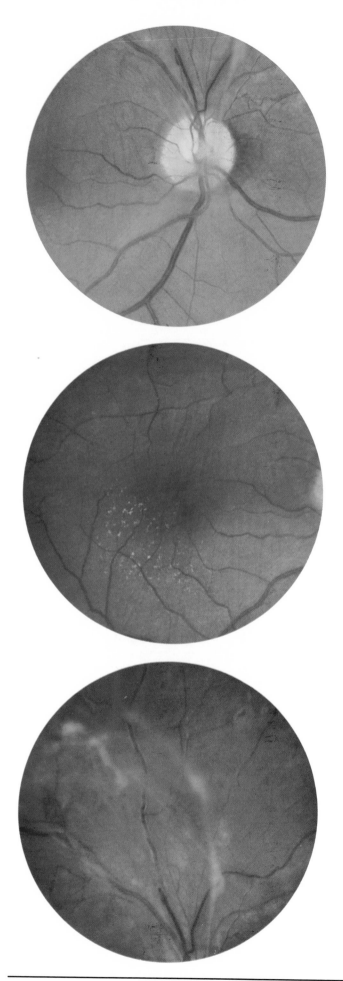

There has been complete clearing of the vitreous hemorrhage. An area of fibrous proliferation can be seen extending superiorly from the optic nerve. The superior temporal vessels appear irregular.

The macular region of the right eye shows deposition of fine intraretinal hard exudate. There are very fine vertical striae of the sensory retina secondary to the fibrotic tissue, causing some slight traction.

There has been a marked reduction in the density of the fibrous tissue and complete regression of the neovascular component. Argon laser photocoagulation scars can be seen beyond the fibrovascular proliferation.

Fluorescein angiography of the left posterior pole shows some fine intraretinal microvascular abnormalities, dilatation of the capillary bed, and microaneurysmal change. Collaterals along the superior temporal arcade can also be seen.

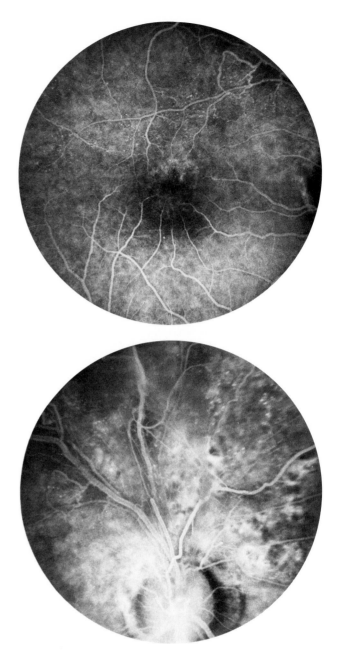

Later in the angiogram there is no evidence of significant leakage of fluorescein. There has been complete regression of the vascular component of the proliferative tissue. There is some hyperfluorescent change due to staining of the fibrous component.

AUTHOR'S NOTE

After bed rest there was some inferior settling of the vitreous hemorrhage. It was obvious that the patient had sustained a major branch vein occlusion with extensive fibrovascular proliferation and tractional changes on the sensory retina along the superior temporal arcade. Therefore, argon laser photocoagulation was applied to the quadrant involved in the occlusion without focal treatment to the elevated fibrovascular tissue. Approximately 8 weeks after treatment, there was almost complete regression of the proliferative tissue with clearing of the vitreous hemorrhage.

Proliferative Retinopathy
(secondary to long-standing retinal detachment)

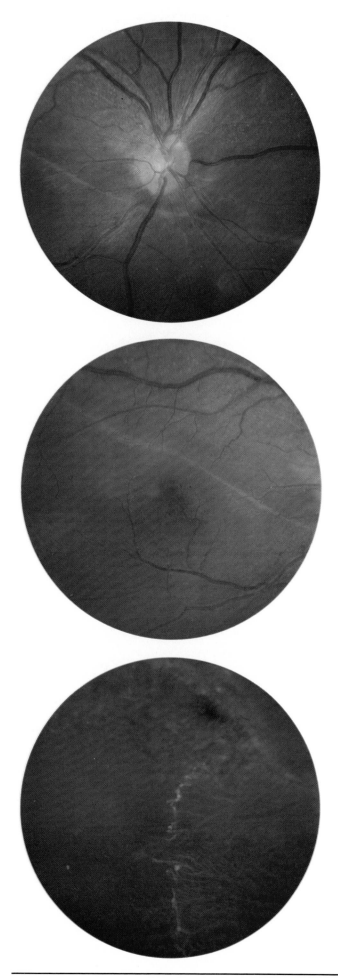

The optic nerve of the right eye eppears normal. An inferior retinal detachment with a demarcation line extending below the optic nerve and into the temporal and nasal quadrant can be seen.

In the posterior pole, the demarcation line extends superior to the fovea, and inferiorly there is a rhegmatogenous retinal detachment.

In the inferior temporal periphery, elevated neovascularization in association with the detached retina can be seen. Superior to the proliferative tissue is marked thinning of the retina with multiple retinal holes.

Along the inferior temporal arcade, there is hyper-fluorescence due to fluorescein leakage from the smaller caliber retinal vessels and also diffuse leakage from neovascular fronds peripherally.

Further out in the inferior temporal quadrant there is diffuse leakage of fluorescein into the vitreous from the fine neovascularization.

A large area of nonperfused retina can be seen. Small tufts of neovascularization as well as a larger neovascular frond superiorly leak fluorescein into the vitreous.

AUTHOR'S NOTE

This patient sustained trauma to the right eye and noted blurred vision for approximately 8 months, which was ignored. At the time of initial examination, there was a long-standing rhegmatogenous retinal detachment with peripheral proliferative tissue. A complete systemic work-up and careful ocular examination revealed no other cause for the proliferative retinopathy. It is assumed that the long-standing detachment resulted in a extensive amount of retinal nonperfusion, which, in turn, stimulated the development of neovascularization within the area of detachment.

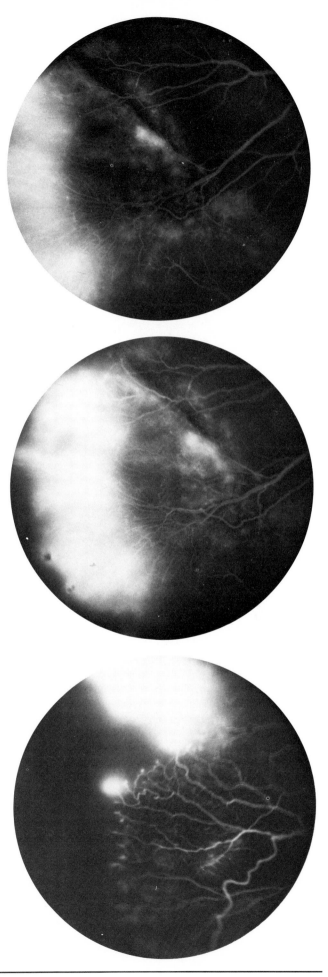

Eales' Sarcoid Disease

A. Sheathing of the veins
B. Areas of nonperfusion and neovascularization
C. Elevated fibrovascular tissue with slight traction on the peripheral retina

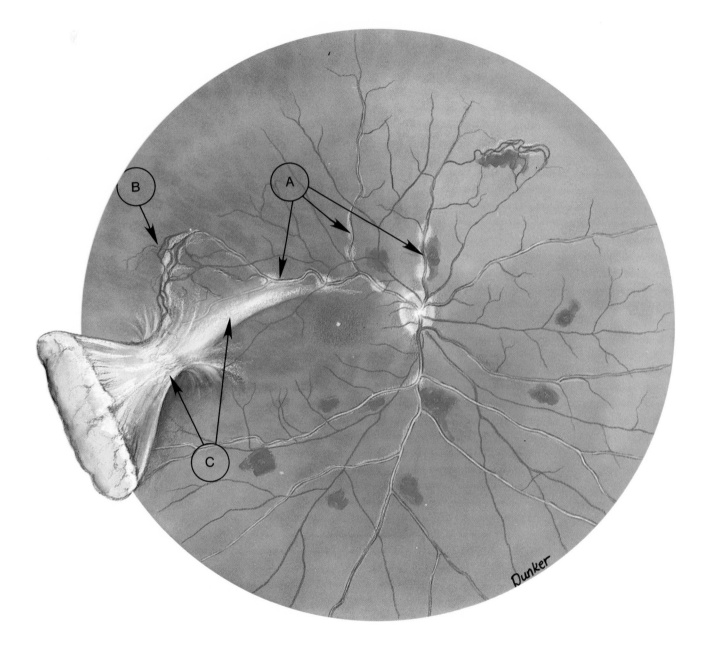

Eales' Disease (periphlebitis retinae with probable disc neovascularization)

The left optic nerve is hyperemic, and there is suspicion of very fine surface neovascularization. The retinal veins are slightly engorged. There is sheathing of the retinal vessels at the superior pole of the optic nerve.

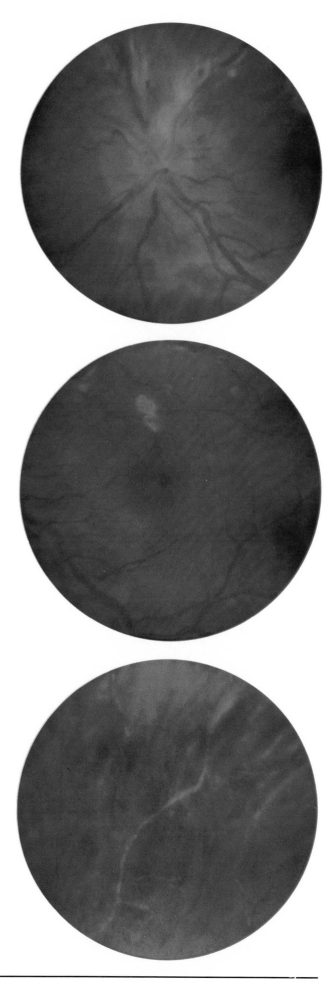

In the posterior pole, there is deposition of intra-retinal inflammatory material.

In the superior temporal mid-periphery, occlusion of the more peripheral branches can be seen. There are also numerous intraretinal blotch hemorrhages.

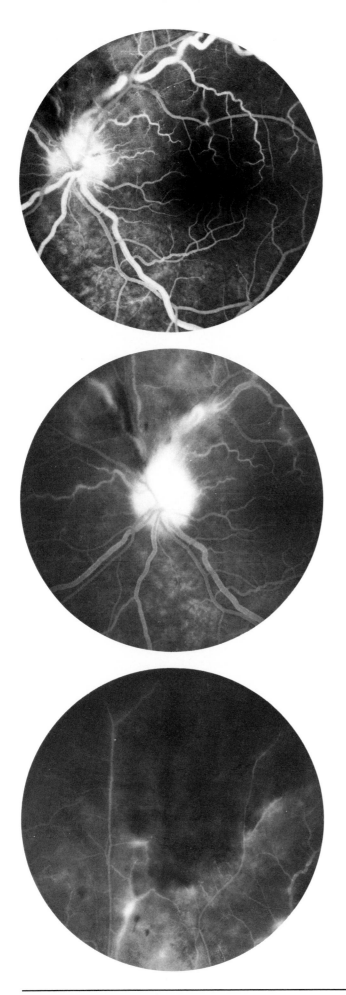

During the venous phase of the fluorescein angiogram there is increased hyperfluorescence on the surface of the optic nerve. The retinal veins appear to be slightly engorged.

Later in the angiogram there is leakage of fluorescein from both dilated capillaries on the surface of the nerve and probable fine disc neovascularization. There is staining of the superior temporal branch retinal vein secondary to a loss of endothelial cell junction integrity. The intraretinal hemorrhages superior to the optic nerve block the background choroidal fluorescence.

In the superior mid-periphery, there is a large, wedge-shaped area of nonperfusion secondary to a small caliber vascular occlusion. There is also some staining of the walls of the branch retinal veins.

AUTHOR'S NOTE

Clinically, it was difficult to determine whether this patient had definite disc neovascularization or whether there was merely leakage of fluorescein from dilated capillaries on the surface of the optic nerve associated with the hyperemia. However, the patient did have a small vitreous hemorrhage, and it was therefore assumed that there was, indeed, very fine disc neovascularization present. A complete medical workup was negative and therefore a diagnosis of Eales' disease was made primarily by exclusion.

Sarcoidosis (proliferative retinopathy with disc neovascularization—pre- and post-photocoagulation)

The optic nerve of the right eye is markedly hyperemic. On the surface of the nerve is fine neovascularization. The retinal arteries are narrowed and show irregularity in their caliber. There is also irregularity in the major branches of the central retinal vein. There is some deposition of intraretinal hard exudate in the vicinity of the macula.

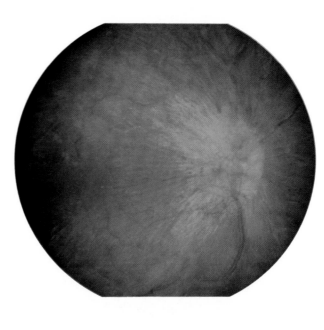

In the temporal mid-periphery of the right eye, there is evidence of vascular occlusion with perfused and nonperfused retina. The larger caliber occluded vessels appear as white cords.

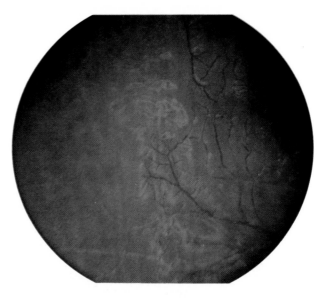

After panretinal photocoagulation there is less hyperemia of the optic nerve. There is also marked regression of the disc neovascularization with residual fibrous tissue. Fine striae throughout the posterior pole at the level of the internal limiting membrane are apparent.

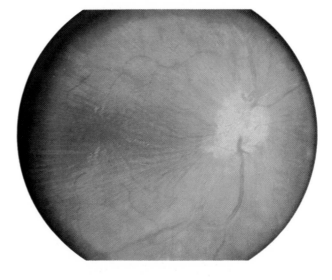

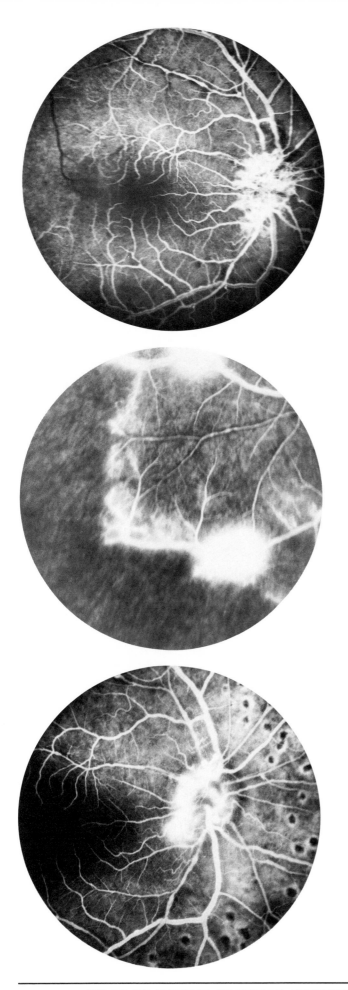

Fluorescein angiography of the right eye shows the disc neovascularization. There is marked irregularity in the fluorescein flow within the arterial and venous branches. Temporal to the macula there is a branched vessel which shows no evidence of fluorescein, indicating a marked delay in filling or occlusion.

In the temporal mid-periphery there is a sharp border between vascular and avascular retina. Fronds of neovascularization diffusely leak fluorescein into the vitreous. This neovascularization is along a branched vein at the junction between the vascular and avascular retina.

After panretinal photocoagulation, there is subtle leakage of fluorescein into the vitreous from the residual regressed proliferative tissue on the optic nerve. The panretinal photocoagulation scars nasal to the optic nerve stain with the fluorescein dye in a typical fashion.

AUTHOR'S NOTE

This patient was found to have systemic sarcoidosis. In addition to the systemic findings, there was evidence of proliferative retinopathy secondary to significant retinal ischemia from vascular occlusive disease. Panretinal photocoagulation with specific treatment being applied to the avascular areas resulted in marked regression of the disc neovascularization.

Sarcoidosis (proliferative retinopathy with disc neovascularization—pre- and post-corticosteroid treatment)

The left optic nerve is hyperemic with fine neovascularization on its surface. There are a few scattered intraretinal hemorrhages just temporal to the optic nerve. Branches of the central retinal artery appear to be narrowed. In the macular region are several small intraretinal hard exudates. Superior to the macula is a small area of preretinal hemorrhage.

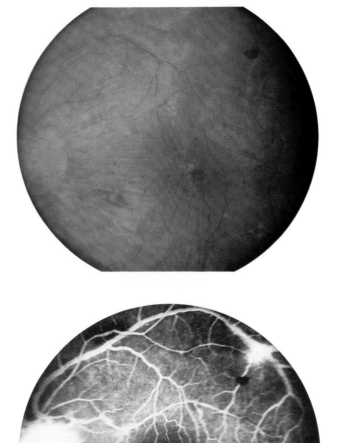

Fluorescein angiography of the left eye shows hyperfluorescence from the disc neovascularization. The intraretinal hemorrhage just temporal to the optic nerve blocks the background choroidal fluorescence. In the macular region there are several hyperfluorescent changes secondary to mottling of the retinal pigment epithelium. Superior temporal to the macula there is blockage of the background fluorescence by the small preretinal hemorrhage overlying one of the retinal vessels. Just superior to this hemorrhage is a small frond of neovascularization extending from the superior temporal branch vein and leaking fluorescein into the vitreous.

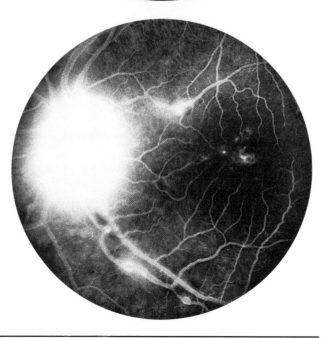

The late angiogram of the left eye shows diffuse leakage into the vitreous of the fluorescein dye from the disc neovascularization. There is irregularity and "sausaging" change of the inferior temporal artery and vein. These vessels stain slightly with the fluorescein dye, indicating a breakdown in the blood-retinal barrier. The window defects in the macular region persist late in the angiogram.

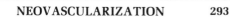

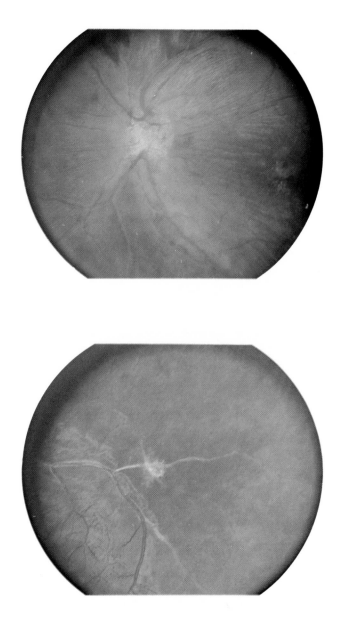

After systemic corticosteroid treatment, there is marked regression of the disc neovascularization with less hyperemia of the optic nerve. There is an intraretinal blotch hemorrhage superior to the nerve. The retinal arteries are irregular in their caliber. There is still some residual hard exudate in the macular region, as well as mottling of the retinal pigment epithelium. Fine striae can be seen in the posterior pole.

In the temporal periphery of the left eye, the occluded branches of the retinal vasculature and sheathing of the retinal vein are obvious. The avascular retina has lost its normal sheen as compared to the vascularized sensory retina.

AUTHOR'S NOTE

This is the fellow eye of the previous case presented with sarcoidosis and disc neovascularization responding to photocoagulation treatment. This eye showed a similar response to systemic corticosteroids. This patient demonstrates a prominent retinal sheen where the retina is vascularized because of her young age. A possible hypothesis to explain the proliferative changes in this patient with sarcoidosis is the development of large areas of nonperfused retina secondary to vascular occlusion from inflammation. The possibility that inflammation may play a role in causing neovascularization must be considered in this case. Apparently the systemic corticosteroids reduced the amount of intraocular inflammation, and there was also a dramatic regression of the proliferative retinopathy.

Choroidal Retinal Vitreal Neovascularization

Neovascularization extends from the choroid, through a break in Bruch's membrane, through the sensory retina and into the vitreous.

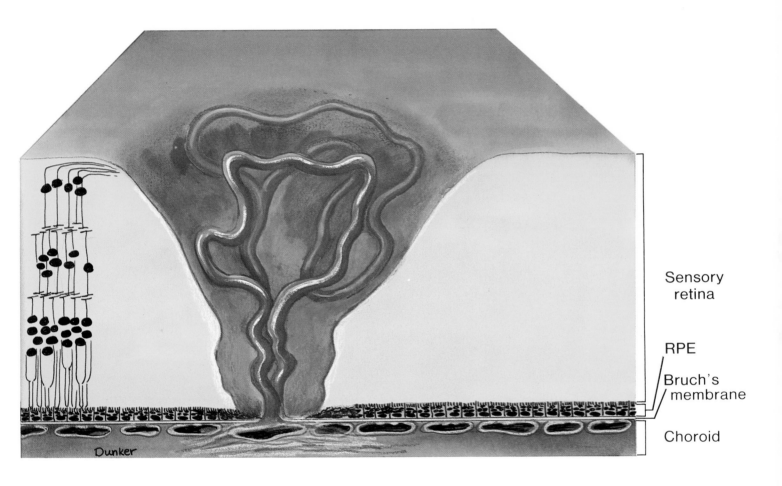

Sensory retina

RPE

Bruch's membrane

Choroid

Dunker

Choroidal Retinal Vitreal Neovascularization (post-photocoagulation)

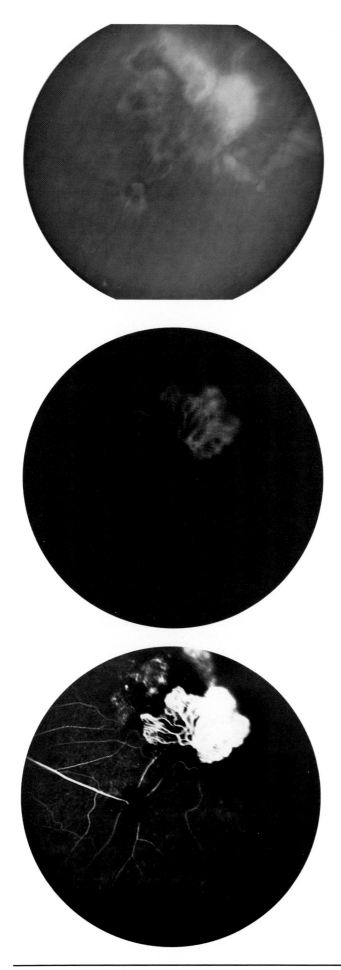

The color photograph of the temporal periphery of the left eye reveals photocoagulation scars and evidence of some preretinal hemorrhage. Fresh photocoagulation scars can also be seen extending into the avascular retina. Adjacent to the larger fresh photocoagulation scar is a lacy network of neovascularization.

Several seconds after the injection of the fluorescein dye, there is filling of the neovascular frond in the far temporal periphery prior to any evidence of fluorescein within the retinal vasculature.

Later in the angiogram, as the peripheral retinal vasculature is filled with fluorescein dye, there is evidence of further filling of the neovascularization with leakage of fluorescein into the vitreous. The junction between perfused and nonperfused retina is clearly visible. Several of the photocoagulation scars block the background fluorescence due to the hyperpigmentation involved in the scar formation.

AUTHOR'S NOTE

This patient had proliferative sickle cell retinopathy with "sea fans" in the temporal periphery of the left eye. After photocoagulation treatment, choroidal vitreal neovascularization developed, most likely secondary to breaks in Bruch's membrane from the photocoagulation. The initial fluorescein demonstrates that the neovascularization does originate at the level of the choroid with choroidal filling in view of the fact that there is no fluorescein dye which has reached the retinal vasculature.

I am grateful to Timothy P. Flood, M.D. and Lee Jampol, M.D. for permitting me to publish this case.

Choroidal Retinal Vitreal Neovascularization
(post-photocoagulation)

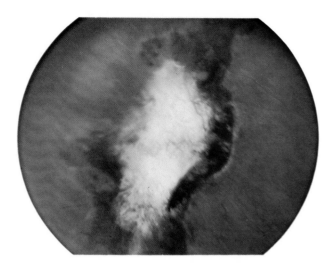

The color photograph of the far periphery of the left eye shows a heavily pigmented and fibrotic photocoagulation scar at the junction between normal vascularized sensory retina and avascular retina. Within the photocoagulation scar, very fine neovascular twigs can be seen.

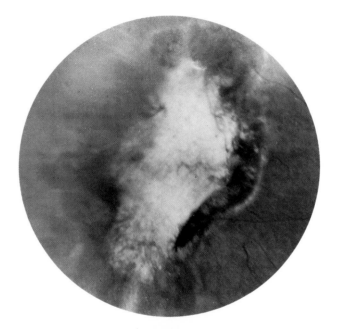

The red-free photograph shows the heavy fibrotic photocoagulation scar and fine neovascularization within the scar.

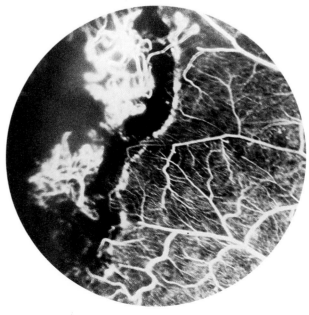

The fluorescein angiogram shows the filling of the peripheral retinal vasculature and capillary bed. The pigmented portion of the photocoagulation scar blocks the background choroidal fluorescence. Fronds of neovascularization can be seen as hyperfluorescent and originating within the substance of the photocoagulation scar without any continuity to the normal retinal vasculature.

AUTHOR'S NOTE

This is a case of a patient with sickle cell proliferative retinopathy who was treated with heavy photocoagulation. The finding of neovascularization emanating from within the scar without any origin from the retinal vasculature is highly indicative of this being choroidal vitreal neovascularization. This type of complication has also been seen in patients with diabetic proliferative retinopathy treated with panretinal photocoagulation.

I am grateful to Lee Jampol, M.D. for permitting me to publish this case.

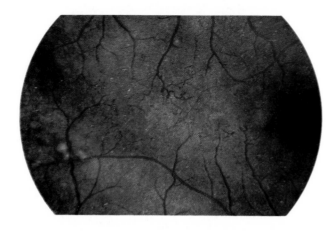

Talc Retinopathy (capillary occlusion; larger caliber vascular occlusion with proliferative retinopathy)

The left posterior pole shows multiple punctate glistening talc emboli along the small end arterioles. There are multiple irregular intraretinal microvascular abnormalities. Deep to the sensory retina there appeared to be round, yellowish lesions at the level of the choroid.

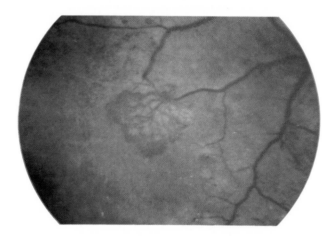

In the periphery there is evidence of neovascularization in the form of a "sea fan." There are several intraretinal dot hemorrhages and microaneurysms.

Fluorescein angiography of the left posterior pole shows a loss of integrity of the perifoveal capillaries due to capillary dropout from talc embolization. There are also some fine intraretinal microvascular abnormalities as well as dilatation of the capillary bed. There is some staining of the emboli as well as microaneurysmal changes.

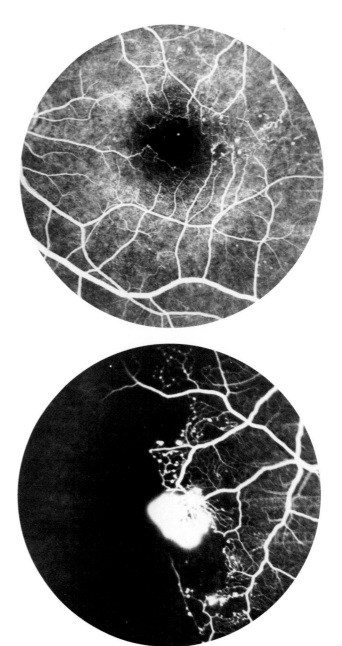

Fluorescein angiography of the peripheral retina reveals a sharp zone of perfused and nonperfused retina. At this junction there is leakage of fluorescein into the vitreous from the neovascular frond. The capillaries are dilated and show microaneurysm-like dots.

AUTHOR'S NOTE

Special thanks to David Tse, M.D., and Richard R. Ober, M.D., for permitting the publication of this case of talc retinopathy. It demonstrates the spectrum of involvement which can take place in those patients with talc retinopathy. The changes can cause occlusion at the capillary level and, in more severe cases, peripheral vascular occlusion with neovascularization, similar to that seen in sickle cell retinopathy and in proliferative retinopathy secondary to intraocular inflammation.

Bibliography

Aaberg TM: Pars plana vitrectomy for diabetic traction retinal detachment. *Ophthalmology* 88:639–642, 1981.

Aiello LM, Beetham W, Baladimos MC, et al: Ruby laser photocoagulation in treatment of proliferative diabetic retinopathy. In Goldberg M, Fine S: *Symposium on Treatment of Diabetic Retinopathy*. Washington DC, United States Department of Health, Education and Welfare, Publication no. 1890, 1968.

Aiello LM, Briones JC: Ruby laser photocoagulation of proliferative diabetic retinopathy: Five-year follow-up. *Int Ophthalmol Clin* 16:4, 1976.

Aiello LM, Rand LI, Briones JC, et al: Diabetic retinopathy in Joslin Clinic patients with adult-onset diabetes. *Ophthalmology* 88:619–623, 1981.

Algvere P: Fluorescein studies of retinal vasculitis in sarcoidosis: Report of a case. *Acta Ophthalmol* 48:1129–1139, 1970.

Alm A, Bill A: Ocular and optic nerve blood flow at normal and increased intraocular pressures in monkeys: A study with radioactively labelled microspheres including flow determinations in brain and some other tissues. *Exp Eye Res* 15:15–29, 1973.

Arribas NP, Johnston GP, Okun E: Photocoagulation in diabetic retinopathy. *Int Ophthalmol Clin* 16:59–77, 1976.

Asdourian GK, Goldberg MF, Busse BJ: Peripheral retinal neovascularization in sarcoidosis. *Arch Ophthalmol* 93:787–791, 1975.

Asdourian GK, Nagpal KC, Busse B, et al: Macular and perimacular vascular remodeling in sickling haemoglobinopathies. *Br J Ophthalmol* 60:431–453, 1976.

Ashton N: Pathological basis of retrolental fibroplasia. *Br J Ophthalmol* 38:385–396, 1954.

Ashton N: Oxygen and the growth and development of retinal vessels. *Am J Ophthalmol* 62:412–435,1966.

Ashton N: The mode of development of the retinal vessels in man. In Cant JS: *The William MacKenzie Centenary Symposium on the Ocular Circulation in Health and Disease*. London, Henry Kimpton, 1969, pp 7–25.

Ashton N: The pathogenesis of retrolental fibroplasia. *Ophthalmology* 86:1695–1699, 1979.

Ashton N, Ward B, Serpell G: Role of oxygen in the genesis of retrolental fibroplasia: A preliminary report. *Br J Ophthalmol* 37:513, 1953.

Auerbach R, Kubai L, Sidky Y: Angiogenesis induction by tumors, embryonic tissues, and lymphocytes. *Cancer Res* 36:3435–3440, 1976.

Bamford CR, Ganley JP, Sibley WA, et al: Uveitis, perivenous sheathing and multiple sclerosis. *Neurology* 28:119–124, 1978.

Baum JL, Martola EL: Corneal edema and corneal vascularization. *Am J Ophthalmol* 65:881–884, 1968.

Bedrossian RH, Carmichael P, Ritter J: Retinopathy of prematurity (retrolental fibroplasia) and oxygen. Clinical study: Further observations on disease. *Am J Ophthalmol* 37:78, 1965.

Beetham WP, Aiello LM, Balomides MC, et al: Ruby laser photocoagulation of early diabetic neovascular retinopathy. *Arch Ophthalmol* 83:261–272, 1970.

BenEzra D: Neovasculogenic ability of prostaglandins, growth factors, and synthetic chemoattractants *Am J Ophthalmol* 86:455–461, 1978.

BenEzra D: Neovasculogenesis: Triggering factors and possible mechanisms. *Surv Ophthalmol* 24:167–176, 1979.

Brem S, Preis I, Langer R, et al: Inhibition of neovascularization by an extract derived from vitreous. *Am J Ophthalmol* 84:323–328, 1977.

British Multicentric Photocoagulation Trial: Proliferative diabetic retinopathy: Treatment with xenon arc photocoagulation. *Br Med J* 1:739–741, 1977.

Brockhurst RJ, Schepens CL, Okamura ID: Uveitis. II. Peripheral uveitis: Clinical description, complications, and differential diagnosis. *Am J Ophthalmol* 49:1257–1266, 1960.

Brucker AJ: Disk and peripheral retinal neovascularization sec-ondary to talc and cornstarch emboli. *Am J Ophthalmol* 88:864–867, 1979.

Busse BJ, Mittelman D: Use of the astigmatism correction device on the Zeiss fundus camera for peripheral retinal photography. *Int Ophthalmol Clin* 16:63–74, 1976.

Campbell K: Intensive oxygen therapy as a possible cause of retrolental fibroplasia: A clinical approach. *Med J Aust* 2:48–50, 1951.

Canny CLB, Oliver GL: Fluorescein angiographic findings in familial exudative vitreoretinopathy. *Arch Ophthalmol* 94:1114–1120, 1976.

Chandra SR, Bresnick GH, David MD, et al: Choroidovitreal neovascular ingrowth after photocoagulation for proliferative diabetic retinopathy. *Arch Ophthalmol* 98:1593–1609, 1980.

Condon PI, Serjeant GR: Ocular findings in elderly cases of homozygous sickle-cell disease in Jamaica. *Br J Ophthalmol* 60:361–364, 1976.

Condon PI, Serjeant GR: Ocular findings in sickle cell haemoglobin O Arab disease. *Br J Ophthalmol* 63:839–841, 1979.

Criswick VG, Schepens CL: Familial exudative vitreoretinopathy. *Am J Ophthalmol* 68:578–594, 1969.

Cross VM, Evans PJ: Prevention of retrolental fibroplasia. *Arch Ophthalmol* 48:83, 1952.

Cunha-Vaz JG, Faria de Abreu JR: Physiopathogenesis of retinal new vessel formation. *Exp Ophthalmol* 3:21–34, 1977.

Davis MD: Natural course of diabetic retinopathy. In R Kimura and WM Caygill: *Vascular Complications of Diabetes Mellitus*. St Louis, CV Mosby, 1967, p 139.

Davis MD: Definition, classification, and course of diabetic retinopathy. In Lynn JR, Snyder WB, Vaiser A: *Diabetic Retinopathy*. New York, Grune and Stratton, 1974, pp 7–33.

Deckert T, Simonsen SVE, Paulson JE: Prognosis of proliferative retinopathy in juvenile diabetics. *Diabetes* 16:728, 1967.

Diabetic Retinopathy Study Research Group: Preliminary report on effects of photocoagulation therapy. *Am J Ophthalmol* 81:383–396, 1976.

Diabetic Retinopathy Study Research Group: Photocoagulation treatment of proliferative diabetic retinopathy: The second report of diabetic retinopathy study findings. *Ophthalmology* 85:82–106, 1978.

Diabetic Retinopathy Study Research Group: A modification of the Airlie House classification of diabetic retinopathy. *Invest Ophthalmol* 21:210–226, 1981.

Diabetic Retinopathy Study Research Group: Baseline monograph: DRS report #6. *Invest Ophthalmol* 21:149–195, 1981.

Diabetic Retinopathy Study Research Group: Photocoagulation treatment of proliferative diabetic retinopathy: Clinical application of Diabetic Retinopathy Study: (DRS) Findings, DRS report #8. *Ophthalmology* 88:583–600, 1981.

Diabetic Retinopathy Study Research Group: Photocoagulation treatment of proliferative diabetic retinopathy: Relationship of adverse treatment effects to retinopathy severity: DRS report #5. *Dev Ophthalmol* 2:248–261, 1981.

Diabetic Retinopathy Study Research Group: Photocoagulation treatment of proliferative diabetic retinopathy: A short report of long range results: DRS report #4. In *Proceedings, 10th Congress International Diabetes Foundation*. Amsterdam, Excerpta Medica, 1980, pp 789–794.

Dizon-Moore RV, Jampol LM, Goldberg MF: Chorioretinal and choriovitreal neovascularization: Their presence after photocoagulation of proliferative sickle cell retinopathy. *Arch Ophthalmol* 99:842, 1981.

Dobree JH: Proliferative diabetic retinopathy: Evolution of the retinal lesions. *Br J Ophthalmol* 48:637–649, 1964.

Doxanas MT, Kelley JS, Prout TE: Sarcoidosis with neovascularization of the optic nerve head. *Am J Ophthalmol* 90:347–351, 1980.

Eales H: Cases of retinal hemorrhage associated with epistaxis and constipation. *Birmingham Med Rev* 9:262–273, 1980.

Elliot AJ: 30-year observation of patients with Eales' disease. *Am*

J Ophthalmol 80:404–408, 1975.

Engerman RL, Meyer RK: Development of retinal vasculature in rats. *Am J Ophthalmol* 60:628–641, 1965.

Felton SM, Brown GC, Felberg NT, et al: Vitreous inhibition of tumor neovascularization. *Arch Ophthalmol* 97:1710–1713, 1979.

Fletcher MC, Brandon S: Myopia of prematurity. *Am J Ophthalmol* 40:474–481, 1955.

Flynn JT, Cassady J, Zesking J, et al: Fluorescein angiography in retrolental fibroplasia: Experience from 1969–1977. *Ophthalmology* 86:1700–1723, 1979.

Flynn J, O'Grady GE, Herrera J, et al: Retrolental fibroplasia: I. Clinical observations. *Arch Ophthalmol* 95:217–223, 1977.

Folkman J: Tumor angiogenesis factor. *Cancer Res* 34:2109–2113, 1974.

Folkman J: The vascularization of tumors. *Sci Am* 234:58–73, 1976.

Folkman J: Tumor angiogenesis. In Becker FF: *Cancer: A Comprehensive Treatise*, vol 3: *Biology of Tumors: Cellular Biology and Growth*. New York, Plenum Press, 1976, pp 355–388

Folkman J, Merler E, Abernathy C, et al: Isolation of a tumor factor responsible for angiogenesis. *J Exp Med* 133:275–288, 1971.

Foos RY: Acute retrolental fibroplasia. *Albrecht von Graefes Arch Klin Ophthalmol* 195:87–100, 1975.

Frank RN, Cronin MA: Posterior pole neovascularization in a patient with hemoglobin SC disease. *Am J Ophthalmol* 88:680–682, 1979.

Frank RN, Ryan SJ, Jr: Peripheral retinal neovascularization with chronic myelogenous leukemia. *Arch Ophthalmol* 87:585–589, 1972.

Franks EP, Kasprzyk JS, McMeel JW: Computer-enhanced studies of diabetic retinopathy. 1. *Ophthalmology* 88:624–629, 1981.

Freidenwald JS, Owens WC, Owens EU: Retrolental fibroplasia in premature infants. III. The pathology of the disease. *Trans Am Ophthalmol Soc* 49:207–234, 1951.

Fromer CH, Klintoworth GK: An evaluation of the role of leukocytes in the pathogenesis of experimentally induced corneal neovascularization. I. Comparison of experimental models of corneal vascularization. *Am J Pathol* 79:537–554, 1975.

Galinos SO, Asdourian GK, Woolf MB, et al: Choroidovitreal neovascularization after argon laser photocoagulation. *Arch Ophthalmol* 93:524–530, 1975.

Garoon I, Epstein G, Segall M, et al: Vascular tufts in retrolental fibroplasia. *Ophthalmology* 87:1128–1132, 1980.

Gitter KA, Rothschild H, Wlatman DD, et al: Dominantly inherited peripheral retinal neovascularization. *Arch Ophthalmol* 96:1601–1605, 1978.

Goldbaum MH, Fletcher RC, Jampol LM, et al: Cryotherapy of proliferative sickle retinopathy. II. Triple freeze-thaw circle. *Br J Ophthalmol* 63:97–101, 1979.

Goldbaum MH, Galinos SO, Apple D, et al: Acute choroidal ischemia as a complication of photocoagulation. *Arch Ophthalmol* 94:1025–1035, 1976.

Goldbaum MH, Goldberg MF, Nagpal K, et al: Proliferative sickle retinopathy. In L'Esperance FA: *Current Diagnosis and Management of Chorioretinal Diseases*. St Louis, CV Mosby, 1977, pp 132–145.

Goldberg MF: Classification and pathogenesis of proliferative sickle retinopathy. *Am J Ophthalmol* 71:649–665, 1971.

Goldberg MF: Natural history of untreated proliferative sickle retinopathy. *Arch Ophthalmol* 85:428–437, 1971.

Goldberg MF, Tso MOM: Rubeosis iridis and glaucoma associated with sickle cell retinopathy: A light and electron microscopic study. *Ophthalmology* 85:1028–1041, 1978.

Gordon HH, Lubchenco L, Hix I: Observations on the etiology of retrolental fibroplasia. *Bull Johns Hopkins Hosp* 94:34, 1954.

Gospodarowicz D, Bialecki H, Thakral TK: The angiogenic activity of the fibroblast and epidermal growth factor. *Exp Eye Res* 28:501–514, 1979.

Gospodarowicz D, Moran JS; Growth factors in mammalian cell culture. *Annu Rev Biochem* 45:531–558, 1979.

Gospodarowicz D, Rudland P, Lindstrom J, et al: Fibroblast growth factor. Its localization, purification, mode of action, and physiologic significance. *Adv Metab Disord* 8:301–335, 1975.

Grunwald E, Yassur Y, Ben-Sira I: Buckling procedures for retinal detachment caused by retrolental fibroplasia in premature babies. *Br J Ophthalmol* 64:98–101, 1980.

Gyllensten LJ, Hellstrom BE: Retrolental fibroplasia: Animal experiments—the effect of intermittently administered oxygen on the postnatal development of the eyes of fullterm mice: A preliminary report. *Acta Paediatr* 41:577, 1952.

Gyllensten LJ, Hellstrom BE: Experimental approach to the pathogenesis of retrolental fibroplasia: Changes of eye induced by exposure of newborn mice to concentrated oxygen. *Acta Paediatr* 43:131, 1954.

Hedges TR: The aortic arch syndromes. *Arch Ophthalmol* 71:28–34, 1964.

Henkind P: Ocular neovascularization. *Am J Ophthalmol* 85:287–301, 1978.

Henkind P, DeOliveira LF: Development of retinal vessels in the rat. *Invest Ophthalmol* 6:520–530, 1967.

Hercules BL, Gayes II, Lucas SB, et al: Peripheral retinal ablation in the treatment of proliferative diabetic retinopathy: A three-year interim report of a randomised, controlled study using the argon laser. *Br J Ophthalmol* 61:555–563, 1977.

Imre G: Studies on the mechanism of retinal neovascularization. *Br J Ophthalmol* 48:75–82, 1964.

James LS, Lanman JT: Committee on fetus and newborn. American Academy of Pediatrics. History of oxygen therapy and retrolental fibroplasia. *Pediatrics* (Suppl 2) 57:591–642, 1976.

James LS, Lanman JT: History of oxygen therapy and retrolental fibroplasia. *Pediatrics* (Suppl) 57:591–642, 1976.

James WA, L'Esperance FH: Treatment of diabetic optic nerve neovascularization by extensive retinal photocoagulation. *Am J Ophthalmol* 78:939–947, 1974

Jampol LM: Ocular manifestations of selected systemic disease. In Peyman G, Sanders DR, Goldberg MD: *Principles and Practice of Ophthalmology*. Philadelphia, WB Sanders, 1980.

Jampol LM, Goldbaum MH: Peripheral proliferative retinopathies. *Surv Ophthalmol* 25:1–14, 1980.

Jampol LM, Goldberg MF: Retinal breaks after photocoagulation of proliferative sickle cell retinopathy. *Arch Ophthalmol* 98:676–679, 1980.

Jampol LM, Goldberg MF, Busse B: Peripheral retinal microaneurysms in chronic leukemia. *Am J Ophthalmol* 80:242–248, 1975.

Jampol LM, Isenberg SJ, Goldberg MF: Occlusive retinal arteriolitis with neovascularization. *Am J Ophthalmol* 81:583–589, 1976.

Johnson DR, Swan KC: Retrolental fibroplasia—a continuing problem. *Trans Pac Coast Otoophthalmol Soc Annu Meet* 47:129–133, 1966.

Johnson L, Schaffer DB, Boggs TR: The premature infant, vitamin E deficiency and retrolental fibroplasia. *Am J Clin Nutr* 27:1158–1173, 1974.

Kalina RE: Examination of the premature infant. *Ophthalmology* 86:1690–1694, 1979.

Kalina RE, Kelly WA: Proliferative retinopathy after treatment of carotid-cavernous fistulas. *Arch Ophthalmol* 96:2058–2060, 1978.

Kelley JS, Randall HG: Peripheral retinal neovascularization in rheumatic fever. *Arch Ophthalmol* 97:81–83, 1979.

Kelly PJ, Weiter JJ: Resolution of optic disk neovascularization associated with intraocular inflammation. *Am J Ophthalmol* 90:545–548, 1980.

King MJ: Retrolental fibroplasia. A clinical study of two hundred and thirty-eight cases. *Arch Ophthalmol* 43:694–711, 1950.

Kingham JD: Acute retrolental fibroplasia. *Arch Ophthalmol* 95:39–47, 1977.

Kinsey VE: Retrolental fibroplasia: Cooperative study of retrolental fibroplasia and the use of oxygen. *Arch Ophthalmol* 56:481–543, 1956.

Kinsey VE, Arnold HJ, Kalina RE, et al: PaO2 levels and retrolental fibroplasia: A report of the cooperative study. *Pediatrics* 60:655–668,1977.

Kinsey VE, Hemphill, FM: Etiology of retrolental fibroplasia and preliminary report of co-operative study of retrolental fibroplasia. *Trans Am Acad Ophthalmol* 59:OP-15, 1955.

Kresca L, Goldberg MF, Jampol LM: Talc emboli and retinal neovascularization in a drug abuser. *Am J Ophthalmol* 87:334–339, 1979.

Krill AE, Archer FRCS, Newell FW, et al: Photocoagulation in diabetic retinopathy. *Am J Ophthalmol* 72:299–321, 1971.

Lee CB, Woolf MB, Galinos SO, et al: Cryotherapy of proliferative sickle cell retinopathy. I. Single freeze-thaw cycle. *Ann Ophthalmol* 7:1299–1308, 1975.

L'Esperance FH: Argon laser photocoagulation in diabetic lesions. In Lynn JR, Snyder WB, Vaiser A: *Diabetic Retinopathy*. New York, Grune and Stratton, 1974, pp 145–169.

L'Esperance FH: Focal photocoagulation of retinovitreal neovascularization. *Int Ophthalmol Clin* 16:79–103, 1976.

Letocha CE, Shields JA, Goldberg RE: Retinal changes in sarcoidosis. *Can J Ophthalmol* 10:184–192, 1975.

Little HL: Retinal neovascularization in diabetes mellitus and the role of fluorescein angiography in argon laser photocoagulation. In Lynn JR, Snyder WB, Vaiser A: *Diabetic Retinopathy*. New York, Grune and Stratton, 1974, pp 133–144.

Little HL: Argon laser photocoagulation of proliferative diabetic retinopathy. *Int Ophthalmol Clin* 16:79–103, 1976.

Little HL: Alterations in blood elements in the pathogenesis of diabetic retinopathy. *Ophthalmology* 88:647–654, 1981.

Little HL, Rosenthal AR, Dellaporta A, et al: The effect of panretinal photocoagulation on rubeosis iridis. *Am J Ophthalmol* 81:804–809,1976.

Little HL, Zweng HC, Jack RL, et al: Techniques of argon laser photocoagulation of diabetic disc new vessels. *Am J Ophthalmol* 82:675–683, 1976.

Machemer R, Blankenship G: Vitrectomy for proliferative diabetic retinopathy associated with vitreous hemorrhage. *Ophthalmology* 88:643–646, 1981.

Madigan JC, Jr, Gragoudas ES, Schwartz PL, et al: Peripheral retinal neovascularization in sarcoidosis and sickle cell anemia. *Am J Ophthalmol* 83:387–391, 1977.

McCormick AQ: Retinopathy of prematurity. *Curr Probl Pediatr* 7:3–28, 1977.

McMeel JW, Franks EP: Computer-enhanced studies of diabetic retinopathy. I. *Ophthalmology* 88:630–634, 1981.

McPherson A, Hittner HM: Scleral buckling in 2½ to 11 month-old premature infants with retinal detachment associated with acute retrolental fibroplasia. *Ophthalmology* 86:819–835,1979.

Michaelson IC: The mode of development of the vascular system of the retina with some observations on its significance for certain retinal diseases. *Trans Ophthalmol Soc UK* 68:137–180, 1948.

Morse PH: Retinal venous sheathing and neovascularization in disseminated sclerosis. *Ann Ophthalmol* 7:949–952, 1975.

Morse PH, McCready JL: Peripheral retinal neovascularization in chronic myelocytic leukemia. *Am J Ophthalmol* 72:975–978,1971.

Moschandreou M, Galinos S, Valenzuela R, et al: Retinopathy in hemoglobin C trait (AC hemoglobinopathy). *Am J Ophthalmol* 77:465–471, 1974.

Mousel DK, Hoyt CS: Cryotherapy for retinopathy of prematurity. *Ophthalmology* 87:1121–1127,1980.

Muraoka K, Kobayashi Y, Kitagawa M: Involvement of the mid-peripheral fundus in diabetic retinopathy. *Jpn J Clin Ophthalmol* 33:425–439, 1979.

Nagpal KC, Asdourian GK, Patrianakos D, et al: Proliferative retinopathy in sickle cell trait. *Arch Intern Med* 37:325–328, 1977.

Nagpal KC, Goldberg MF, Rabb MF: Ocular manifestations of

sickle hemoglobinopathies. *Surv Ophthalmol* 29:391–411, 1977.

Nagpal KC, Patrianakos D, Asdourian GK, et al: Spontaneous regression (autoinfarction) of proliferative sickle cell retinopathy. *Am J Ophthalmol* 80:885–892, 1975.

Neupert JR, Brubaker RF, Kearns TP, et al: Rapid resolution of venous stasis retinopathy after carotid endarterectomy. *Am J Ophthalmol* 81:600–602, 1976.

Noth JM, Vygantas C, Cunha-Vaz JGF: Vitreous fluorophotometry evaluation of xenon photocoagulation. *Invest Ophthalmol* 17:1206–1209, 1978.

Ober RR, Michels RG: Optic disk neovascularization in hemoglobin SC disease. *Am J Ophthalmol* 85:711–714, 1978.

Okun E: The effectiveness of photocoagulation in the therapy of proliferative diabetic retinopathy (PDR): A controlled study in 50 patients. *Trans Am Acad Ophthalmol Otolaryngol* 72:253–258, 1968.

Okun E: Selection of cases for photocoagulation by xenon or argon. In Lynn JR, Synder WB, Vaiser A: *Diabetic Retinopathy*. New York, Grune and Stratton, 1974, pp 127–132.

Orth DH, Patz A: Retinal branch vein occlusion. *Surv Ophthalmol* 22:357–376, 1978.

Ostler RH: Pulseless disease (Takayasu's disease). *Am J Ophthalmol* 43:583–589, 1957.

Owens WC: Clinical course: Symposium: Retrolental fibroplasia (retinopathy of prematurity). *Am J Ophthalmol* 40:159–162, 1955.

Owens WC, Owens EU: Retrolental fibroplasia in premature infants. *Am J Ophthalmol* 32:1–21, 1949.

Owens WC, Owens EU: Retrolental fibroplasia in premature infants: Studies on prophylaxis of disease: Use of alphatocopheral acetate. *Am J Ophthalmol* 32:1631–1637, 1949.

Palmberg P, Smith M, Waltman S, et al: The natural history of retinopathy in insulin-dependent juvenile-onset diabetes. *Ophthalmology* 88:613–617, 1981.

Palmer AE: Optimal timing of examination for acute retrolental fibroplasia. *Ophthalmology* 88:662–666, 1981.

Pascual RS, Gee LBL, Finch SC: Usefulness of serum lysozyme in diagnosis and evaluation of sarcoidosis. *N Engl J Med* 289:1074–1076, 1973.

Patz A: Retrolental fibroplasia. *Surv Ophthalmol* 14:1–29, 1969.

Patz A: Photocoagulation of diabetic disc neovascularization. In Lynn JR, Synder WB, Vaiser A: *Diabetic Retinopathy*. New York, Grune and Stratton, 1974, pp 241–249

Patz A, Berkow J: Visual prognosis in advanced diabetic retinopathy. In Goldberg M, Fine S: *Symposium on Treatment of Diabetic Retinopathy*. Washington DC, United States Department of Health, Education and Welfare, Publication No. 1890, 1968, pp 87–91.

Patz A, Berkow JW: Visual and systemic prognosis in diabetic retinopathy. *Trans Am Acad Ophthalmol Otolaryngol* 72:253–257, 1968.

Patz A, Eastham A, Higgenbotham DH, et al: Oxygen studies in retrolental fibroplasia: Production of the microscopic changes of retrolental fibroplasia in experimental animals. *Am J Ophthalmol* 36:1511, 1953.

Patz A, Hoeck LE, de la Cruz E: Studies on the effect of high oxygen administration in retrolental fibroplasia: Nursery observations. *Am J Ophthalmol* 35:1248, 1952.

Payne JW, Patz A: Current status of retrolental fibroplasia, the retinopathy of prematurity. *Ann Clin Res* 11:205–221, 1979.

Pender PM, Benson WE, Compton H, et al: The effects of panretinal photocoagulation on dark adaptation in diabetics with proliferative retinopathy. *Ophthalmology* 88:634–638, 1981.

Peyman GA, Bok D: Peroxidase diffusion in the normal and laser-coagulated primate retina. *Invest Ophthalmol* 11:35–45, 1972.

Phelps DL, Rosenbaum AL: The role of tocopherol in oxygen-induced retinopathy: Kitten model. *Pediatrics* 59 (Suppl): 998–1005, 1977.

Phelps DL, and Rosenbaum AL: Observations of vitamin E in experimental oxygen-induced retinopathy. *Ophthalmology* 86:1741–1748, 1979.

Preston FE, Sokol RJ, Lilleyman JS, et al: Cellular hyperviscosity as a cause of neurologic symptoms in leukemia. Br Med J 1:476–478,1978.

Raichand M, Goldberg MF, Nagpal KC, et al: Evolution of neovascularization in sickle cell retinopathy. Arch Ophthalmol 95:1543–1552, 1977.

Raymond LA, Spaulding AG, Vitter RW: Peripheral retinal neovascularization in sarcoidosis with α-thalassemia. Ann Ophthalmol 10:745–748, 1978.

Reese AB, Blodi F: Retrolental fibroplasia: 5th Francis I. Proctor lecture. Am J Ophthalmol 34:1–24, 1951.

Schaffer DB, Johnson L, Quinn GE, et al: A classification of retrolental fibroplasia to evaluate vitamin E therapy. Ophthalmology 86:1749–1760, 1979.

Schatz H, Drake M: Self-injected retinal emboli. Ophthalmology 86:468–483, 1979.

Schoefl GI: Studies on inflammation. III. Growing capillaries: Their structure and permeability. Virchows Arch (Pathol Anat) 337:97–141, 1963

Schulman J, Jampol LE, Schwartz H: Peripheral proliferative retinopathy without oxygen therapy in a full-term infant. Am J Ophthalmol 90:509–514, 1980.

Shabo AL, Maxwell DS: Experimental immunogenic proliferative retinopathy in monkeys. Am J Ophthalmol 83:471–480, 1977.

Shakib M, de Oliveira LF, Henkind P: Development of retinal vessels. II. Earliest stages of vessel formation. Invest Ophthalmol 7:689–700,1968.

Shimizu K, Kobayashi Y, Muraoka K: Midperipheral fundus involvement in diabetic retinopathy. Ophthalmology 88:601–602, 1981.

Shorb SR, Irvine AR, Kimura SJ, et al: Optic disk neovascularization associated with chronic uveitis. Am J Ophthalmol 82:175–178,1976.

Spencer R, McMeel W, Franks EP: Visual outcome in moderate and severe proliferative diabetic retinopathy. Arch Ophthalmol 99:1551–1554, 1981.

Spitznas M, Meyer-Schwickerath G, Stephan B: The clinical picture of Eales' disease. Albrecht von Graefes Arch Klin Exp Ophthalmol 194:73–85, 1975.

Spitznas M, Meyer-Schwickerath G, Stephan B: Treatment of Eales' disease with photocoagulation. Albrecht von Graefes Arch Klin Exp Ophthalmol 194:193–198, 1975.

Studdy P, Bird R, James DG, et al: Serum angiotensin-converting enzyme (SACE) in sarcoidosis and other granulomatous disorders. Lancet 2:1331–1334, 1978.

Szewczyk TS: Retrolental fibroplasia: Etiology and prophylaxis: A preliminary report. Am J Ophthalmol 34:1648–1650, 1951.

Szewczyk TS: Retrolental fibroplasia: Etiology and prophylaxis. Am J Ophthalmol 35:301–310, 1952.

Taniguchi Y: Ultrastructure of newly formed blood vessels in diabetic retinopathy. Jpn J Ophthalmol 20:19–31, 1976.

Tasman W: Late complications of retrolental fibroplasia. Ophthalmology 86:1724–1740, 1979.

Taylor E, Dobree JH: Proliferative diabetic retinopathy: Site and size of initial lesions. Br J Ophthalmol 54:11, 1970.

Terry TL: Extreme prematurity and fibroblastic overgrowth of persistent vascular sheath behind each crystalline lens: I. Preliminary report. Am J Ophthalmol 25:203–204, 1942.

Tolentino FI, Lapus JV, Novalis G, et al: Fluorescein angiography of degenerative lesions of the peripheral fundus and rhegmatogenous retinal detachment. Int Ophthalmol Clin 16:13–29, 1976.

Toussaint D, Kuwabara T, Cogan DG: Retinal vascular pattern. II. Human retinal vessels studied in three dimensions. Arch Ophthalmol 65:575, 1961.

Tse DT, Ober RR: Talc retinopathy. Am J Ophthalmol 90:624–640, 1980.

Valone JA, McMeel W, Franks EP: Unilateral proliferative diabetic retinopathy. I. Initial Findings. Arch Ophthalmol 99:1357–1366, 1981.

Versari R: Morfologia dei vasi sanguigni arteriosi dell'occhio dell' unomo et di altri mammiferi. Ric Labor Anat Norm (Rome) 5:181, 1900.

Versari R: La morfogenesi dei vasi sanguigni della retina umana. Ric Labor Anat Norm (Rome) 10:25, 1904.

Watzke RC, Stevens TS, Carney RG, Jr: Retinal vascular changes of incontinentia pigmenti. Arch Ophthalmol 94:743–746, 1976.

Wessing A, Meyer-Schwickerath G: Results of photocoagulation in diabetic retinopathy. In Goldberg MF, Fine SL: Symposium on Treatment of Diabetic Retinopathy. Washington DC, United States Department of Health, Education and Welfare, Publication No. 1890, 1968, pp 569–592.

Wise GN: Retinal neovascularization. Trans Am Ophthalmol Soc UK 54:729, 1956.

Wise GN: Factors influencing retinal new vessel formation. Am J Ophthalmol 52:637–650, 1961.

Worthen DM, Fenton BM, Rosen P, et al: Morphometry of diabetic conjunctival blood vessels. Ophthalmology 88:655–657, 1981.

Yassur Y, Pickle LW, Fine SL, et al: Optic disc neovascularization in diabetic retinopathy. I. A system for grading proliferation at the optic nerve head in patients with proliferative diabetic retinopathy. Br J Ophthalmol 64:69–76, 1980.

Yassur Y, Pickle LW, Fine SL, et al: Optic disc neovascularization in diabetic retinopathy. II. Natural history and results of photocoagulation treatment. Br J Ophthalmol 64:77–86,1980.

Zweng HC: Selection of cases of diabetic retinopathy for treatment by argon laser slit lamp photocoagulation. In Lynn JR, Snyder WB, Vaiser A: Diabetic Retinopathy. New York, Grune and Stratton, 1974, pp 109–125.

Zweng HC, Little HL, Peabody RR: Further observations on argon laser photocoagulation of diabetic retinopathy. Trans Am Acad Ophthalmol Otolaryngol 76:990, 1972.

Zweng HC, Little HL, Vassiliadis A: Argon laser photocoagulation. St Louis, CV Mosby, 1977, pp 180–217.

CHAPTER 5

Telangiectasis

Differential Diagnosis

A. LEBER'S MILIARY ANEURYSMS
B. COATS' DISEASE

Retinal telangiectasis is a term that can be used to encompass the complete spectrum of minimal retinal vascular changes as in Leber's miliary aneurysms or massive retinal vascular abnormalities as seen in Coats' disease.

Coats' disease is usually unilateral, and 80% of those affected are young males. Frequently, there is a white pupillary reflex due to organized hard exudate or a fibrous disciform scar at the macular region associated with peripheral retinal vascular abnormalities.

Leber's miliary aneurysms also may show lipid deposition in the retina, cystoid macular edema, and retinal hemorrhage.

For peripheral telangiectatic changes, xenon arc or argon laser photocoagulation treatment can be effective in reducing the intraretinal edema and hard exudate in the posterior pole. Frequently, more than one treatment is necessary. Because Leber's miliary aneurysms are frequently in the paramacular region, argon laser photocoagulation with a slit lamp delivery system can be used in the hopes of reducing the amount of hard exudate and intraretinal hemorrhage when it is present. The differential diagnosis in a patient who has telangiectatic vessels in the macular region is as follows: (1) macular branch vein occlusion, (2) sickle cell maculopathy, (3) diabetic retinopathy, (4) radiation retinopathy, (5) familial retinal capillary telangiectasis, and (6) bilateral familial idiopathic obliterative parafoveal retinal angiopathy.

Retinal Telangiectasis
(juxtafoveal)

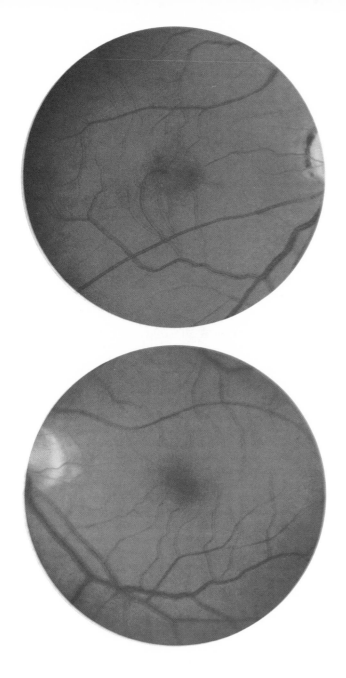

In the macular region of the right eye there is some slight thickening of the sensory retina. Several punctate intraretinal hard exudates can be seen. In addition, very fine telangiectatic changes are present.

The macular region of the left eye is entirely normal.

During the late laminar phase of the fluorescein angiogram, the telangiectatic changes around the perifoveal capillaries and, more predominantly, temporal to the retinal avascular zone can be seen.

The late angiogram shows diffuse intraretinal accumulation of fluorescein dye, indicating macular edema.

The left posterior pole is entirely normal.

AUTHOR'S NOTE

This patient was diagnosed as having juxtafoveal retinal telangiectasis. A complete medical work-up was negative. There was no evidence of intraocular inflammation in either eye, and the peripheral retinal examination was entirely normal. The macular edema in the right eye is secondary to a breakdown of the endothelial cell tight junctions within the telangiectatic small caliber vessels.

Retinal telangiectasis with macular edema is frequently diagnosed by exclusion after all other causes for possible macular edema and microaneurysmal formation or capillary dilatation have been eliminated.

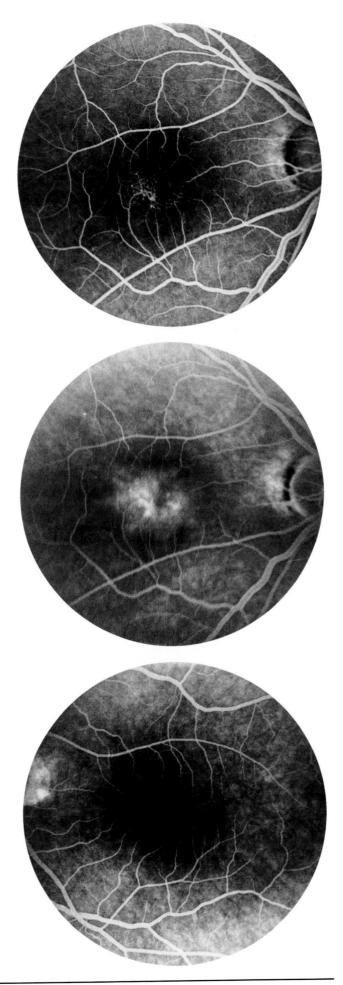

Retinal Telangiectasis
(juxtafoveal—bilateral)

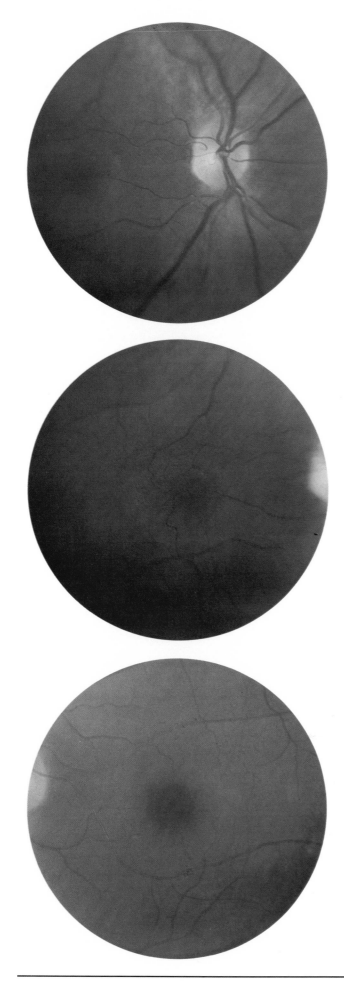

The optic nerve of this right aphakic eye appears normal.

In the macular region, there is some thickening of the sensory retina.

The posterior pole of the left phakic eye reveals some slight thickening of the retina just temporal to the center of the macula, i.e. fovea. The retinal arteries show some sclerotic changes.

Fluorescein angiography of the right eye shows fine telangiectatic changes at the temporal aspect of the retinal avascular zone. The remainder of the perifoveal capillaries appear normal.

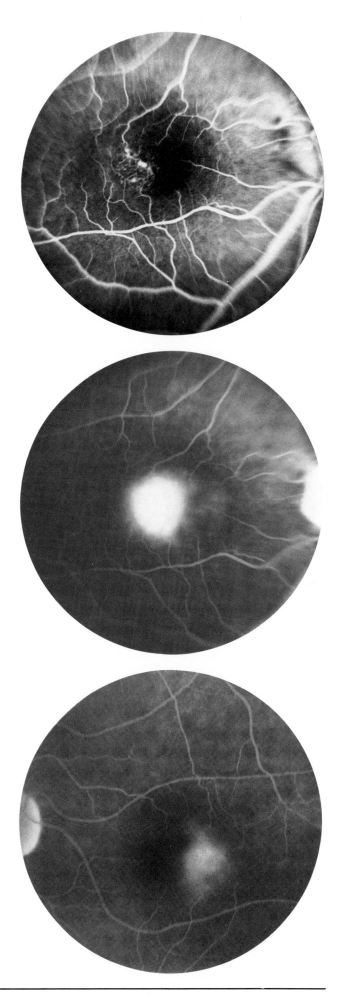

The late angiogram shows diffuse leakage of fluorescein intraretinally with significant hyperfluorescence, indicating macular edema.

Late frames of the left eye show intraretinal leakage of fluorescein involving the temporal macula, indicating macular edema.

AUTHOR'S NOTE

This interesting patient presented initially with macular edema in the right eye on clinical examination. Because the patient was aphakic, a preliminary diagnosis of aphakic cystoid macular edema, or Irvine-Gass syndrome, was made. However, fluorescein angiography of both eyes revealed bilateral macular edema. A diagnosis of retinal telangiectasis was made due to the bilaterality and the distribution of the telangiectatic vessels, primarily at the temporal aspect of the fovea. Complete medical work-up was negative, and there was no other cause for the bilateral cystoid edema. Vision in the right eye is 20/200, and vision in the left eye is 20/40.

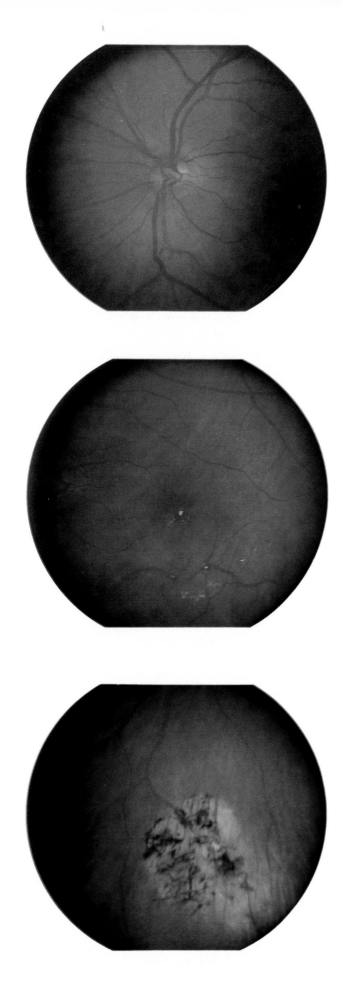

Retinal Telangiectasis (with lipid and arterial aneurysmal formation)

The optic nerve and the major vessels in the vicinity of the left disc appear normal.

In the macular region there is deposition of intraretinal hard exudate. Fine telangiectatic vessels can be seen inferior to the fovea. There are definite aneurysmal changes of the branch artery coursing below the macula. In the vicinity of these aneurysmal dilatations is deposition of intraretinal hard exudate. The branch artery coursing above the macula shows irregularity in its caliber.

Inferior to the left optic nerve there is an area of chorioretinal scarring with both atrophy and pigmentary migration into the sensory retina. The branch retinal artery extending into the area of scarring appears to be occluded. There are two round, whitish lesions along the course of this occluded vessel, which may be previous arterial aneurysmal changes.

During the arterial phase of the fluorescein angiogram two oval aneurysmal outpouchings of the branch artery can be seen.

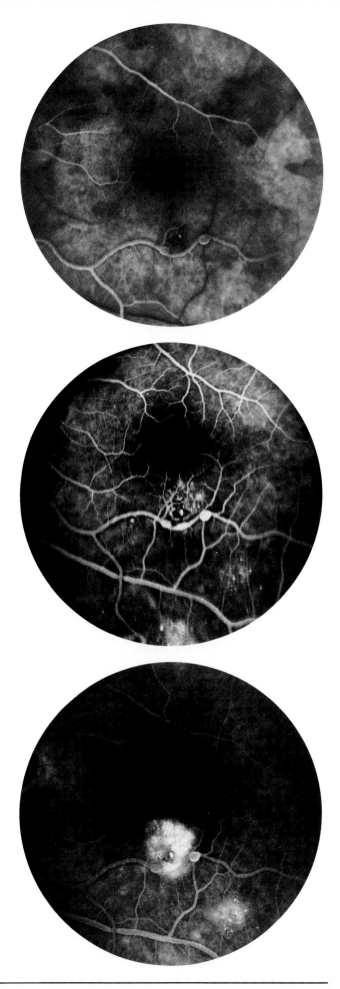

Later in the angiogram, the aneurysmal changes within the inferior temporal branch artery fill and stain with the fluorescein dye. Above this artery are multiple telangiectatic changes. Small telangiectatic vessels leaking fluorescein can be seen inferior to the artery with the aneurysms.

The late angiogram shows intraretinal accumulation of fluorescein dye from the telangiectatic vessels in the vicinity of the inferior temporal branch artery. This leakage of fluorescein extends toward the center of the fovea. There is also some subtle intraretinal accumulation of fluorescein from the retinal vascular abnormalities inferior temporal to the macula.

AUTHOR'S NOTE

This patient showed a very interesting spectrum of retinal vascular disease consisting of retinal telangiectasis, arterial aneurysmal formation, and spontaneous closure of arterial aneurysms. Arterial macroaneurysms are frequently isolated findings in patients who usually have hypertensive disease. This patient definitely shows aneurysmal changes along the inferior temporal artery with associated leakage from the capillary bed. It is frequently impossible to distinguish what is termed telangiectatic changes of the retinal capillaries from actual microaneurysms.

This patient also shows an interesting finding of chorioretinal scarring which is related to closure of previously existing arterial aneurysms. Although no history or clinical information is available, it is possible that these aneurysms hemorrhaged and eventually scarred down, leaving the present clinical picture.

Retinal Telangiectasis
(juxtafoveal with pigment— bilateral)

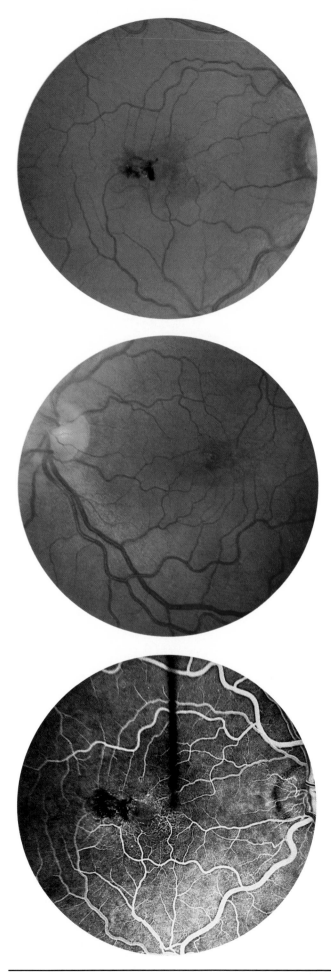

In the macular region of the right eye, there is evidence of hyperpigmentation in the perifoveal region. There is also some slight mottling of the retinal pigment epithelium.

In the left macular region, there is some slight thickening of the sensory retina with hypopigmented changes at the level of the pigment epithelium. Small pinpoint reddish dots can be seen in the perifoveal region, indicating either microaneurysmal or telangiectatic changes.

During the laminar phase of the fluorescein angiogram in the right eye, there is blockage of the background choroidal fluorescence by the pigment temporal to the retinal avascular zone. There appears to be some dilatation of the capillary bed with telangiectatic and microaneurysmal changes.

Later in the angiogram, there is evidence of early leakage from the telangiectatic changes as well as apparent dilatation of the perifoveal capillaries.

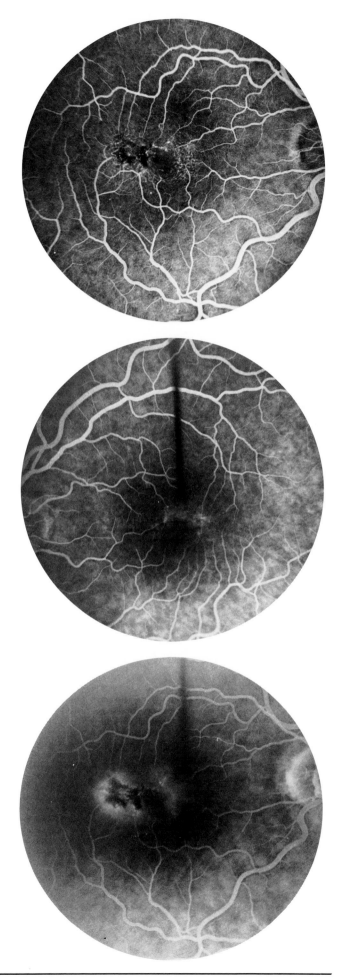

The left eye shows perifoveal leakage of fluorescein dye, indicating macular edema.

The late angiogram of the right eye shows intraretinal leakage of fluorescein from the telangiectatic and microaneurysmal changes. This leakage involves the center of the fovea as well as the area surrounding the pigment.

AUTHOR'S NOTE

This 46-year-old white male stated that he has been amblyopic in the right eye since early childhood. Vision in the right eye was 20/200. The patient had noticed intermittent fluctuations in the central vision in the left eye for the past 10 years. The vision in the left eye was 20/30 best corrected. The patient shows evidence of bilateral juxtafoveal telangiectasis with macular edema. There is also evidence of pigment in the perifoveal region of the right eye which can be seen with this entity. The patient has never had laser treatment to either eye. The exact cause for seeing pigment with this particular entity is unknown. However, one could hypothesize that the pigment is present secondary to long-standing irritation of the pigment epithelium from intraretinal and, perhaps, subretinal serous fluid.

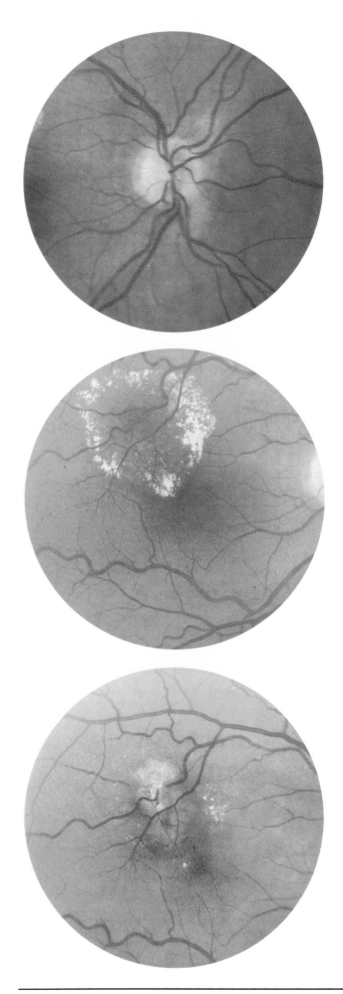

Retinal Telangiectasis (with hard exudate—pre- and post-treatment)

The right optic nerve and major branches of the central retinal artery and vein appear normal.

In the macular region there is a ring of hard exudate with the exudate encroaching toward the center of the fovea. Along the course of the branched superior temporal artery, in the center of the hard exudate, there is a slight bulging of the vessel wall with an increased reflex.

Treatment to areas of vascular abnormality within the center of the ring of hard exudate has caused reduction in the amount of intraretinal hard exudate and less density of the exudate near the center of the fovea.

In the pretreatment laminar phase of the fluorescein angiogram, the dilatation of the capillary bed and the retinal telangiectatic vessels can be seen. There is some very faint blockage of the background fluorescence, corresponding to the circinate area of exudate. There is some slight leakage of fluorescein from the branch retinal artery in the center of the ring of exudate. On each side of this slightly dilated artery is some blockage of the background fluorescence by very faint intraretinal hemorrhage.

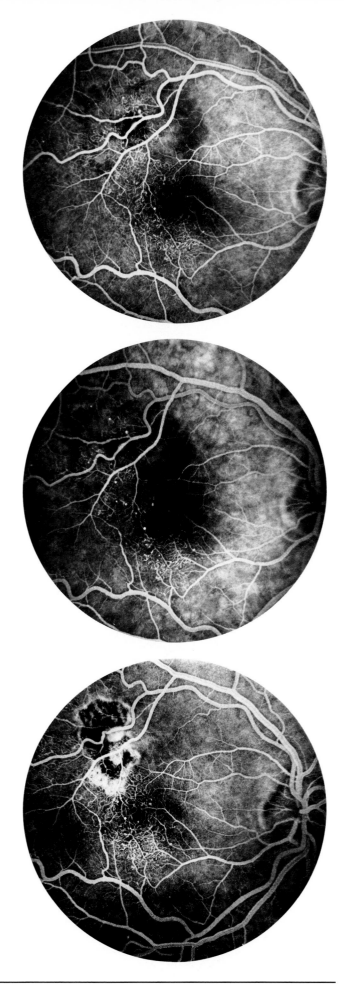

Later in the angiogram, more of the telangiectatic vessels, dilatation of the capillary bed, and aneurysmal changes can also be seen.

There is blockage of the background choroidal fluorescence from the argon laser photocoagulation to the telangiectatic vessels within the center of the ring of exudate. There is less blockage of the background choroidal fluorescence, because there has been absorption of the intraretinal hard exudate. A smaller than normal retinal avascular zone can be seen. The perifoveal capillaries are very prominent with telangiectatic changes and microaneurysmal changes. An arterial macroaneurysm is clearly seen.

AUTHOR'S NOTE

This patient was treated with argon laser photocoagulation because the vision was 20/80 in the right eye and the deposition of hard exudate was in close proximity to the fovea. The treatment was carried out predominantly within the center of the ring of exudate, with significant clearing of the exudate and improvement of vision to 20/25. Treatment was also applied over the slightly dilated branched retinal artery which coursed through the center of the exudative ring. The only indications for photocoagulation are risk of loss of central vision secondary to either exudate or hemorrhage from retinal telangiectasis.

Coats' Disease (with organized exudative maculopathy)

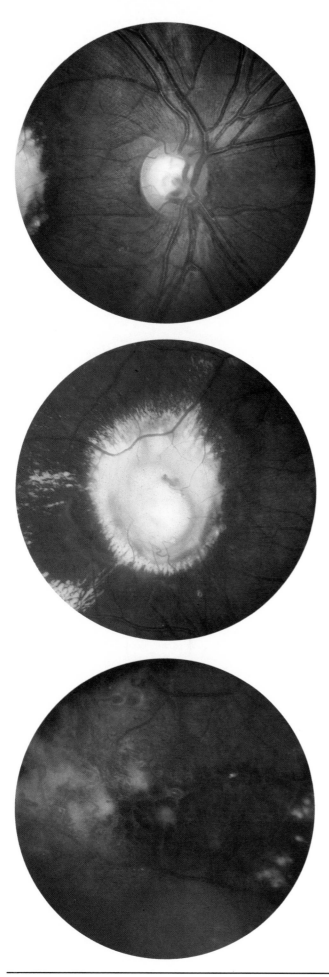

The right optic nerve and major branches of the central retinal artery and vein appear normal. A prominent nerve fiber layer can be seen.

In the macular region, there is a whitish, organized scar surrounded by a ring of intraretinal hard exudate. The exudate extends into the superior and inferior temporal quadrants.

In the temporal periphery, there are multiple telangiectatic vessels coursing intraretinally with aneurysmal dilatation. Yellowish intraretinal exudate can also be seen.

Fluorescein angiography of the temporal periphery shows the multiple telangiectatic vessels with saccular and microaneurysmal dilatation. There is dilatation of the capillary bed and multiple areas of capillary dropout and nonperfusion.

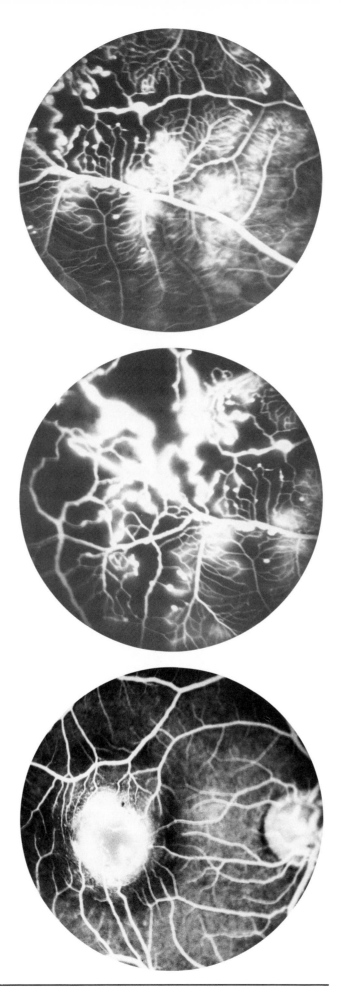

Later in the angiogram there is intraretinal leakage of fluorescein from the telangiectatic vessels and marked hyperfluorescence of the saccular and aneurysmal changes. Additional large areas of nonperfusion and avascularity can be seen.

In the posterior pole of the right eye, there is hyperfluorescence due to staining of the fibrotic scar tissue. Very fine telangiectatic changes can be seen around the periphery of the hyperfluorescent disciform scar.

AUTHOR'S NOTE

This 9-year-old black male presented with a unilateral picture of retinal telangiectasis with exudative maculopathy in the right eye. The left eye was entirely normal. Therefore, a diagnosis of Coats' disease was made. The patient also showed a right esotropia. The diagnosis of Coats' disease must be considered in the differential diagnosis of leukocoria.

Bibliography

Archer D, Krill AE: Leber's miliary aneurysms and optic atrophy. *Surg Ophthalmol* 15:384, 1971.

Coats G: Forms of retinal disease with massive exudation. *R Lond Ophthalmol Hosp Rep* 17:440, 1908.

Coats G: Uber retinitis exudativa. *Albrecht von Graefes Arch Ophthalmol* 18:275, 1912.

Egerer I, Tasman W, Tomer TL: Coats' disease. *Arch Ophthalmol* 92:109–112, 1974.

Ehlers N, Jensen VA: Hereditary central retinal angiography. *Acta Ophthalmol* 51:171–178, 1973.

Farkas TG, Potts AM, Boone C: Some pathological and biochemical aspects of Coats' disease. *Am J Ophthalmol* 75:289–301, 1973.

Harris GS: Coats' disease: Diagnosis and treatment. *Can J Ophthalmol* 5:311, 1970.

Harris GS: Coats' disease: Diagnosis and treatment. *Mod Probl Ophthalmol* 10:277–285, 1972.

Leber T: Uber eine durch Vorkommen multipler Miliaraneurysmen Charakteristik. Form von Retinaldegeneration. *Albrecht von Graefes Arch Ophthalmol* 18:1, 1912.

Maggi C: Leber's retinal degeneration with miliary aneurysms. *Am J Ophthalmol* 56:901, 1963.

Manschot WA, deBruijn WC: Coats' disease: Definition and pathogenesis. *Br J Ophthalmol* 51:145, 1967.

McGrand JC: Photocoagulation in Coats' disease. *Trans Ophthalmol Soc UK* 40:47–56, 1970.

Morgan WE III, Crawford JB: Retinitis pigmentosa and Coats' disease. *Arch Ophthalmol* 79:146–149, 1968.

Reese AB: Telangiectasis of the retina and Coats' disease. *Am J Ophthalmol* 42:1, 1956.

Sugar HS: Coats' disease: Telangiectatic or multiple vascular origin? *Am J Ophthalmol* 45:408, 1958.

Tour RL: Miliary retinal aneurysms. *Am J Ophthalmol* 43:426, 1957.

Tripathi R, Ashton N: Electron microscopical study of Coats' disease. *Br J Ophthalmol* 55:289, 1971.

von Hippel E: Angiomatosis retinae und retinitis exudativa Coats'. *Albrecht von Graefes Arch Ophthalmol* 127:27, 1931.

Wise GN: Coats' disease. *Arch Ophthalmol* 58:735, 1957.

CHAPTER 6

Aneurysm (Arterial and/or Capillary)

Differential Diagnosis

A. ARTERIAL MACROANEURYSM
B. DIABETES MELLITUS
C. VENOUS OCCLUSION

D. RACEMOSE OR CIRSOID ANEURYSM (WYBURN-MASON)
E. OTHER

Arterial macroaneurysms are characterized by a single or multiple aneurysmal outpouchings of the larger caliber retinal arteries. Arteriosclerosis and hypertension are frequently associated findings. This condition is usually unilateral. The macular vision is reduced secondary to hemorrhage, hard exudate, and/or intraretinal edema. The hemorrhage may be located beneath the pigment epithelium, sensory retina, preretinal, or in the vitreous. Conservative management is recommended when no visual impairment occurs; however, with recurrent bleeding or maculopathy secondary to serous fluid or hard exudate, photocoagulation can be considered. The differential diagnosis includes: (1) diabetic retinopathy, (2) venous occlusive disease, (3) retinal telangiectasis, (4) cavernous hemangioma of the retina, and (5) retinal angiomatosis.

AUTHOR'S NOTE

The author has a group of patients who have typical arterial macroaneurysms, are under the age of 40, and have no history of arteriosclerosis or systemic hypertension. In all of these patients there has also been evidence of associated retinal telangiectasis or miliary aneurysms. Therefore, there may be a spectrum between the disease entities known as retinal telangiectasis (Leber's miliary aneurysms), Coats' disease, and arterial macroaneurysms.

Congenital retinal arterio-venous malformation has been described using several different terms. These terms include racemose angioma, arterio-venous aneurysm, and cirsoid aneurysm. Patients who also have arterio-venous malformations involving the central nervous system are said to have the syndrome of Wyburn-Mason. This type of malformation frequently has one or more arterio-venous anastomoses. The vessels are frequently very dilated and tortuous. Clinically, it is often impossible to distinguish the arterial from the venous side of the circulation. Fortunately, there is infrequently hemorrhage or deposition of hard exudate from this type of malformation. The Wyburn-Mason syndrome includes arterio-venous malformation of the retina along with arterio-venous malformation in any of the following possible locations: (1) the posterior fossa midbrain; (2) the orbit; (3) the optic nerve, optic chiasm, or both; (4) the ipsilateral maxilla, mandible, and pterygoid fossa; or (5) the ipsilateral basal-frontal area.

A definite difference exists between the vascular lesions found in the retina and central nervous system in the Wyburn-Mason syndrome and the von Hippel-Lindau syndrome. In the Wyburn-Mason syndrome, the malformation is arterio-venous, both in the retina and central nervous system. In the von Hippel-Lindau syndrome, the retinal vascular malformation is an angioma and the central nervous system vascular lesion is a hemangioblastoma. Patients with Wyburn-Mason syndrome should be warned about dental care and, in particular, tooth extractions, because of the possibility of a vascular malformation being present in the maxilla or mandibular regions.

Arterial Macroaneurysm

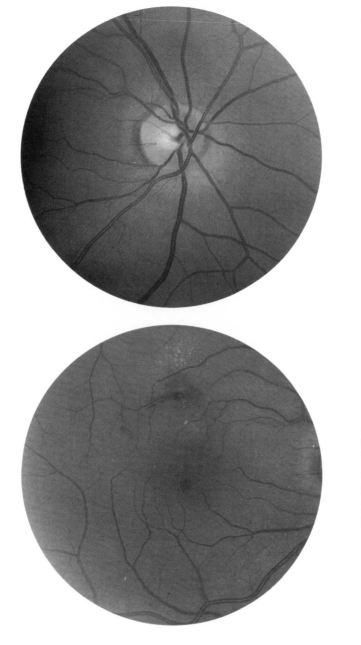

The optic nerve and the major branches of the central retinal vein and artery appear normal.

Along one of the branches of the superior temporal artery a round, red macroaneurysm can be seen. There is some slight intraretinal hemorrhage surrounding the macroaneurysm. In addition to the intraretinal hemorrhage, there is deposition of intraretinal hard exudate. The foveal region appears to be clear.

During the early arterial phase of the angiogram, there is blockage of the background choroidal fluorescence by the intraretinal hemorrhage above the macula.

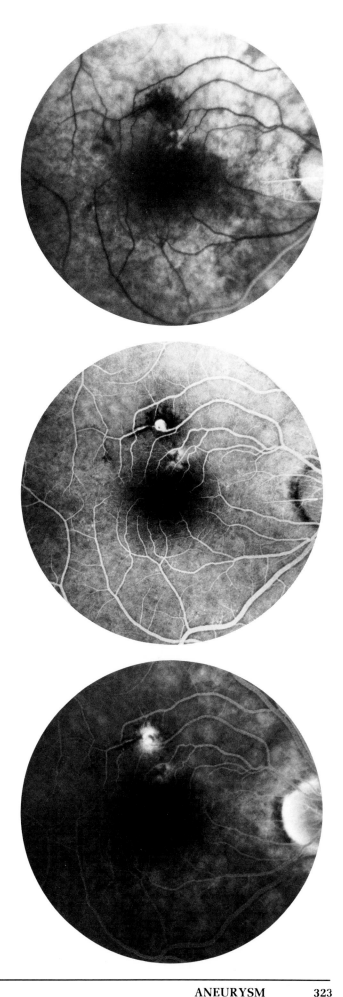

Later in the angiogram the arterial macroaneurysm is hyperfluorescent. The blockage of background fluorescence around the macroaneurysm continues and is secondary to the intraretinal hemorrhage. Just above the foveal region and below the macroaneurysm there appears to be some hyperfluorescent change due to pigment epithelial mottling.

The late angiogram shows the arterial macroaneurysm to be markedly hyperfluorescent with slight leakage of fluorescein intraretinally around the arterial aneurysmal formation.

AUTHOR'S NOTE

Photocoagulation was not considered in this case because there did not seem to be any direct threat to macular vision, either from hemorrhage or hard exudate. The hemorrhage and exudate eventually cleared with the arterial macroaneurysm undergoing fibrotic change.

Arterial Macroaneurysm (deep intraretinal hemorrhage and preretinal hemorrhage)

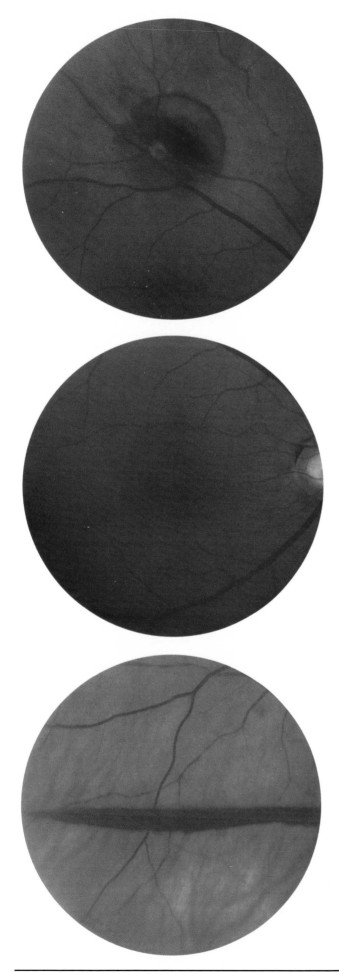

Along one of the branches of the superior temporal artery there is a whitish "light bulb" dilatation surrounded by deep intraretinal hemorrhage. The whitish lesion is an arterial macroaneurysm. Part of the intraretinal hemorrhage is greenish in color and is undergoing some organization and absorption.

The posterior pole of the right eye is normal.

A linear streak of preretinal hemorrhage can be seen along the superior temporal arcades. There is marked attenuation and irregularity of the arterial branches. The venous side of the circulation appears normal.

During the early laminar phase of the fluorescein angiogram, blockage of the background choroidal fluorescence by the deep intraretinal hemorrhage can be seen. The roundish area of hyperfluorescence along the superior temporal branched artery indicates the location of the arterial macroaneurysm.

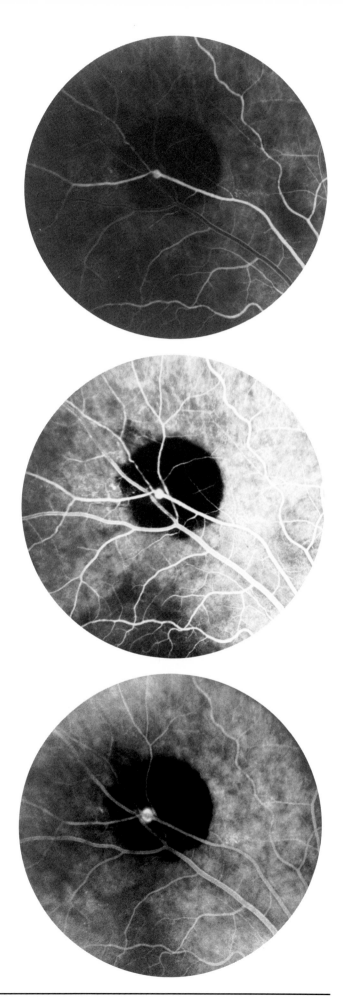

Later in the angiogram there is increased hyperfluorescence of the arterial macroaneurysm. The branches of the artery beyond the macroaneurysm are markedly narrowed and irregular. The intraretinal hemorrhage continues to block the background choroidal fluorescence.

The late angiogram shows slight leakage of fluorescein from the arterial macroaneurysm.

AUTHOR'S NOTE

Although there was some preretinal hemorrhage in this eye, it was decided to consider further observation without photocoagulation treatment. Fortunately, the intraretinal and preretinal hemorrhages cleared, and the arterial macroaneurysm appeared to be sclerotic, and no photocoagulation treatment was necessary.

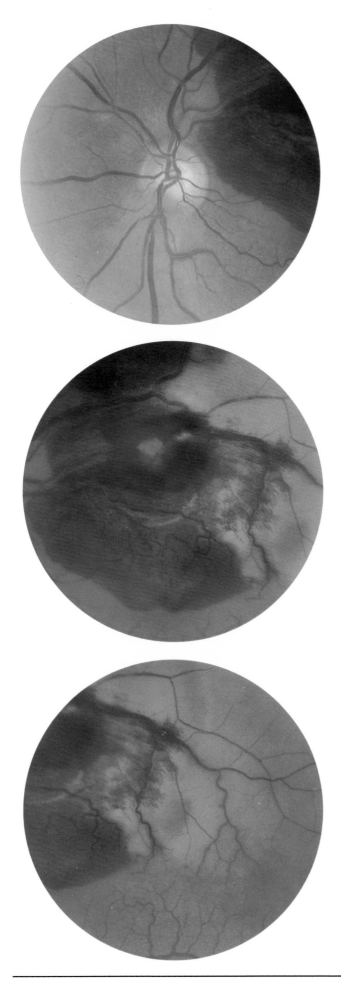

Arterial Macroaneurysm (large intraretinal hemorrhage with macular involvement)

The optic nerve of the left eye appears normal. The retinal arteries are slightly narrowed. Temporal to the optic nerve and along the superior temporal arcade there is extensive intraretinal hemorrhage.

The hemorrhage extends into the center of the macula and into the superior temporal quadrant. Within the reddish hemorrhage, along the branch of the superior temporal artery, there appears to be a round, yellowish lesion.

There is hemorrhage extending into the superior temporal quadrant. The hemorrhage is both superficial and deep. Just beyond the hemorrhage there is whitish discoloration to the sensory retina, which may indicate the presence of some ischemic retinal whitening secondary to arterial insufficiency or occlusion.

During the laminar phase of the fluorescein angiogram, there is extensive blockage of the background choroidal fluorescence by the large intraretinal hemorrhage. The capillaries in the superior aspect of the macula appear more prominent because of the black background from the hemorrhage.

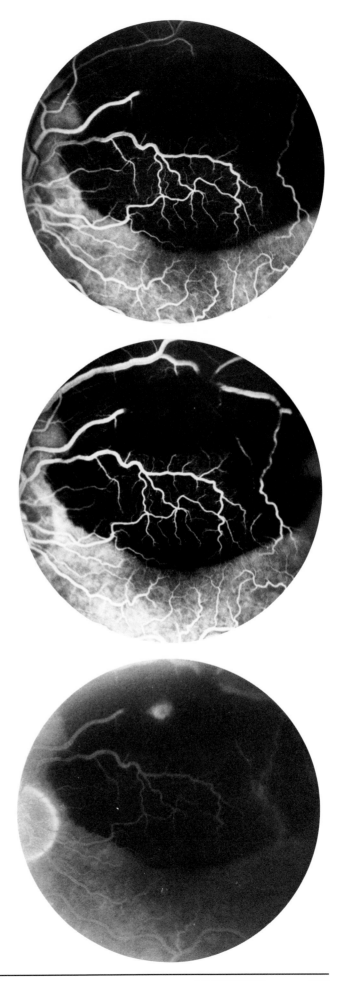

Later in the angiogram there is further blockage of the background fluorescence by the intraretinal hemorrhage. The hemorrhage extends through the center of the fovea. Part of the superior temporal branch artery is obscured by the superficial intraretinal hemorrhage. There is a slight suggestion of a roundish faint area of hyperfluorescence along this branch artery within the hemorrhagic region.

The late phase of the angiogram shows continued blockage of the background choroidal fluorescence by the hemorrhage. However, along the course of the superior temporal branch artery there is a round area of hyperfluorescence and leakage of fluorescein dye, indicating the origin of the hemorrhage to be an arterial macroaneurysm.

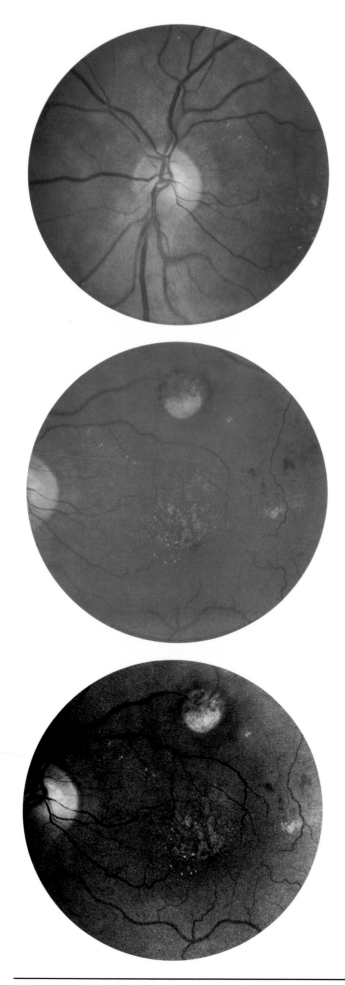

The optic nerve appears normal. There has been dramatic clearing of the intraretinal hemorrhage temporal to the optic nerve.

In the posterior pole there has also been dramatic clearing of the surface and deep intraretinal hemorrhage. There is residual intraretinal hard exudate. Just temporal to the macula there is some hyperpigmentation. Along the superior temporal artery a large, yellow macroaneurysm is clearly evident.

The red-free photograph of the left eye shows the pigment epithelial mottling change secondary to irritation of the pigment epithelium by the deep intraretinal hemorrhage. In addition, the round arterial macroaneurysm is clearly evident.

During the early laminar phase of the fluorescein angiogram there is definite irregularity of the superior temporal artery as it courses in the vicinity of the macroaneurysm. There is some slight blockage of the background fluorescence in the area of the arterial macroaneurysm. Throughout the posterior pole there are multiple hypo- and hyperfluorescent changes due to mottling of the pigment epithelium.

Later in the angiogram very fine vessels can be seen around the arterial macroaneurysm and connecting the branch artery where it enters and exits the macroaneurysm. The diffuse mottling of the pigment epithelium is demonstrated by an irregular hypo- and hyperfluorescent pattern.

The late angiogram shows some very slight hyperfluorescence and leakage of the sclerotic arterial macroaneurysm.

AUTHOR'S NOTE

The initial clinical impression by the referring physician on this patient was hemorrhagic macular degeneration because of the extensive hemorrhage and the fact that the patient was 78 years old. However, the late angiogram during the hemorrhagic stage revealed what appeared to be an arterial macroaneurysm. Due to the extensive intraretinal hemorrhage, it was decided that photocoagulation treatment should be withheld because of secondary changes which could occur within the retina from heating up the blood. Three months after initial examination, there had been nearly total absorption of the intraretinal hemorrhage and the arterial macroaneurysm was clinically evident. On angiography, the fine vessels coursing through the arterial macroaneurysm could be considered arterial to arterial collaterals.

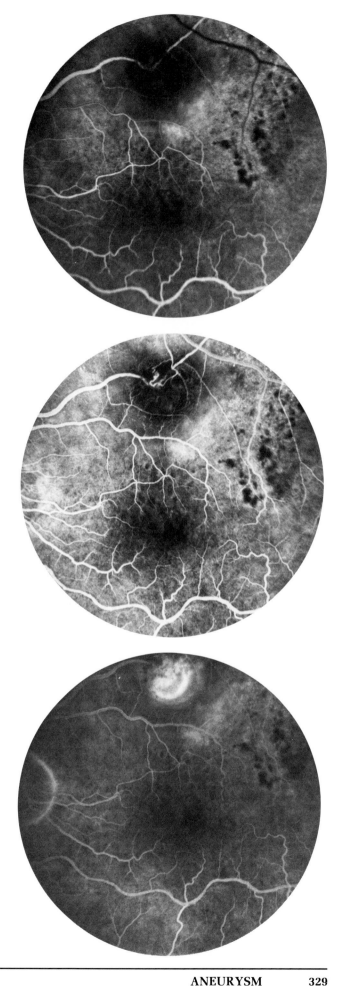

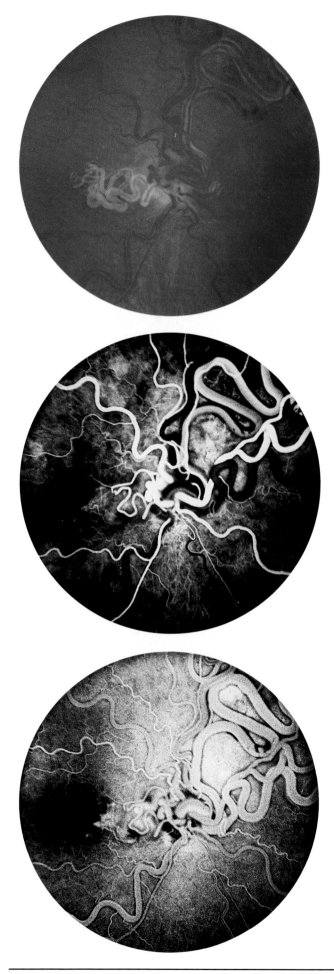

Racemose Aneurysm
(Wyburn-Mason syndrome)

The right eye shows a complex retinal vascular abnormality consisting of large dilated and markedly tortuous vessels which completely obscure the optic nerve. The abnormal vessels extending from the temporal aspect of the disc toward the macula appear to be void of blood.

During the early phase of the fluorescein angiogram, the arterial side of this vascular retinal malformation is clearly evident as the fluorescein dye passes through the lumen. The venous side of the malformation shows no fluorescein dye. This malformation is predominantly over the right optic nerve.

Later in the angiogram both the arterial and venous sides of the vascular malformation are filled with the fluorescein dye. The macular region can be seen and shows no significant vascular abnormality. There is no evidence of intraretinal fluorescein leakage from this arterio-venous malformation.

AUTHOR'S NOTE

I am indebted to Jerry A. Shields, M.D. and R. D. Mulburger, M.D. for permitting me to publish this case. This is a patient who was initially seen at the age of 9 and followed for a period of 17 years. The patient was diagnosed as having Wyburn-Mason syndrome because of the presence of the retinal arterio-venous malformation and also vascular malformation of the central nervous system. One can speculate that the reason there is no leakage of fluorescein from this arterio-venous malformation is the fact that this malformation is congenital in origin and, therefore, has normal endothelial cell tight junctions.

Racemose Aneurysm
(Wyburn-Mason syndrome)

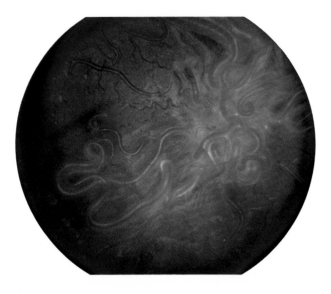

The right optic nerve is obscured by the arterio-venous malformation. The vessels are markedly engorged and tortuous.

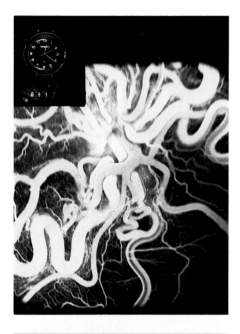

The fluorescein angiogram demonstrates the extensive arterio-venous malformation overlying the optic nerve. One of the retinal vessels shows laminar flow and is on the venous side of the malformation.

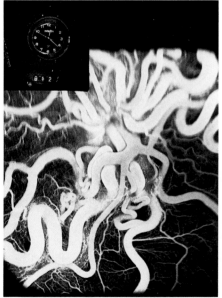

Later in the angiogram there is filling of both the arterial and venous sides of the retinal vascular malformation. However, there is no leakage of fluorescein.

AUTHOR'S NOTE

I am indebted to Stuart L. Fine, M.D., and Neil Miller, M.D. for permitting me to publish this case. This case appears in *Sights and Sounds in Ophthalmology*, vol 3: *The Ocular Fundus in Neuro-ophthalmologic Diagnosis*. St Louis, CV Mosby, 1977.

Bibliography

Asdourian GK, Goldberg MF, Jampol L, et al: Retinal macroaneurysms. *Arch Ophthalmol* 95:624, 1977.

Cleary PR, Kohner EM, Hamilton AM, et al: Retinal macroaneurysms. *Br J Ophthalmol* 59:355, 1975.

Francois J: Acquired macroaneurysms of the retinal arteries. *Int Ophthalmol* 1:153, 1979.

Hudomel J, Imre G: Photocoagulation treatment of solitary aneurysm near the macula lutea. *Acta Ophthalmol* 51:633–638, 1973.

Lewis RA, Norton EWD, Gass JDM: Acquired arterial macroaneurysms of the retina. *Br J Ophthalmol* 60:21, 1976.

Nadel AJ, Gupta KK: Macroaneurysms of the retinal arteries. *Arch Ophthalmol* 94:1092, 1976.

Nouhuys FV, Deutman AF: Argon laser treatment of retinal macroaneurysms. *Int Ophthalmol* 2:45, 1980.

Palestine AG, Robertson DM, Goldstein BG: Macroaneurysms of the retinal arteries. *Am J Ophthalmol* 93:164–171, 1982.

Robertson DM: Macroaneurysms of the retinal arteries. *Trans Am Acad Ophthalmol Otolaryngol* 77:OP55, 1973.

Shults WT, Swan KC: Pulsatile aneurysms of the retinal arterial tree. *Am J Ophthalmol* 77:304–309, 1974.

CHAPTER 7

Vascular Tumors

Differential Diagnosis

A. ANGIOMATOSIS RETINAE (VON HIPPEL'S DISEASE)
B. CAVERNOUS HEMANGIOMA OF THE RETINA
C. ASTROCYTIC HAMARTOMA OF THE RETINA

Angiomatosis retinae (von Hippel's disease) is a congenital, hereditary, capillary angiomatous hamartoma of the optic nerve and/or retina. These lesions have been described as being both endophytic, i.e. arising from the inner retinal layers, or exophytic, i.e. arising from the outer layers of the sensory retina. The mode of transmission is autosomal dominant with a complete penetrance and variable expressivity. The angiomas can be bilateral in approximately 50% of patients. When there is central nervous system involvement and other organ involvement, the condition is referred to as von Hippel-Lindau disease. Approximately 20% to 25% of the patients with retinal angiomas develop clinical evidence of central nervous system involvement.

The larger peripheral vascular tumors are often associated with dilated, tortuous feeder and collector vessels (A). The tumors can cause circinate maculopathy and exudative elevations of the sensory retina. Depending on the duration of the exudation, treatment of a peripheral angioma can, in some cases, improve the central vision by causing a reduction of the intraretinal hard exudate in the macular region.

Astrocytic hamartomas are usually developmental tumors which are discovered in the second or third decades of life. In many cases, they are associated with tuberous sclerosis or Bourneville's disease. The lesions are usually globular, white, and well circumscribed (B). They are usually slightly elevated, arising from the inner surface of the retina, and, in some cases, in close proximity to the optic nerve. Optic nerve head drusen have also been seen associated with astrocytic hamartomas and with tuberous sclerosis. The retinal astrocytic hamartomas rarely show evidence of growth and usually cause no secondary damage, such as exudation or detachment. If diagnosed early in life, the lesions may be semitranslucent, and a differentiation from retinoblastoma must be made. The nodular calcific areas within the lesion give it a "mulberry" appearance. Skull x-rays in adult patients may reveal radiodense, calcified cerebral hamartomas, often referred to as "brain stones."

Astrocytic hamartomas are the second most frequent retinal finding causing autofluorescence. The most common cause for autofluorescence is optic nerve head drusen. Autofluorescence is the emission of fluorescent light from ocular structures without the presence of the sodium fluorescein dye. These structures, i.e. astrocytic hamartomas and optic nerve head drusen, naturally emit a fluorescence when exposed to the blue light from the fundus camera. The lesions are excited by the blue light, and a green-yellow light is emitted through the barrier filter. Therefore, when autofluorescence is suspected, several photographs should be taken with the blue light prior to the injection of fluorescein dye.

Cavernous hemangioma of the retina is a sessile tumor that consists of thin-walled saccular aneurysms with dark venous blood (Figure). This tumor is considered a hamartoma. Clinically, this lesion has been described as having the appearance of a "cluster of grapes." Occasionally, patients also have cavernous hemangiomas involving the central nervous system with symptoms of seizures. The skin can also show angiomatous lesions. For the most part, cavernous hemangiomas are relatively isolated from the retinal circulation and, therefore, rarely cause exudation or hemorrhage. The differential diagnosis of this hamartoma includes retinal telangiectasis or Leber's miliary aneurysms, retinal angiomatosis (von Hippel's disease), and racemose angioma of the retina.

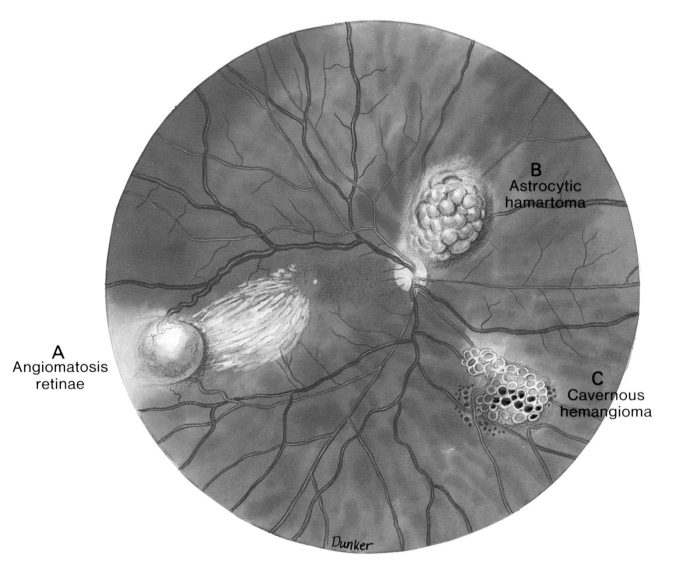

A
Angiomatosis
retinae

B
Astrocytic
hamartoma

C
Cavernous
hemangioma

Reader's Notes

Angiomatosis Retinae
(von Hippel's disease)

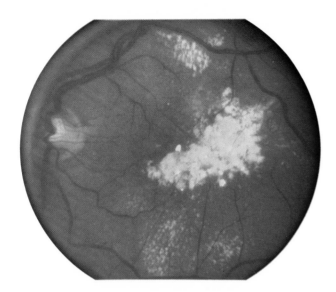

In the macular region of the left eye, there is evidence of intraretinal yellowish hard exudate.

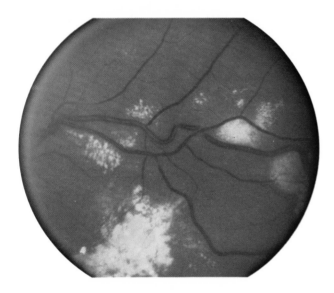

The intraretinal hard exudate extends along the superior temporal arcade and into the superior temporal peripheral quadrant.

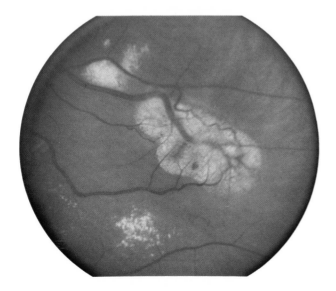

A yellowish, well circumscribed tumor can be seen. A large, draining retinal vein can be seen at the superior medial aspect of the tumor.

During the laminar phase of the angiogram, there is rapid shunting of the fluorescein dye through the tumor mass.

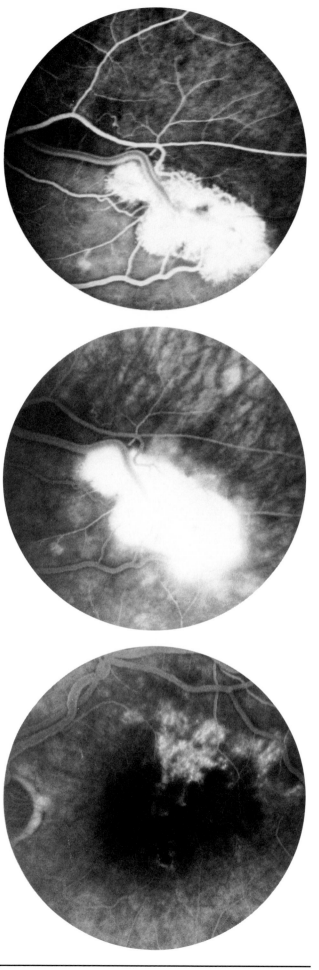

Later in the angiogram, there is slight leakage of fluorescein from the vessels within the tumor. Some of the leakage also comes from dilatation of the retinal capillary bed surrounding the angioma.

The late angiogram of the posterior pole shows some intraretinal leakage of fluorescein dye. There is also some slight blockage of the background choroidal fluorescence from the concentrated deposition of hard exudate.

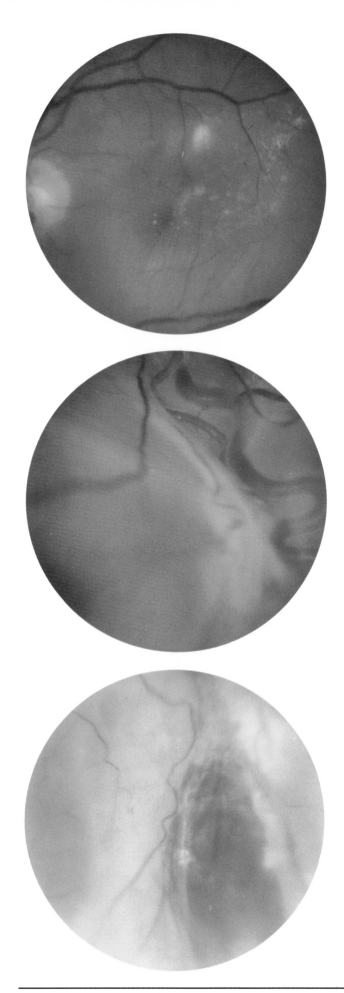

Retinal Angioma
(with associated bullous retinal detachment)

The left posterior pole demonstrates a serous and exudative retinal detachment. This detachment involves the inferior portion of the macula and extends through the fovea.

In the inferior temporal quadrant, there is an enlarged, tortuous retinal artery and vein. The associated large bullous retinal detachment is evident.

Further out into the inferior temporal periphery, a large, reddish, elevated angioma is apparent.

The enlarged and tortuous retinal artery and vein are evident. The retinal vein can be differentiated from the artery by its laminar flow. A large area of hypofluorescence can be seen in the region of the bullous retinal detachment.

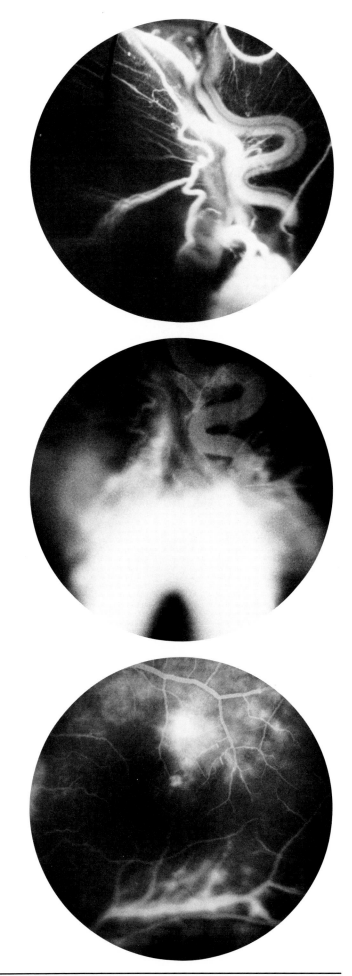

Later in the angiogram, there is marked hyperfluorescence from the tumor, with leakage of fluorescein into the surrounding area.

Late in the angiogram there is leakage of fluorescein in the superior aspect of the macula as well as along one of the inferior temporal retinal vessels. The leakage from the walls of the vessel indicates a breakdown in the blood-retinal barrier secondary to loss of endothelial cell junction integrity.

Retinal Angioma (with optic nerve involvement)

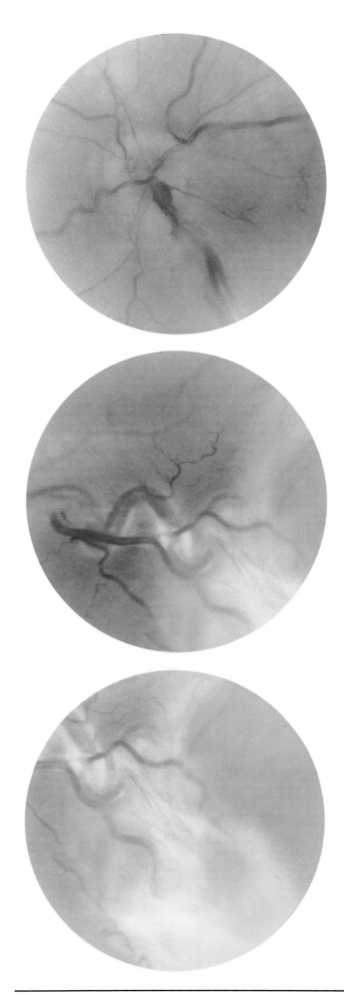

The left optic nerve is hyperemic. The disc margins are slightly blurred. The inferior temporal artery and vein are engorged.

The feeding retinal artery to the angioma and the draining vein are significantly dilated. The retinal vein is markedly engorged. Intraretinal, yellowish exudative material can be seen extending into the inferior temporal quadrant.

An orange-colored angioma is visible surrounded by the yellowish, intraretinal exudate. There also is serous fluid beneath the sensory retina surrounding the angioma.

The arterial phase of the angiogram clearly shows the dilated artery. The enlarged, tortuous, draining vein is void of the fluorescein dye. There is some blockage of the background choroidal fluorescence by the serous fluid beneath the sensory retina.

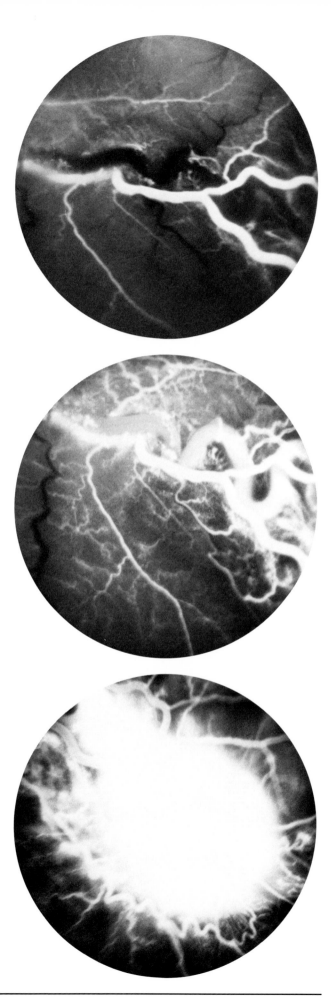

Later in the angiogram there is rapid filling of the dilated draining vein. One of the more proximal small caliber veins is still void of fluorescein dye. The capillary bed shows some irregularity and slight intraretinal leakage of fluorescein.

There is diffuse leakage of fluorescein from the retinal angioma. There is also some intraretinal leakage of fluorescein around the tumor from the abnormal leaking retinal vasculature.

AUTHOR'S NOTE

This patient was unusual from the point of view that the optic nerve in the left eye was hyperemic and the dilated tortuous vessels extended from the nerve to the inferior temporal periphery, where the retinal angioma could be localized.

Cavernous Hemangioma of the Retina

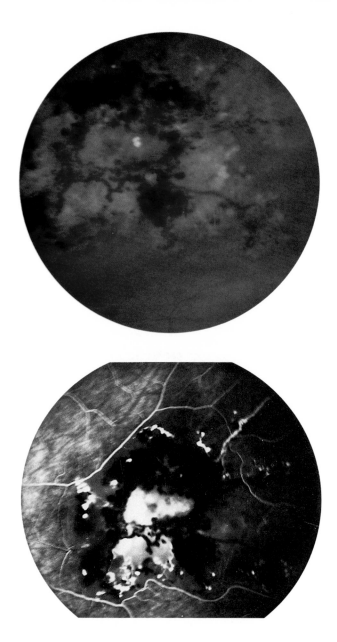

In the temporal periphery of the left eye there is an irregularly elevated vascular mass. There are multiple dilated, round, thin-walled saccular blood vessels which give the appearance of a "cluster of grapes." It appears that there may be some intraretinal blotch hemorrhages associated with the vascular tumor.

During the fluorescein angiogram, there is an irregular filling pattern of some of the saccular aneurysms. This indicates a sluggish blood flow within the tumor. The small blotch hemorrhage in the vicinity of the inferior portion of the tumor blocks the background choroidal fluorescence.

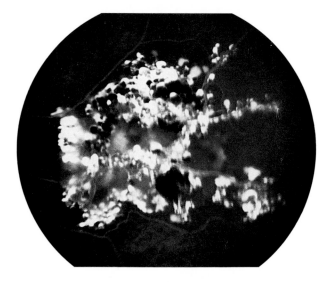

The late angiogram still shows incomplete perfusion of the tumor. The inferior blotch hemorrhage continues to block the background fluorescence. There is evidence of plasma layering in many of the aneurysms. The more confluent areas of hyperfluorescence represent fluorescein dye within cystic spaces which are part of the overall tumor mass.

AUTHOR'S NOTE

Many portions of this vascular tumor show incomplete perfusion because the lesion is relatively isolated from the retinal circulation. Plasma erythrocytic layering within the saccular aneurysms is a very characteristic finding with these vascular tumors. Usually, the fluorescein pattern within the saccular aneurysm shows an area of hypofluorescence with the superior aspect of the aneurysm being hyperfluorescent.

I am indebted to Drs. J. A. Shields and N. Schatz for contributing this case.

Cavernous Hemangioma of the Retina

Involving the inferior temporal quadrant of the left eye is a slightly elevated, irregular vascular mass. The lesion is composed of slightly dilated, round or oval saccular vessels which are difficult to differentiate from intraretinal dot hemorrhages or microaneurysms. These give the appearance of a "cluster of grapes." Extending through the center of the saccular vessels is a slightly dilated branch retinal vein. Certain areas of the sensory retina have lost their normal transparency as evidenced by the whitish discoloration.

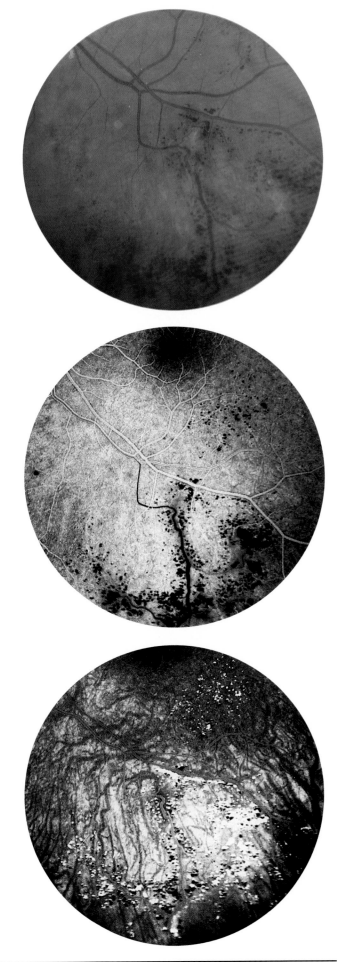

During the arterio-venous phase of the angiogram there is a lack of perfusion of the vascular tumor. Extension of the small, oval saccular portions of the tumor can be seen extending toward the macula.

A very late frame of the fluorescein angiogram shows many portions of the hemangioma to still be void of the fluorescein dye while others contain fluorescein. Careful examination of the fluorescein pattern indicates the typical plasma layering within some of the individual oval portions of the tumor. There is an obvious lack of intraretinal fluorescein leakage. The choroidal vessels can be clearly identified deep to the sensory retina and vascular tumor.

AUTHOR'S NOTE

At the time of the ocular examination this patient gave a history of grand mal seizures and was, therefore, referred for a neurologic work-up for a possible cerebral vascular tumor in conjunction with the cavernous hemangioma of the retina.

Astrocytic Hamartoma of the Retina

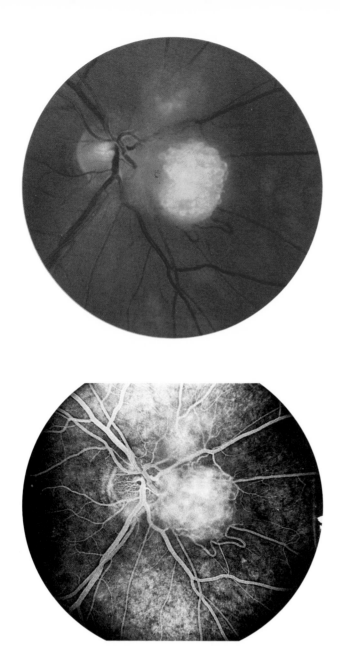

At the nasal aspect of the right optic nerve, there is an elevated astrocytic hamartoma. The inferior portion of the lesion is calcified and has a "mulberry" appearance. A slightly abnormal vascular channel can be seen at the inferior portion of the calcified lesion. Superior to the calcified portion, there is a more translucent area.

The fluorescein angiogram shows a fine extensive capillary network within the hamartoma. Retinal vessels can be seen extending into the tumor mass and around the the edges of the lesion.

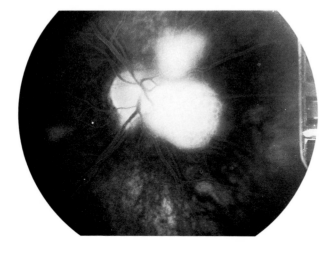

The late angiogram shows hyperfluorescence of both the calcified and translucent portions of the hamartoma. Small, round, slightly hypofluorescent areas can be seen at the peripheral portion of the calcified mass, indicating multiple small cystic spaces.

AUTHOR'S NOTE

I am indebted to Drs. J. A. Shields and A. L. Schein for contributing this case.

Reader's Notes

Astrocytic Hamartoma
(demonstration of autofluorescence)

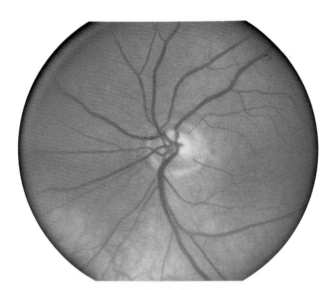

The left optic nerve and retinal vasculature appear normal.

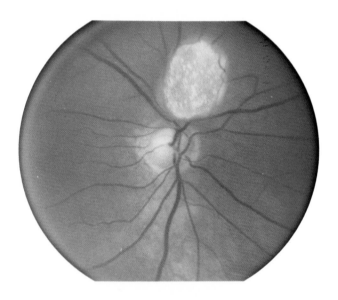

Superior to the right optic nerve there is a yellowish, "mulberry-like" lesion. The more calcific portions of the lesion appear as small, round, punctate, yellowish deposits.

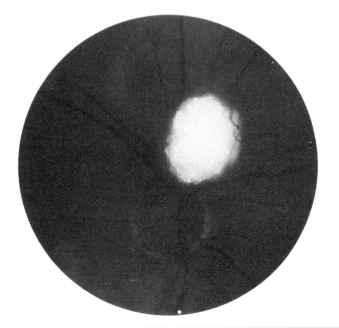

Autofluorescence is demonstrated prior to the injection of the fluorescein dye using the blue excitor filter. The scalloped edges of the tumor mass are evident.

During the arterial phase of the angiogram, there is increased hyperfluorescence within the center of the astrocytic hamartoma. Branches of the retinal arterial tree course around the lesion.

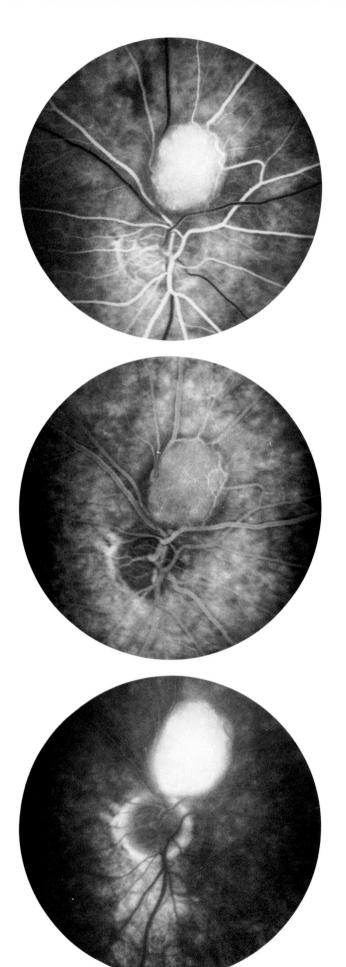

Later in the angiogram there is slight fading of the fluorescence associated with the hamartoma.

The late angiogram reveals late staining of the tumor mass with the fluorescein dye. There is essentially no leakage of fluorescein into the surrounding region.

Bibliography

Apple DJ, Goldberg MF, Wyhinny GJ: Argon laser treatment of von Hippel-Lindau retinal angiomas. II. Histopathology of treated lesions. *Arch Ophthalmol* 92:126–130, 1974.

Archer DB, Deutman A, Ernest JT, et al: Arteriovenous communications of the retina. *Am J Ophthalmol* 75:224–241, 1973.

Cardoso RD, Brockhurst RJ: Perforating diathermy coagulation for retinal angiomas. *Arch Ophthalmol* 94:1702–1715, 1974.

Cordes FC, Hogan MJ: Angiomatosis retinae (von Hippel's disease): 11 years after irradiation. *Am J Ophthalmol* 36:1362–1366, 1953.

Davies WS, Thumin M: Cavernous hemangioma of the optic disc and retina. *Trans Am Acad Ophthalmol Otolaryngol* 60:217–218, 1956.

Gass JDM: Cavernous hemangioma of the retina: A neuro-oculocutaneous syndrome. *Am J Ophthalmol* 71:799–814, 1971.

Gautier-Smith PC, Sanders MD, Sanderson KV: Ocular and nervous system involvement in angioma serpiginosum. *Br J Ophthalmol* 55:433–443, 1971.

Goldberg MF, Duke JR: von Hippel-Lindau disease: Histopathologic findings in a treated and an untreated eye. *Am J Ophthalmol* 66:693–705, 1968.

Jakobiec FA, Font RL, Johnson RB: Angiomatosis retinae: An ultrastructural study and lipid analysis. *Cancer* 38:2042–2056, 1976.

Kirby TJ: Ocular phakomatoses. *Am J Med Sci* 222:227, 1951.

Lewis RA, Cohen MH, Wise GN: Cavernous hemangioma of the retina and optic disc: A report of three cases and a review of the literature. *Br J Ophthalmol* 59:422–434, 1975.

Lindau A: Zur Frage Angiomatosis retinae und inher Hirnkoplicationen. *Acta Ophthalmol* 4:193–226, 1926.

Lindau A, Sargent P, Collins ET: Discussion on vascular tumours of the brain and spinal cord. *Proc R Soc Med* 24:363–382, 1930.

Lowenstein A, Stell J: Retinal tuberous sclerosis (Bourneville's disease). *Am J Ophthalmol* 24:731, 1941.

Moller, PM: Another family with von Hippel-Lindau's disease. *Acta Ophthalmol* 30:155, 1952.

Neame H: Angiomatosis retinae, with report of pathological examination. *Br J Ophthalmol* 32:677–689, 1948.

Pinkerton OD: Angioma of the retina: Report of two cases with fundus photographs. *Am J Ophthalmol* 29:711–712, 1946.

Schwartz PL, Beards JA, Maris PJG: Tuberous sclerosis associated with a retinal angioma. *Am J Ophthalmol* 90:485–488, 1980.

Spencer WH: Primary neoplasms of the optic nerve and its sheaths: Clinical features and current concepts of pathogenetic mechanism. *Trans Ophthalmol Soc UK* 70:490–528, 1972.

Thomas JV, Schwartz PL, Gragoudas ES: von Hippel's disease in association with von Recklinghausen's neurofibromatosis. *Br J Ophthalmol* 62:604, 1978.

Van de Hoeve J.: Doyne memorial lecture on symptoms in phakomatoses. *Trans Ophthalmol Soc UK* 43:534, 1923.

Watzke RC, Weingeist TA, Constantine JB: Diagnosis and management of von Hippel-Lindau disease. In Peyman GA, Apple DJ, Sanders DR: *Intraocular Tumors.* New York, Appleton-Century-Crofts, 1977, pp 199–217.

Wing GL, Weiter JJ, Kelly PJ, et al: von Hippel-Lindau disease: Angiomatosis of the retinal and central nervous system. *Ophthalmology* 88:1311–1314, 1981.

CHAPTER 8

Collaterals, Shunts, and Tortuosity

Differential Diagnosis

A. VENOUS OCCLUSION
   (COLLATERALS) (VEIN → VEIN)
B. ARTERIAL OCCLUSION
   (COLLATERALS) (ARTERY →
   ARTERY)
C. ARTERIAL TO VENOUS
   ANASTOMOSIS
D. VON HIPPEL'S DISEASE (SHUNTS)
E. RACEMOSE ANEURYSM (SHUNTS)

F. CONGENITAL TORTUOSITY OF THE
   RETINAL VESSELS
G. PRERETINAL GLIOSIS OR INTERNAL
   LIMITING MEMBRANE
   CONTRACTION (TORTUOSITY)
H. HAMARTOMA OF RETINAL
   PIGMENT EPITHELIUM AND
   SENSORY RETINA
I. VASCULAR LOOP

Collaterals are most frequently seen in patients with venous occlusion. Those patients with central retinal vein occlusions frequently have collaterals in the vicinity of the optic nerve. In retinal branch vein occlusion, the collaterals are usually around the occlusion site, temporal to the macula, across the horizontal raphe, and draining the nasal aspect of the macula.

Although arterial occlusions are not that uncommon, artery to artery collaterals are quite rare.

Congenital tortuosity of the retinal vessels can be differentiated from other retinal vascular disorders by fluorescein angiography. With congenital tortuosity of the retinal vessels, there is usually no abnormal leakage or staining of the vessel walls, because these vessels are normal and have normal endothelial cell junctions.

Preretinal gliosis, epiretinal membrane formation, or internal limiting membrane contraction is fre-

quently idiopathic but can also have secondary causes. The figure on page 350 demonstrates a break in the internal limiting membrane with glial cells migrating from the inner layers of the retina. These cells lay down an epiretinal membrane which contracts and wrinkles the sensory retina.

Causes of preretinal gliosis are (1) idiopathic, (2) inflammatory, (3) retinal holes and/or rhegmatogenous retinal detachment, (4) postscleral buckle, (5) postcryopexy, (6) postvitrectomy, (7) retinal vascular diseases, (8) proliferative retinopathies, (9) intraocular foreign bodies, and (10) combined pigment epithelial and retinal hamartomas.

Combined pigment epithelial and retinal hamartomas usually are in the vicinity of the optic nerve. These lesions involve the pigment epithelium, sensory retina, and frequently the overlying vitreous. In cases where the hamartoma is in the juxtapapillary region, over a period of time there can be distortion of the retina in the macular region secondary to proliferation of glial tissue which begins to contract, causing traction. These hamartomas can also occur within the posterior pole or elsewhere in the fundus. The lesions are usually unilateral. The differential diagnosis is as follows: (1) melanocytoma, (2) choroidal melanoma, (3) choroidal nevus, (4) retinoblastoma, (5) reactive proliferation of the retinal pigment epithelium, and (6) retrolental fibroplasia.

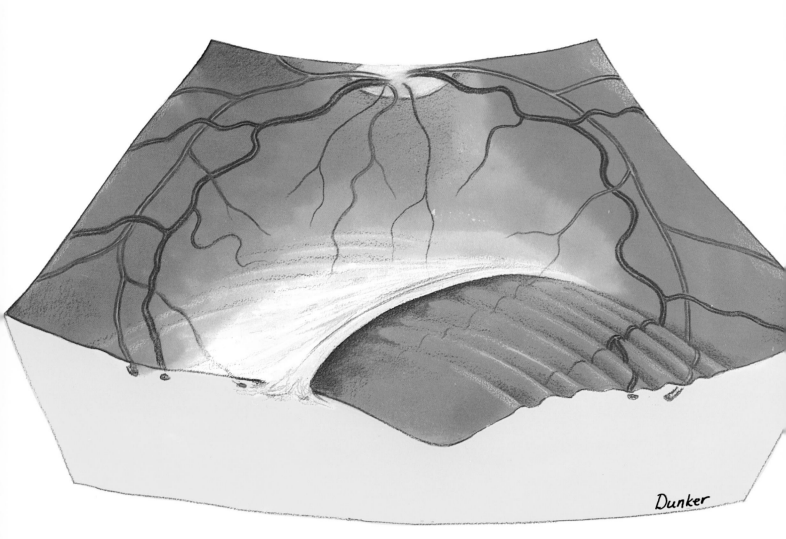

Reader's Notes

Artery → Artery Collaterals
(secondary to branch retinal artery occlusion)

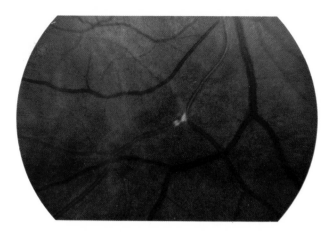

2× magnification reveals an embolus lodged at the bifurcation of the inferior temporal artery.

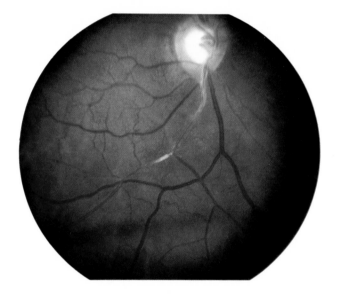

Several months later the embolization has increased through the lumen of the branch retinal artery and extends along the artery toward the optic nerve. Just beyond the embolus, after the bifurcation, arterial to arterial collateralization can be seen.

The artist's schematic represents the area of collateralization seen on the color photograph.

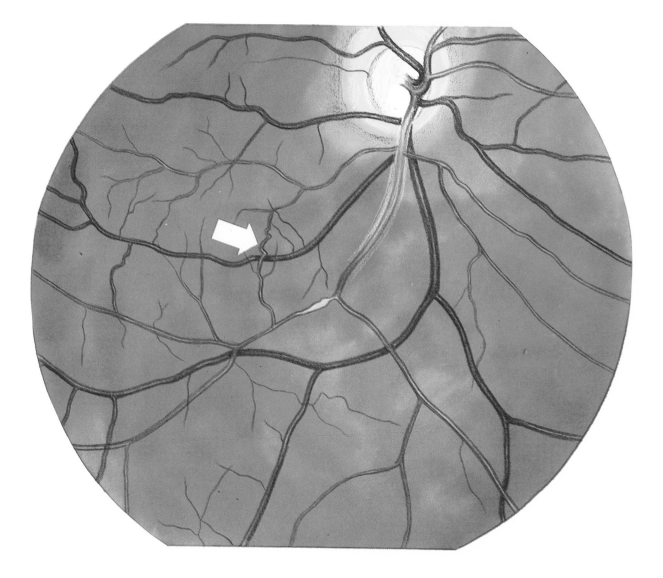

Arterio-venous Anastomoses

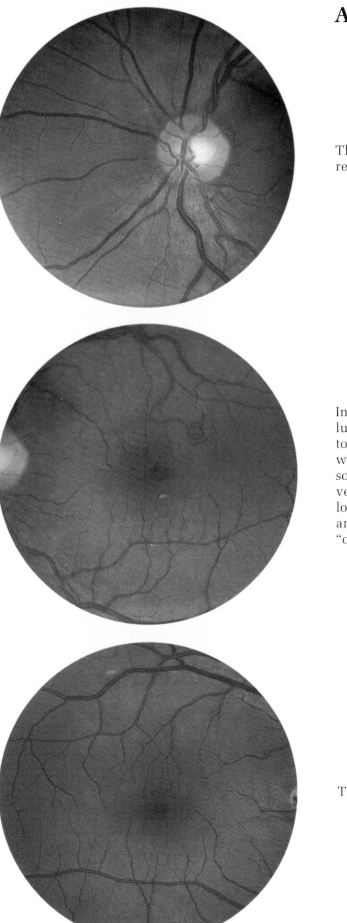

The optic nerve and major branches of the central retinal artery and vein appear normal.

In the macular region, there appears to be a translucent cyst-like area involving the fovea. Superior to the fovea, there is an abnormal vascular pattern which appears to be in the formation of a corkscrew. This anastomosis is between the arterial and venous circulation. There appears to be some yellowish deposition within the temporal aspect of the anastomotic vessel above the area which has a "corkscrew-type" configuration.

The posterior pole of the right eye is entirely normal.

During the early laminar phase of the fluorescein angiogram, it is evident that the anastomosis is between the branches of the superior temporal artery and the superior temporal vein.

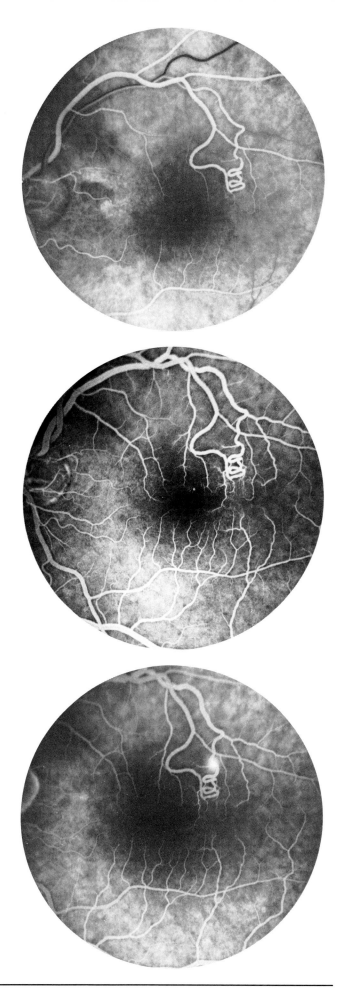

Later in the angiogram, there is complete filling of the anastomotic or collateral vessels between the arterial and venous circulation. There is no evidence of abnormal leakage of fluorescein dye. There is a suggestion that the capillary bed beneath the abnormal vascular pattern is slightly dilated.

The late angiogram shows some very subtle leakage of fluorescein along the anastomotic channel above the area which has a "corkscrew-type" configuration.

AUTHOR'S NOTE

This is a case of a 32-year-old white male who noticed some blurred vision in his left eye. The patient's medical history was negative. The question arises whether the patient may have thrown a small embolus through one of the peripheral arterials, causing an occlusion with this A-V type of collateralization occurring. There is certainly evidence of some vascular wall incompetence as evidenced by the fluorescein leakage. The patient's vision in the left eye was 20/25, whereas the vision in the right eye was 20/20 without symptoms.

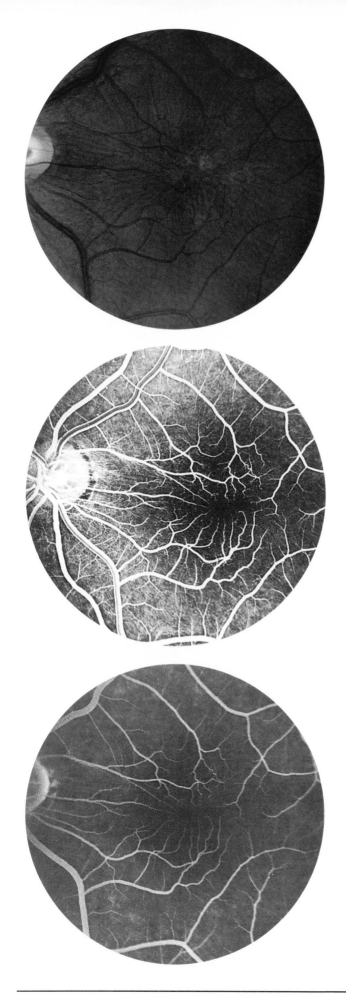

Preretinal Gliosis (minimal contraction without macular edema)

The posterior pole of the left eye shows fine retinal striae. There is a sheen over the macular region, resembling a fine sheet of cellophane.

During the laminar phase of the angiogram, there is tortuosity of the fine perifoveal capillaries with distortion of the normally round perifoveal capillary ring. The vessels in the papillomacular bundle are under stretch.

The late angiogram shows the vessels in the papillomacular bundle being under stretch, as well as the fine tortuosity of the perifoveal vessels. There is no evidence of intraretinal leakage to indicate macular edema.

Preretinal Gliosis (moderate contraction without macular edema)

The vessels in the papillomacular bundle are under stretch. There is definite tortuosity of the paramacular vessels. A fine grayish membrane can be seen just temporal to the fovea with slight traction of the sensory retina temporally.

During the fluorescein angiogram, there is extensive tortuosity of the paramacular capillaries, arterials, and venules. The vessels in the papillomacular bundle are under stretch and dragged temporally.

The late angiogram continues to show the tortuosity of the vessels in the posterior pole. However, there is no evidence of late fluorescein dye leakage.

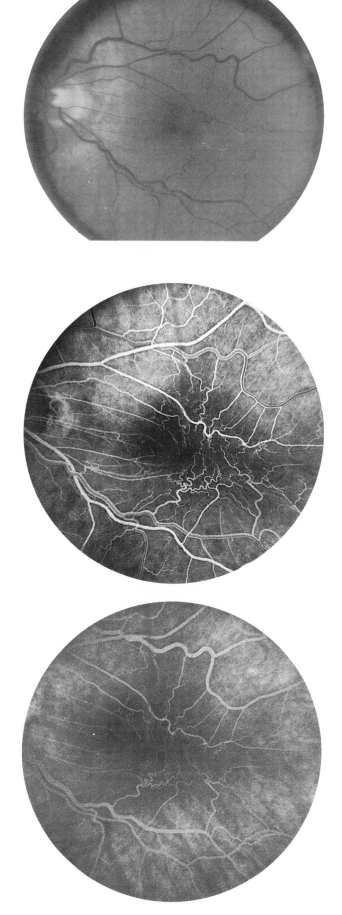

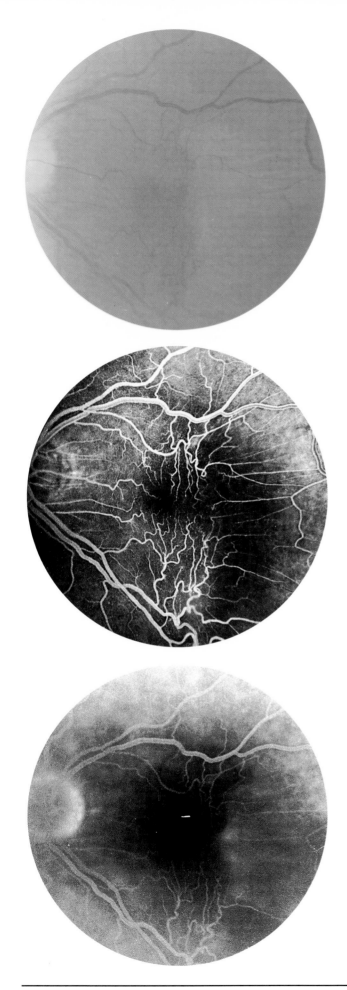

Preretinal Gliosis (moderate contraction with slight macular edema)

The left posterior pole shows a very fine vertical gliotic membrane just temporal to the fovea. The vessels above and below the fovea show tortuosity and are under stretch.

During the fluorescein angiogram, there is distortion of the normally round perifoveal capillary net due to the tortuosity of the vessels. The vessels above and below the fovea are irregular secondary to the contraction of the preretinal membrane.

The late angiogram shows minimal intraretinal accumulation of fluorescein dye temporal to the fovea, indicating slight macular edema.

AUTHOR'S NOTE

In this case, most of the contraction is in a vertical direction. Contraction can be variable, depending on the contraction of the preretinal membrane and location of its epiretinal center.

Preretinal Gliosis (with mild cystoid macular edema)

The posterior pole of the right eye has a grayish color, secondary to the preretinal gliotic membrane. The vessels in the papillomacular bundle appear under stretch.

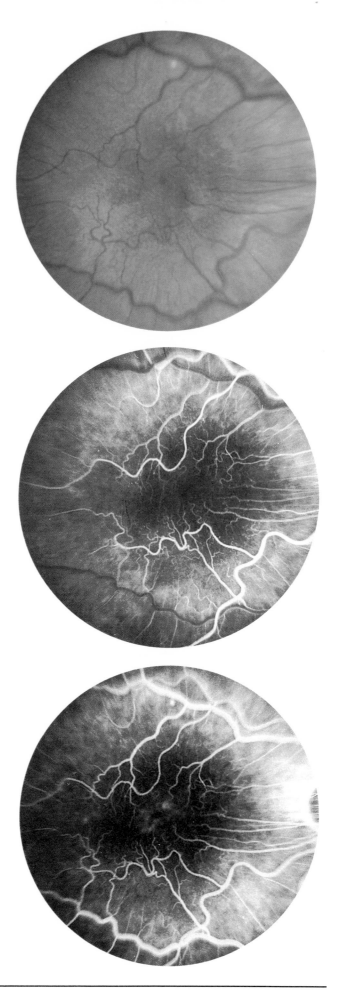

The early laminar phase of the angiogram reveals tortuosity of the fine perifoveal capillaries. The vessels in the papillomacular bundle are under stretch.

The late angiogram shows subtle intraretinal leakage of fluorescein in the perifoveal region, indicating cystoid macular edema.

AUTHOR'S NOTE
The macular edema which occurs in patients with preretinal gliosis is secondary to disruption of the tight endothelial cell junctions being under stretch from the contracting preretinal gliotic membrane.

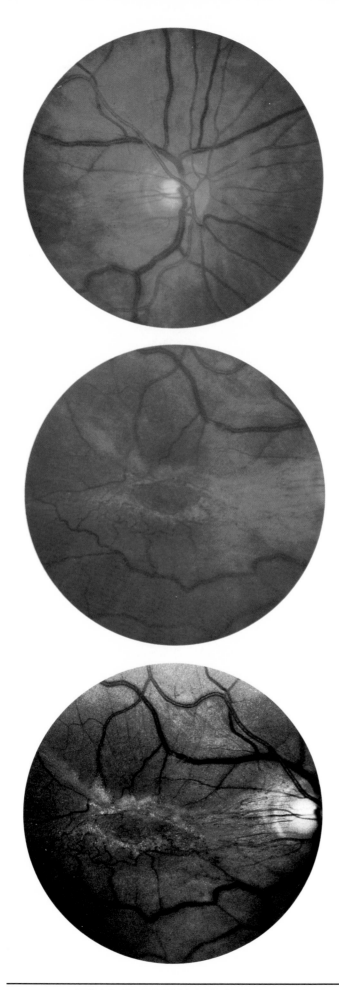

Preretinal Gliosis (with moderate macular edema)

The optic nerve appears normal. The vessels coursing across the temporal edge of the optic nerve and into the papillomacular bundle appear under stretch.

In the posterior pole, a yellowish preretinal membrane can be seen. There is tortuosity of the paramacular vessels, predominantly involving the inferior portion of the macula.

The red-free photograph clearly shows the preretinal or epiretinal membrane.

During the early laminar phase of the fluorescein angiogram, there is tortuosity of the paramacular vessels. The vessels in the papillomacular bundle are under stretch.

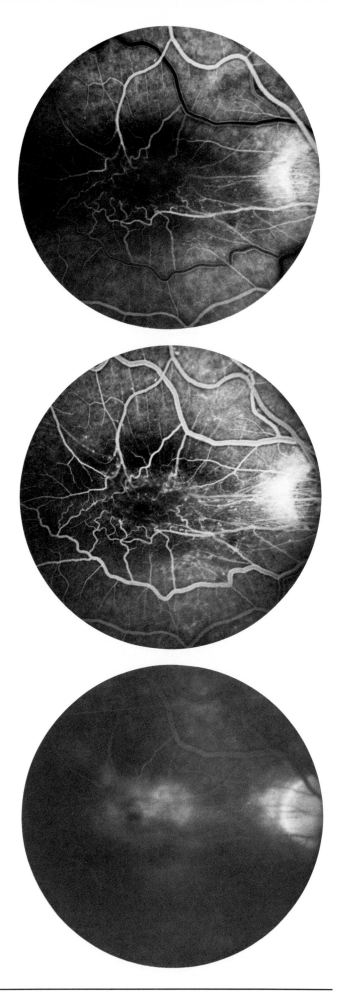

During the venous phase of the angiogram, there is intraretinal leakage of fluorescein from the tortuous small caliber venules and capillaries.

The late angiogram shows intraretinal accumulation of fluorescein dye, indicating macular edema.

AUTHOR'S NOTE

The red-free photograph frequently demonstrates a fine preretinal gliotic membrane which may be difficult to appreciate clinically. This is taken using the green filter of the fundus camera.

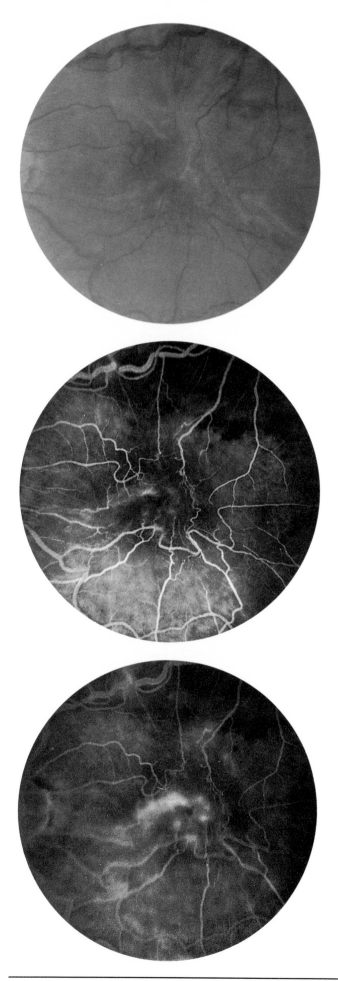

Preretinal Gliosis (with macular edema secondary to previous scleral buckling procedure)

The yellowish preretinal gliotic membrane can be seen wrinkling the sensory retina in the posterior pole. Along the superior temporal arcades, in the subretinal space, is increased pigmentation secondary to pigmentary fallout during the trans-scleral cryopexy as part of the scleral buckling procedure.

There is extensive tortuosity of the paramacular vessels. There is a slight amount of intraretinal fluorescein leakage. The subretinal pigment, superior to the macula, blocks the background choroidal fluorescence.

The late angiogram demonstrates diffuse intraretinal leakage of fluorescein, indicating macular edema. The paramacular vascular tortuosity can still be seen in the late angiogram.

Reader's Notes

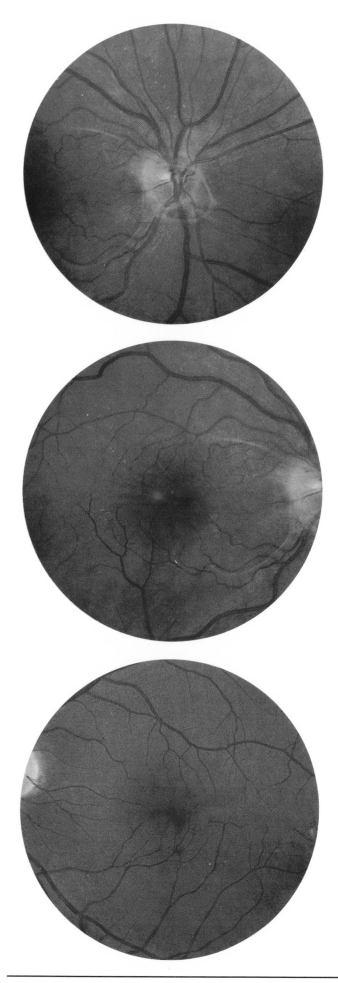

Preretinal Gliosis (etiology unknown; pre- and post-pars plana vitrectomy and membrane peeling)

Overlying the optic nerve is an opacified ring of the posterior hyaloid. Superior to the nerve are pinpoint areas of intraretinal hard exudate.

Extending from the temporal edge of the preretinal ring, overlying the optic nerve, are strands of preretinal membrane. There are very fine striae in the posterior pole. Scattered pinpoint areas of hard exudate can be seen temporal to the macula and along the superior temporal arcades.

The left posterior pole reveals a normal optic nerve and normal retinal vasculature.

During the laminar phase of the fluorescein angiogram, there appears to be some blurriness of the temporal margin of the optic nerve. The retinal vasculature and macular region appear normal.

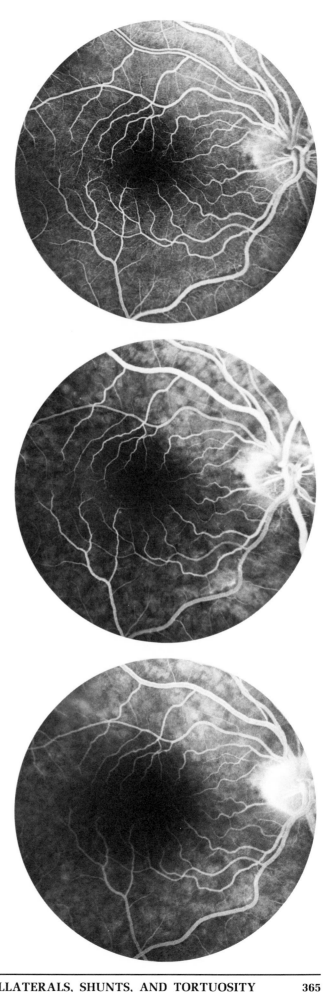

Later in the angiogram, there is some increased hyperfluorescence at the temporal aspect of the nerve. There is no leakage of fluorescein in the posterior pole or significant tortuosity of the vessels in the posterior pole.

Later in the angiogram there is retention of the hyperfluorescence at the temporal aspect of the optic nerve without significant leakage. The macular region and retinal vasculature in the posterior pole appear normal.

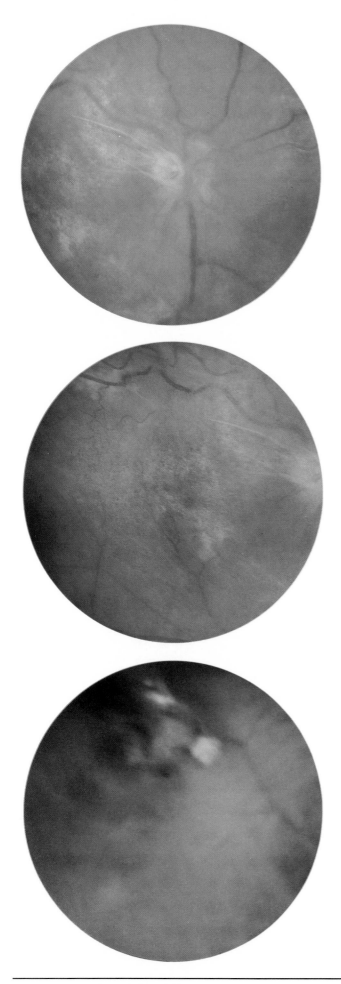

Four months later, there is increased blurriness of the right optic nerve. The previous round ring overlying the optic nerve now appears elliptical, extending temporally.

Overlying the posterior pole is a fairly dense, glistening preretinal membrane. There is some traction on the superior temporal arcade. There also appears to be an increased amount of hard exudate along the superior temporal arcade.

In the far temporal periphery, a slightly elevated pigmented mass can be seen. Associated with the mass is some slight vitreous hemorrhage and yellowish vitreous opacities.

During the laminar phase of the fluorescein angiogram there is some increased tortuosity and irregularity of the vessels along the superior and inferior temporal arcades, extending toward the macula.

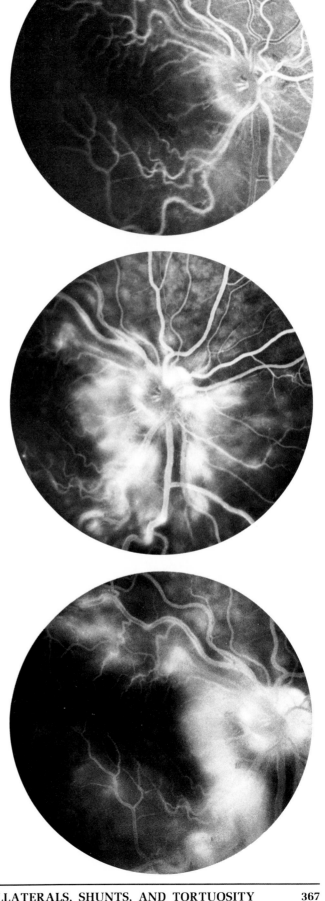

Later in the angiogram, there is diffuse intraretinal leakage of fluorescein around the optic nerve and into the papillomacular bundle.

The late angiogram shows extensive leakage of fluorescein intraretinally in the posterior pole and along the superior and inferior temporal arcades. There are several areas of staining along the superior temporal veins, indicating a breakdown in the blood-retinal barrier.

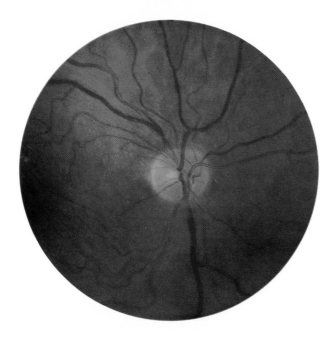

Post-trans pars plana vitrectomy, the optic nerve appears normal. There is no evidence of preretinal membrane formation.

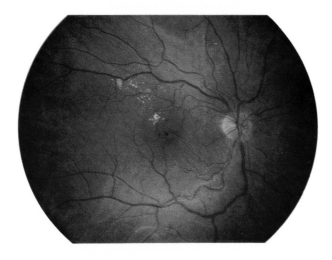

The Canon wide angle photograph gives an overall view of the right posterior pole, showing the postvitrectomy and membrane peeling picture with absence of preretinal membrane and severe contraction of the sensory retina.

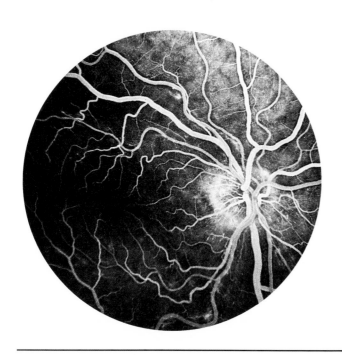

The fluorescein angiogram shows a normal posterior pole and retinal vasculature. There is no significant tortuosity of the vessels or leakage of fluorescein dye. There is a slight increased hyperfluorescence at the level of the pigment epithelium and choroid which does not increase later in the angiogram.

AUTHOR'S NOTE

This is a case of a 32-year-old white female who initially presented with some slight blurriness of vision in the right eye. The patient's ocular history was entirely normal. There was never an injury or history of intraocular foreign body in the right eye. There was initially minimal vitreous reaction in the right eye. The initial vision was 20/25. Over a period of 4 months, the patient's vision decreased dramatically to 20/100 with an increase in the formation of the preretinal gliotic membrane and contraction of the sensory retina. Indirect ophthalmoscopy revealed a peripheral pigmented lesion. All laboratory tests and a complete medical work-up were negative. The patient was referred to Thomas Aaberg, M.D., at the Medical College of Wisconsin, for consultation and possible management. Dr. Aaberg performed a trans-pars plana vitrectomy and membrane peeling with significant improvement of the patient's vision to 20/25. The peripheral lesion, because of its close proximity to the lens, was treated extensively with full-thickness scleral cryopexy. There has been complete resolution of the peripheral lesion, and the patient's vision and posterior pole findings have remained stable.

Hamartoma of the Retinal Pigment Epithelium and Sensory Retina (severe contraction of the sensory retina)

The left macular region and retinal vasculature appear normal.

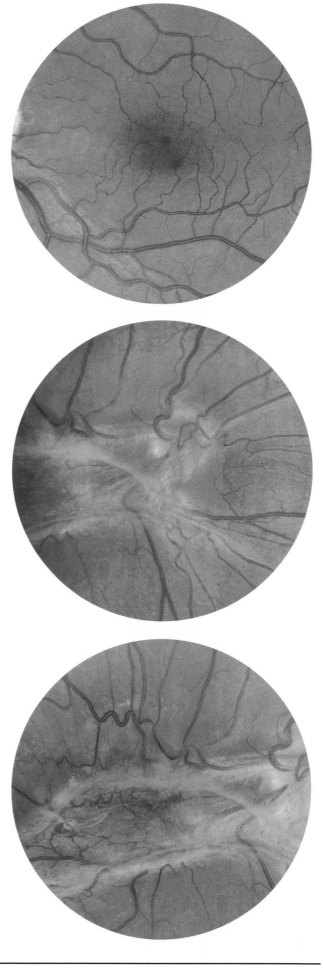

The margins of the optic nerve appear to be slightly blurred. Nasal to the nerve is a vertical area of greenish hyperpigmentation beneath the sensory retina. Extending from the temporal edge of the optic nerve is a coarse preretinal gliotic membrane.

The membrane extends into the macular region with marked tortuosity of the vessels in the posterior pole, along both the superior and inferior temporal arcades. Deep to the gliotic membrane there is a greenish area of hyperpigmentation at the level of the retinal pigment epithelium.

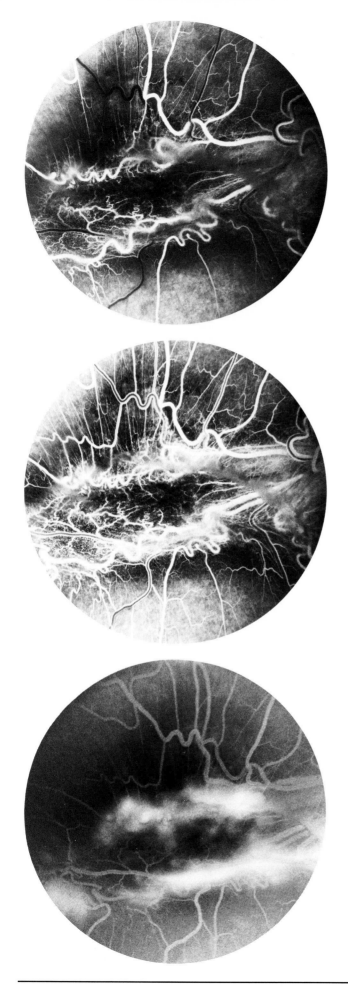

The early laminar phase of the fluorescein angiogram shows marked tortuosity of the smaller caliber vessels in the posterior pole. The superior and inferior temporal arcades are pulled toward the center of the macula by contraction of the preretinal membrane.

Later in the laminar phase of the angiogram there is leakage of fluorescein from the tortuous vessels secondary to a breakdown of the tight endothelial cell junctions. The more dense part of the preretinal membrane, adjacent to the disc, slightly blocks the background choroidal fluorescence.

The late angiogram shows diffuse intraretinal leakage of fluorescein from the smaller caliber vessels which are being disrupted by the preretinal gliotic membrane.

AUTHOR'S NOTE

This is a 12-year-old patient who had a large right esotropia and finger-counting vision. The preliminary diagnosis was retrolental fibroplasia. However, the peripheral retina of the right eye was entirely normal and the left eye was entirely normal. There was also no history of prematurity or oxygen administration. This hamartoma could be considered both macular and juxtapapillary because of the involvement of the optic nerve and the increased hyperpigmentation nasal to the nerve.

Optic Nerve Vascular Loop
(with venous stasis)

The margins of the right optic nerve appear blurred, and there is hyperemia. A tortuous vascular loop can be seen extending from the nasal aspect of the disc into the vitreous. The retinal veins appear slightly engorged. There is dilatation of the capillary bed surrounding the optic nerve.

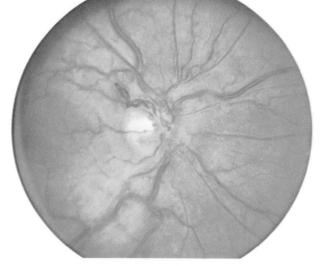

Along the inferior temporal arcade a few pinpoint intraretinal hemorrhages are visible. The retinal veins appear to be slightly engorged. There is some cystic change involving the center of the macula.

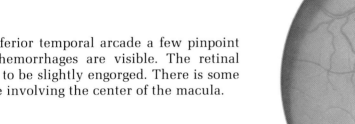

Along the superior temporal arcade a few intraretinal dot hemorrhages and microaneurysms are present.

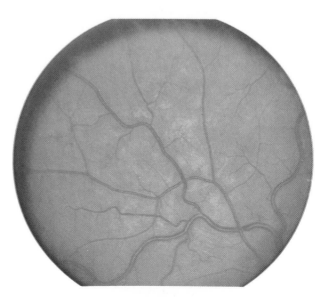

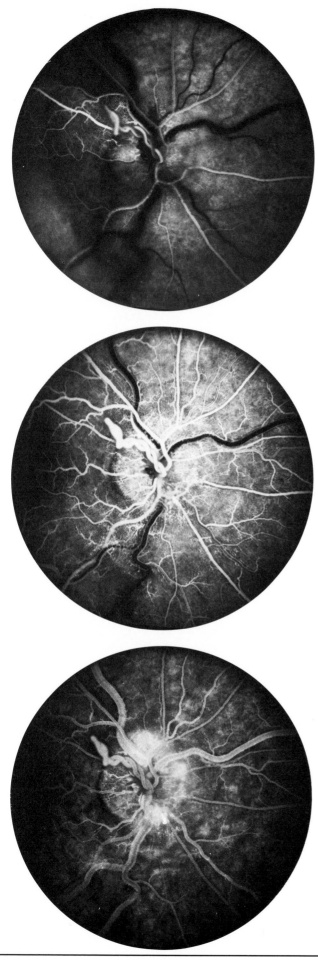

During the arterial phase of the fluorescein angiogram there is filling of the vascular loop which extends into the vitreous. The capillary bed in the superior portion of the papillomacular bundle is also filled with the fluorescein dye.

During the early laminar phase of the angiogram there is complete filling of the vascular loop without evidence of fluorescein leakage. There is an abnormal dilatation of the capillaries surrounding the optic nerve and also the capillaries on the surface of the optic nerve.

The late angiogram shows subtle staining and leakage of fluorescein from the capillaries on the surface of the optic nerve. There is also some staining of the venous walls, indicating a breakdown in the blood-retinal barrier. There is no evidence of leakage from the elevated vascular loop.

AUTHOR'S NOTE

This is a case of a male patient in his late twenties who had a sudden drop of vision in his right eye. It was obvious that the patient had sustained some type of venous compromise with the retinal veins being engorged and slightly tortuous. There were scattered intraretinal hemorrhages 360° around the mid-periphery. Complications secondary to vascular loops of the optic nerve have been reported in the literature. However, the association of a vascular loop with a venous obstructive or venous stasis type of picture is extremely rare. It is conceivable that the vascular loop is completely unrelated to the venous problem. The nonspecific diagnosis of papillophlebitis has also been considered in this particular patient, in view of a completely negative medical evaluation.

Bibliography

Allen AW Jr, Gass JDM: Contraction of perifoveal epiretinal membrane simulating a macular hole. *Am J Ophthalmol* 82:684, 1976.

Anderson DR: Ultrastructure of the optic nerve head. *Arch Ophthalmol* 83:63, 1970.

Archer DD, Deutman A, Ernest JT, et al: Arteriovenous communications of the retina. *Am J Ophthalmol* 75:224, 1973.

Bellhorn MB, Friedman AH, Wise GN, et al: Ultrastructure and clinicopathologic correlation of idiopathic preretinal macular fibrosis. *Am J Ophthalmol* 79:366, 1975.

Brown GC, Magargal L, Augsburger JJ, et al: Preretinal arterial loops and retinal arterial occlusion. *Am J Ophthalmol* 87:646, 1979.

Buettner H: Congenital hypertrophy of the retinal pigment epithelium. *Am J Ophthalmol* 79:177, 1975.

Cardell BS, Starbruck MJ: Juxtapapillary hamartoma of the retina. *Br J Ophthalmol* 45:672, 1961.

Clarkson JG, Green WR, Massof D: A histopathologic review of 168 cases of preretinal membrane. *Am J Ophthalmol* 84:1, 1977.

Curtin VT: Pathologic changes following retinal detachment surgery. In *Symposium on Retina and Retinal Surgery*. St Louis, CV Mosby, 1969, p 147.

Gass JDM: An unusual hamartoma of the pigment epithelium and retina simulating choroidal melanoma and retinoblastoma. *Trans Am Ophthalmol Soc* 71:171, 1973.

Goldstein I, Wexler D: The preretinal artery. An anatomic study. *Arch Ophthalmol* 1:324, 1929.

Hagler WS, Aturaliya U: Macular puckers after retinal detachment surgery. *Br J Ophthalmol* 55:451, 1971.

Harcourt R, Lochet N: Occlusion of a preretinal arterial loop. *Br J Ophthalmol* 51:562, 1967.

Henkind P, Wise GN: Retinal neovascularization, collaterals and vascular shunts. *Br J Ophthalmol* 58:413, 1974.

Jaffe NS: Macular retinopathy after separation of vitreoretinal adherence. *Arch Ophthalmol* 78:585, 1967.

Laqua H, Machemer R: Clinicalpathological correlation in massive periretinal proliferation. *Am J Ophthalmol* 80:913, 1975.

Laqua H, Machemer R: Glial cell proliferation in retinal detachment (massive periretinal proliferation). *Am J Ophthalmol* 80:602, 1975.

Laqua H, Wessing A: Congenital retino-pigment epithelial malformation, previously described as hamartoma. *Am J Ophthalmol* 87:34–42, 1979.

Lobes LA Jr, Burton TC: The incidence of macular pucker after reattachment surgery. *Am J Ophthalmol* 85:72, 1978.

Machemer R: Die primare retinale Pigment-epithelhyperplasie. *Albrecht von Graefes Arch Klin Ophthalmol* 167:1964.

Machemer R: Die chirurgische Entfernung von epiretinalen Makulamembranes (macular puckers). *Klin Monatsbl Augenheilkd* 173:36, 1978.

Machemer R, Laqua H: Pigment epithelial proliferation in retinal detachment (massive periretinal proliferation). *Am J Ophthalmol* 80:1, 1975.

Machemer R, Laqua H: A logical approach to the treatment of massive periretinal proliferation. *Ophthalmology* 85:584, 1978.

Machemer R, Van Horn D, Aaberg TM: Pigment epithelial proliferation in human retinal detachment with massive periretinal proliferation. *Am J Ophthalmol* 85:181, 1978.

Maumenee AE: Further advances in the study of the macula. *Arch Ophthalmol* 78:151, 1967.

McLean EB: Hamartoma of the retinal pigment epithelium. *Am J Ophthalmol* 82:227, 1976.

Michels RG, Gilbert HD: Surgical management of macular pucker after retinal reattachment surgery. *Am J Ophthalmol* 88:925–929, 1979.

Norris JL, Cleasby GW: An unusual case of congenital hypertrophy of the retinal pigment epithelium. *Arch Ophthalmol* 94:190, 1976.

Roth AM, Foos RY: Surface wrinkling retinopathy in eyes enucleated at autopsy. *Trans Am Acad Ophthalmol Otolaryngol* 75:1047, 1971.

Tanenbaum HL, Schepens CL, Elzeneiny I, et al: Macular pucker following retinal detachment surgery. *Arch Ophthalmol* 83:286, 1970.

Theobald GD, Floyd GG, Kirk HQ: Hyperplasia of the retinal pigment epithelium. *Am J Ophthalmol* 45:235, 1958.

Van Horn DL, Aaberg TM, Machemer R, et al: Glial cell proliferation in human retinal detachment with massive periretinal proliferation. *Am J Ophthalmol* 85:181, 1978.

Vogel MH, Wessing A: Die Proliferation des juxtapapillaren retinalen Pigmentepithels. *Klin Monatsbl Augenheilkd.* 162:736, 1973.

Vogel MH, Zimmerman LE, Gass JDM: Proliferation of the juxtapapillary pigment epithelium simulating malignant melanoma. *Doc Ophthalmol* 26:461, 1969.

Wallow IHL, T'so MOM: Proliferation of the retinal pigment epithelium over malignant choroidal tumors. A light and electron microscopic study. *Am J Ophthalmol* 73:914, 1972.

Wise GN: Preretinal macular fibrosis (an analysis of 90 cases). *Trans Ophthalmol Soc UK* 92:131, 1972.

Wise GN: Clinical features of idiopathic preretinal macular fibrosis. *Am J Ophthalmol* 79:349, 1975.

Wise GN: Relationship of idiopathic preretinal macular fibrosis to posterior vitreous detachment. *Am J Ophthalmol* 79:358, 1975.

Reader's Notes

CHAPTER 9

Cystoid Macular Edema

Differential Diagnosis

A. DIABETES MELLITUS
B. VITRITIS
C. TELANGIECTASIS
D. EALES' DISEASE
E. RADIATION RETINOPATHY
F. MACROANEURYSM
G. SOLAR RETINOPATHY
H. VENOUS OCCLUSION
I. ARTERIAL OCCLUSION
J. TUMORS
K. NICOTINIC ACID
L. TOPICAL EPINEPHRINE
M. COLLAGEN VASCULAR DISEASE
N. INTRAOCULAR INFLAMMATION (PARS PLANITIS, SEVERE UVEITIS, ETC.)
O. HYPOTONY

P. IRVINE-GASS SYNDROME
Q. PAPILLITIS
R. OCULAR SURGERY (SCLERAL BUCKLING; KERATOPLASTY, ETC.)
S. INTERNAL LIMITING MEMBRANE CONTRACTION
T. HEREDITARY (RETINITIS PIGMENTOSA)
U. LONG-STANDING ELEVATION OF THE SENSORY RETINA (SUBRETINAL NEOVASCULARIZATION; CHOROIDAL TUMORS)
V. DOMINANT VITREAL RETINOPATHY
W. IDIOPATHIC

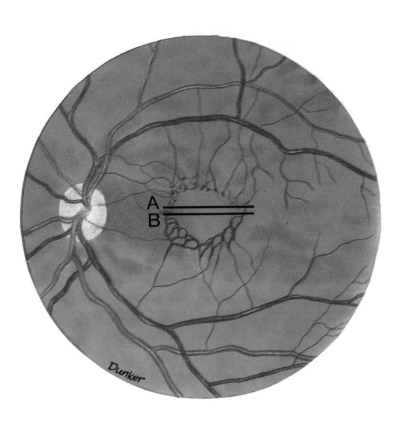

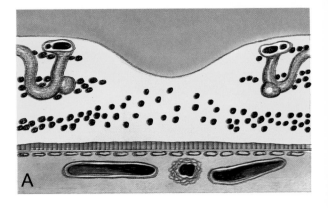

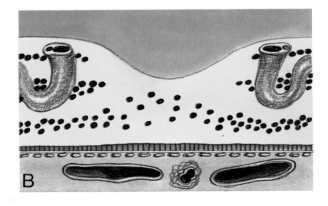

Cystoid macular edema, in many cases, results from a combination of two factors: (1) intraocular inflammation and (2) increased capillary permeability in the paramacular region.

Cystoid macular edema is frequently secondary to microaneurysmal changes seen in such diseases as diabetes mellitus and branch vein occlusion (A). Cystoid macular edema can also be seen in disorders causing dilatation of the perifoveal capillaries resulting in a breakdown in the endothelial cell junctions, leading to leakage of fluorescein dye (B).

The orientation of the outer plexiform layer of the sensory retina in the macular region is responsible for the typical "flower-petal" appearance of cystoid macular edema seen both clinically and on fluorescein angiography.

Cystoid Macular Edema
(secondary to aphakia)

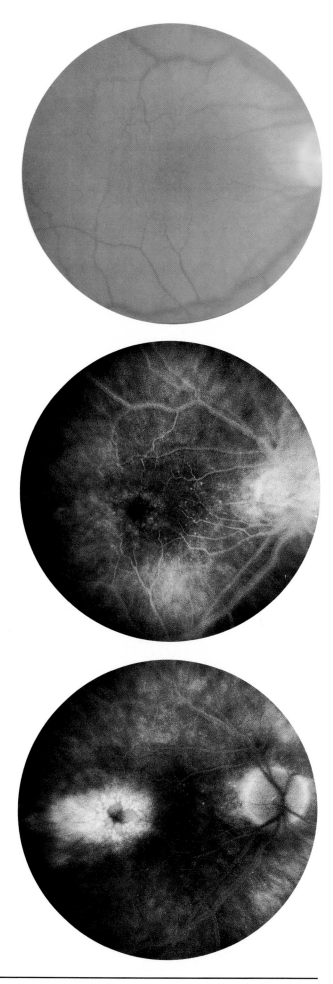

The posterior pole of the right eye shows some slight thickening of the sensory retina in the macular region. There is a loss of the normal foveal reflex and macular ring reflex.

During the venous phase of the fluorescein angiogram, there is definite dilatation of the perifoveal capillaries. A few small punctate areas of hyperfluorescence can also be seen nasal to the foveal region. These areas are secondary to drusen which are hyperfluorescing.

The late angiogram reveals a classic cystoid macular edema pattern with fairly large cystic spaces filling with fluorescein dye around the center of the fovea.

AUTHOR'S NOTE

Aphakic cystoid macular edema is most likely secondary to a low grade inflammation, causing secondary changes in the capillary permeability in the posterior pole.

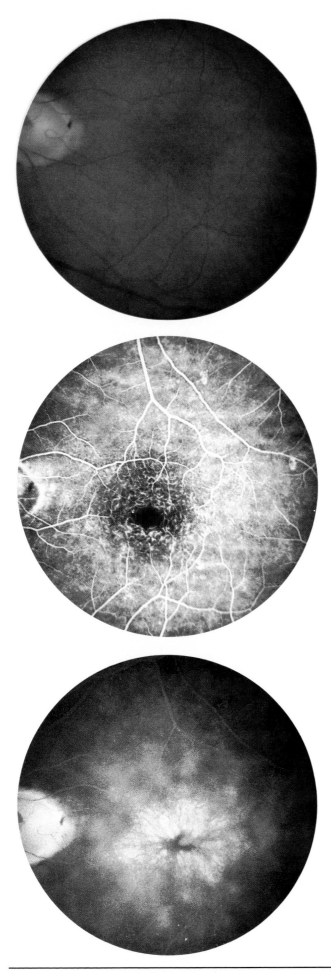

Cystoid Macular Edema
(post-lens extraction with intraocular lens implantation)

There is evidence of peripapillary atrophy. The posterior pole shows an absence of the foveal reflex and the macular ring reflex. Otherwise, no significant abnormality can be seen.

During the venous phase of the fluorescein angiogram, there is definite evidence of dilatation of the perifoveal capillary bed. Two areas of pigment epithelial window defects can be seen at approximately the one o'clock and three o'clock positions.

The late angiogram shows a typical cystoid macular edema pattern, with the cysts pointing toward the center of the fovea. There is also a more diffuse intraretinal edema beyond the cystic changes.

AUTHOR'S NOTE

This patient had an intraocular lens, which was secured in position with an iris suture. As in this particular case, many patients with cystoid macular edema show very little clinical evidence of cystic spaces. However, on fluorescein angiography, the diagnosis is easily made.

Reader's Notes

Cystoid Macular Edema
(secondary to aphakia—
pre- and post-treatment)

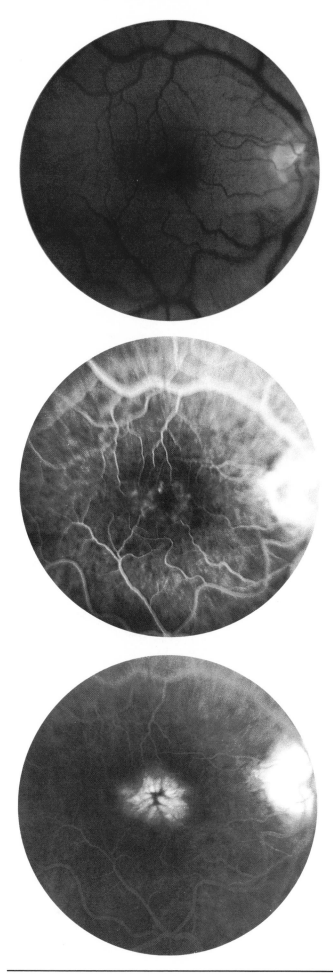

The right eye shows very small cystic spaces in the perifoveal region. The remainder of the posterior pole is normal.

During the venous phase of the angiogram, there is evidence of dilatation of the perifoveal capillaries with slight leakage of fluorescein dye.

The late angiogram shows a classic cystoid macular edema pattern.

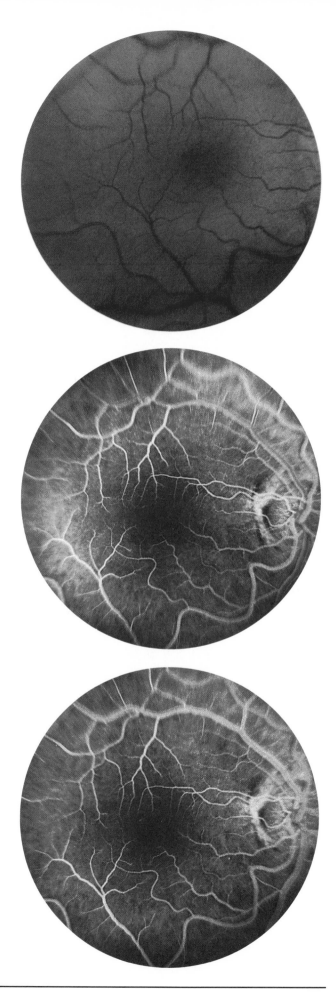

Three weeks after treatment with antiprostaglandin medication, the perifoveal region appears normal.

During the laminar phase of the angiogram, there is no abnormal dilatation of the perifoveal capillary bed.

The later phase of the angiogram shows no leakage of fluorescein and an essentially "dry" macula.

AUTHOR'S NOTE

The patient's initial vision with cystoid macular edema was 20/80. The patient was started on antiprostaglandin medication, i.e. Nalfon, 600 mg t.i.d., for 3 weeks. The post-treatment visual acuity returned to 20/25 with dramatic improvement in the patient's symptoms. Not all patients respond to antiprostaglandin medication. However, if there are no contraindications, it is worthwhile trying to reduce the cystoid macular edema with some type of antiprostaglandin medication.

Cystoid Macular Edema
(secondary to pars planitis)

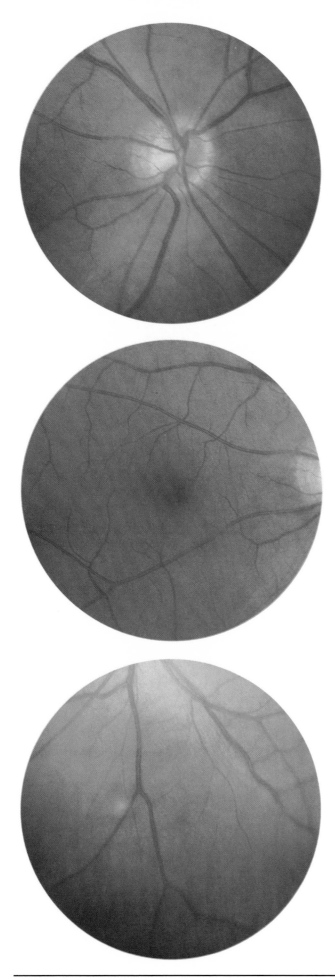

The right optic nerve appears normal. There is a rim of peripapillary atrophic change. The retinal vasculature appears normal.

The macular region shows no significant abnormality. The retinal vasculature in the posterior pole appears normal.

Overlying the inferior retina is a round, intravitreal inflammatory focus.

During the laminar phase of the angiogram, there is dilatation of the perifoveal capillaries.

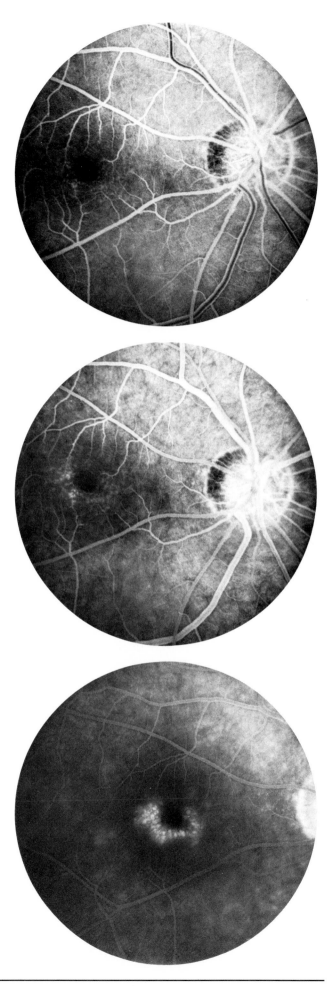

Later in the angiogram, there is intraretinal leakage of fluorescein from the dilated capillaries. The remainder of the retinal vasculature appears normal.

The late fluorescein angiogram shows small intraretinal cystic spaces filling with the fluorescein dye. There is no evidence of a central confluent cyst.

AUTHOR'S NOTE

This is a case of a 23-year-old female who complained of some blurriness of vision in the right eye. Indirect ophthalmoscopy and scleral depression revealed definite peripheral uveitis or pars planitis. The patient's vision was 20/30, probably due to the fact that the cystic spaces were very small and the center of the fovea was uninvolved.

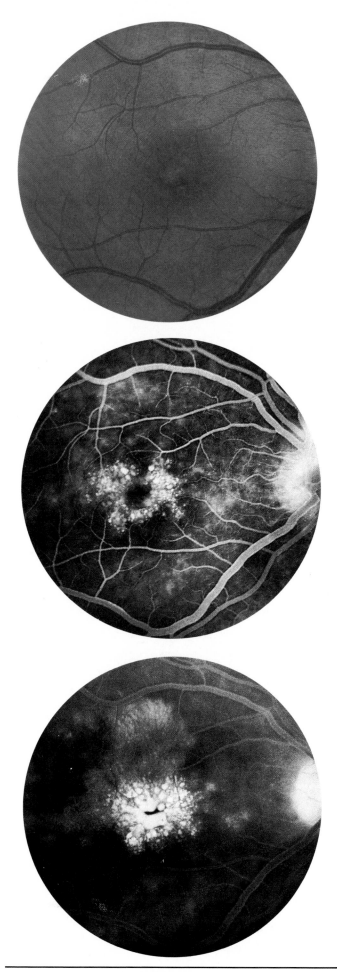

Cystoid Macular Edema
(secondary to intraocular inflammation)

There is hypopigmentation present in the center of the macula. Small intraretinal cystic spaces can be seen in a "honeycomb" type of pattern.

The venous phase of the fluorescein angiogram shows leakage in the paramacular region and throughout the posterior pole. There also appears to be some dilatation of the capillaries with leakage of fluorescein on the temporal aspect of the optic nerve.

The late angiogram shows multiple cystic spaces of different sizes, filling with fluorescein. There is a more diffuse intraretinal leakage of fluorescein dye throughout the sensory retina, extending to the superior and inferior arcades.

The left posterior pole shows hypopigmentation in the center of the macula.

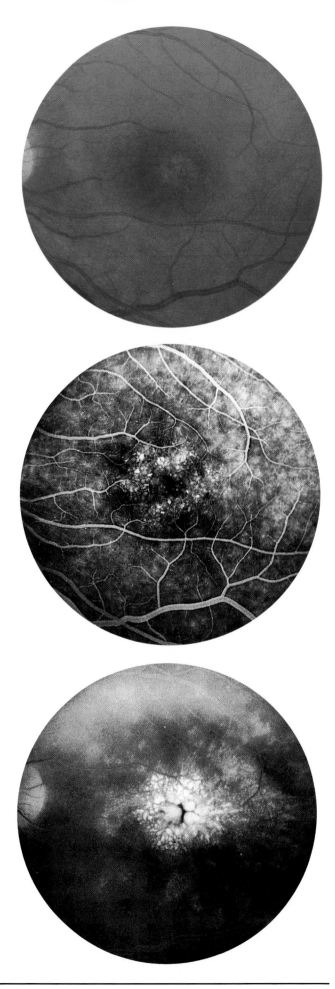

During the venous phase of the angiogram, there is evidence of hyperfluorescence from small cystic spaces filling with fluorescein, as well as dilatation of the perifoveal capillaries.

The late angiogram of the left eye shows large cystic spaces encroaching on the center of the fovea. These large cysts are surrounded by smaller cysts. There is also a diffuse, faint hyperfluorescence throughout the posterior pole, indicating that the sensory retina throughout the posterior pole, and not just the macula, is involved in the leakage of fluorescein dye.

AUTHOR'S NOTE

This is a case of a young white female in her mid-twenties who has had bilateral cystoid macular edema for at least 5 years. No definite etiology can be found. The patient shows no evidence of pars planitis, but she does have a diffuse bilateral vitreal inflammatory reaction. There has been virtually no significant response to any type of periocular or systemic anti-inflammatory medication.

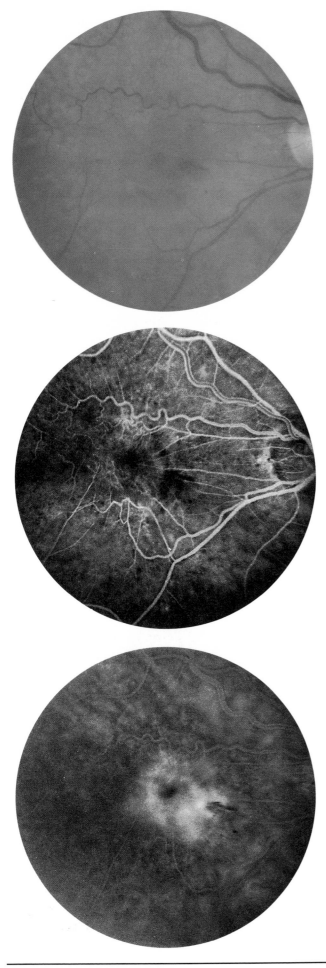

Cystoid Macular Edema
(secondary to idiopathic preretinal gliosis)

In the posterior pole of the right eye there is some tortuosity, or "corkscrewing," of the retinal vessels. This is most obvious with the vessels in the superior aspect of the macula. A few scattered intraretinal hemorrhages can also be seen. The vessels in the papillomacular bundle appear to be under stretch, as evidenced by their straight course.

The laminar phase of the fluorescein angiogram shows extensive tortuosity and "corkscrewing" of the paramacular vessels. The retinal vessels appear to be pulled toward the center of the macula.

The late angiogram shows definite intraretinal accumulation of fluorescein. There is some blockage of the background choroidal fluorescence by the small, punctate intraretinal hemorrhages.

AUTHOR'S NOTE

The cystoid macular edema as evidenced by fluorescein leakage is most likely secondary to a break in the tight endothelial junctions secondary to direct traction on the vessels by the epiretinal membrane. These small punctate hemorrhages are secondary to direct trauma to the capillary bed by the membrane. No cause for the epiretinal membrane formation could be determined; therefore, a diagnosis of idiopathic preretinal gliosis was made.

Cystoid Macular Edema
(secondary to severe epiretinal membrane formation)

The posterior pole of the right eye shows extensive tortuosity and "corkscrewing" of the retinal vessels above and below the horizontal raphe. Very fine linear striae of the sensory retina can also be seen.

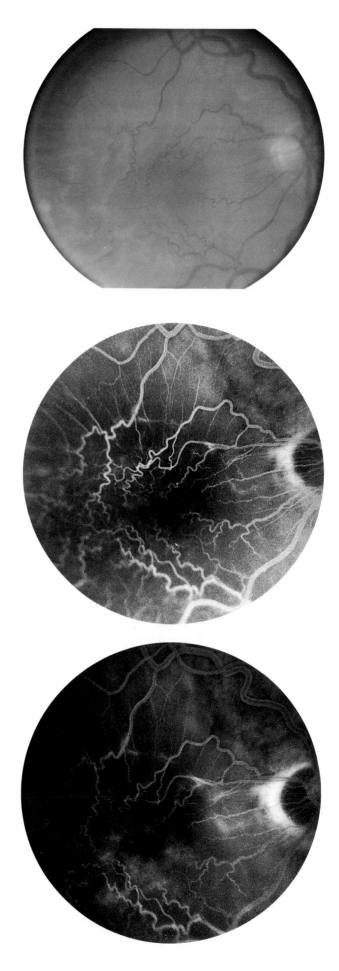

During the venous phase of the angiogram, the amount of vascular tortuosity is apparent. The retinal vessels in the papillomacular bundle appear under stretch.

The late angiogram shows faint leakage of fluorescein in the macular region in a cystic pattern. Several of the retinal vessels show staining changes.

AUTHOR'S NOTE

The amount of tortuosity of the vessels and the epiretinal membrane formation does not always indicate that there will be extensive macular edema. The amount of edema does not necessarily depend on the tortuosity, but rather on the disruption of the tight endothelial junctions and zonula occludens.

Cystoid Macular Edema
(associated with retinitis pigmentosa)

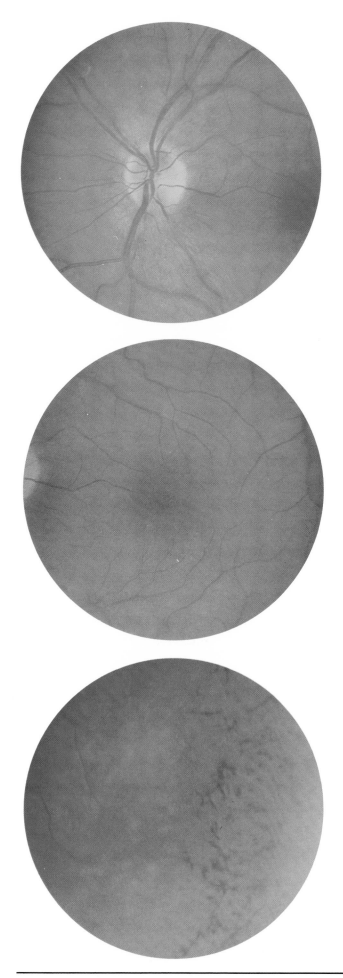

The left optic nerve reveals a slight waxy pallor.

The retinal arteries are definitely narrowed. The posterior pole is essentially normal.

In the temporal periphery of the left eye there is pigmentary migration into the sensory retina in a bone spicule pattern.

During the venous phase of the fluorescein angiogram, there appears to be some abnormal dilatation of the perifoveal capillaries. There is increased hyperfluorescence from the choroid along the inferior temporal arcade.

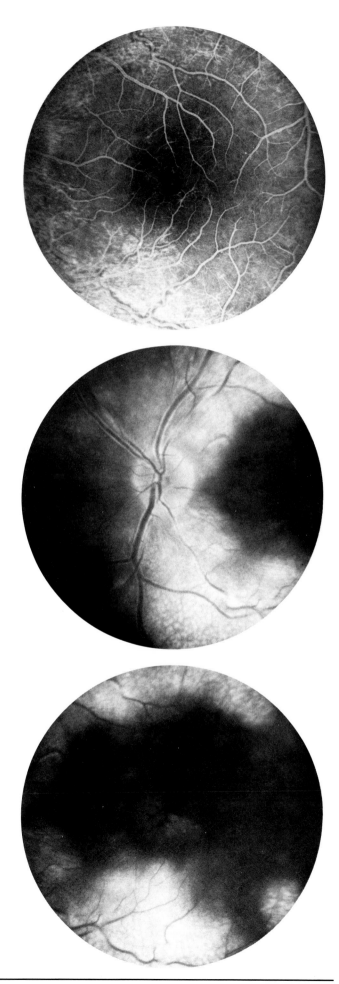

The late angiogram reveals diffuse hyperfluorescence extending from the superior and inferior poles of the optic nerve and along the temporal arcades. This is secondary to retinal pigment epithelial atrophy giving the appearance of a window defect.

The late angiogram also shows a typical cystoid macular edema pattern. There is obvious late hyperfluorescence along the temporal arcades secondary to the pigment epithelial atrophy.

AUTHOR'S NOTE

This patient shows bilateral fundus findings compatible with retinitis pigmentosa, which was documented with electrophysiologic testing. Only the left eye showed evidence of cystoid macular edema. The hyperfluorescent pattern along the temporal arcades secondary to pigment epithelial atrophy is fairly typical of patients with retinitis pigmentosa.

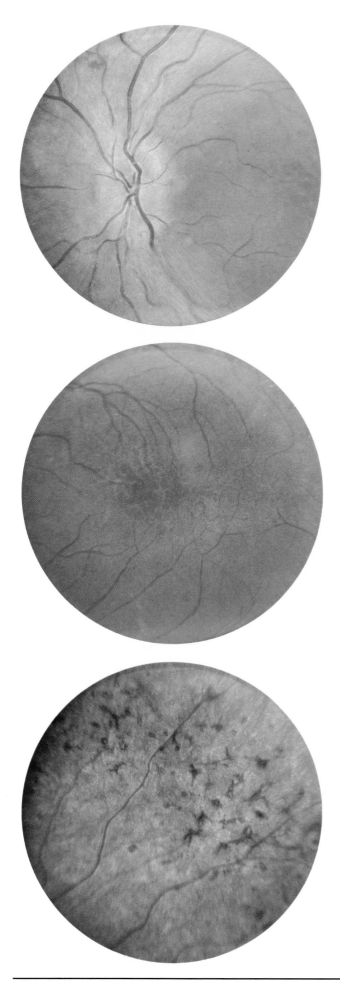

Cystoid Macular Edema— Severe (associated with retinitis pigmentosa)

The optic nerve shows a definite waxy pallor. The branches of the central retinal artery are narrowed. There is some hyperpigmentation superior to the optic nerve.

In the macular region, small intraretinal cystic spaces can be seen.

In the mid-periphery of the left eye, there is pigmentary migration in the typical bone spicule pattern.

During the venous phase of the fluorescein angiogram, there is intraretinal leakage of fluorescein in the perifoveal region, associated with the dilated capillary bed. There are several other areas of pinpoint intraretinal hyperfluorescence from damaged capillaries.

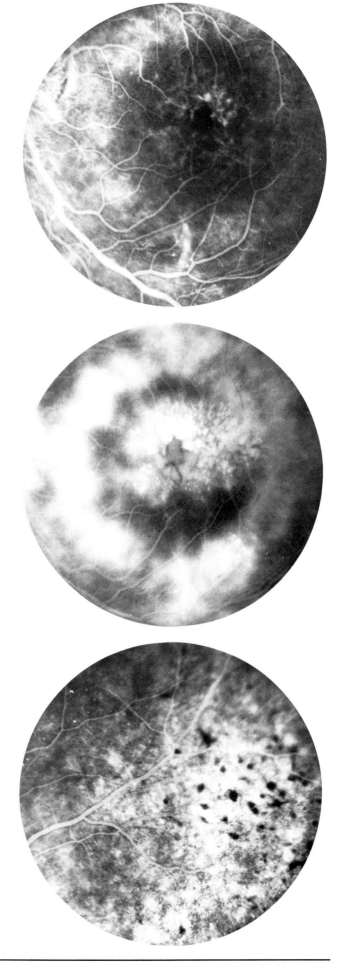

The late angiogram of the left posterior pole shows extensive cystoid macular edema with a large confluent cyst in the center of the fovea. There is increased hyperfluorescence along the superior and inferior temporal arcades at the level of the pigment epithelium. This hyperfluorescent pattern is in a ring-type formation.

The mid-periphery demonstrates an area of diffuse hyperfluorescence deep to the sensory retina secondary to retinal pigment epithelial atrophy. There is blockage of the background fluorescence by the pigmentary migration.

AUTHOR'S NOTE

This patient showed bilateral retinitis pigmentosa with cystoid macular edema. However, the cystoid macular edema was more severe in the left eye. It appears that once there is a confluent cyst in the center of the fovea, no matter what the etiology of the cystoid macular edema might be, the prognosis for return of useful central visual acuity is poor.

Bibliography

Allen A, Jaffe NS: Cystoid macular edema: A preliminary study. *Trans Am Acad Ophthalmol Otolaryngol* 81:133, 1976.

Cocas G, Dhermy P, Bernard JA, et al: Maculopathies osedemateuses, Rapport Annuel. *Bull Soc Ophthalmol Fr (numero special)* 1972.

Delman M, Leubusher K: Transient macular edema due to griseofulvin. *Am J Ophthalmol* 82:540, 1976.

Deutman AF, Pinckers AJLG, Aan De Kerk AL: Dominantly inherited cystoid macular edema. *Am J Ophthalmol* 82:540, 1976.

Ffytche TJ: Cystoid maculopathy in retinitis pigmentosa. *Trans Ophthalmol Soc UK* 42:265, 1972.

Ffytche TJ, Blach RK: The etiology of macular edema. *Trans Ophthalmol Soc UK* 40:637–656, 1970.

Francois J, DeLaey JJ, Verbraeken H: Das Zystoide odem der macula. *Klin Monatsbl Augenheikld* 162:125–138, 1973.

Gass JDM: A fluorescein angiographic study of macular dysfunction secondary to retinal vascular disease. Parts I–VI. *Arch Ophthalmol* 80:535, 1968.

Gass JDM: Fluorescein angiography in endogenous intraocular inflammation. In Aronson SB, Gamble CN, Goodner EK, et al: *Clinical Methods in Uveitis: Fourth Sloan Symposium on Uveitis.* St Louis, CV Mosby, 1968, pp 202–229.

Gass JDM: Nicotinic acid maculopathy. *Am J Ophthalmol* 76:500, 1973.

Gass JDM: Fluorescein angiography: An aid to the retinal surgeon. In Pruett RC, Regan CDJ: *Retina Congress.* New York, Appleton-Century-Crofts, 1974, pp 181–201.

Gass JDM, Norton EWD: Cystoid macular edema and papilledema following cataract extraction: A fluorescein funduscopic and angiographic study. *Arch Ophthalmol* 76:646, 1966.

Gass JDM, Norton EWD: Follow-up study of cystoid macular edema following cataract extraction. *Trans Am Acad Ophthalmol Otolaryngol* 73:665–682, 1969.

Harris W, Taylor BC, Winslow RL: Cystoid macular edema following intraocular lens implantation. *Ophthalmic Surg* 8:134, 1977.

Hitchings RA, Chisholm IH: Incidence of aphakic macular edema. *Br J Ophthalmol* 59:444–450, 1975.

Hitchings RA, Chisholm IH, Bird AC: Aphakic macular edema: Incidence and pathogenesis. *Invest Ophthalmol* 14:68, 1975.

Hyvarinen L, Maumenee IH, Kelly J, et al: Fluorescein angiographic findings in retinitis pigmentosa. *Am J Ophthalmol* 71:17, 1971.

Irvine AR: Cystoid maculopathy. *Surv Ophthalmol* 21:1–17, 1976.

Irvine SR: A newly defined vitreous syndrome following cataract surgery. *Am J Ophthalmol* 36:599–619, 1953.

Jacobson DR, Dellaporta A: Natural history of cystoid macular edema after cataract extraction. *Am J Ophthalmol* 77:445–447, 1974.

Kirsch RE, Steinman W: Spontaneous rupture of the anterior hyaloid membrane following intracapsular cataract surgery. *Am J Ophthalmol* 37:657–665, 1954.

Klein RM, Yannuzzi L: Cystoid macular edema in the first week after cataract extraction. *Am J Ophthalmol* 81:614, 1976.

Kolker AE, Becker B: Epinephrine maculopathy. *Arch Ophthalmol* 79:552–562, 1968.

Mackool RJ, Muldoon T, Fortier A, et al: Epinephrine induced cystoid macular edema in aphakic eyes. *Arch Ophthalmol* 95:791, 1977.

Maumenee AE: Clinical entities in "uveitis." *Am J Ophthalmol* 69:1, 1970.

Meredith T, Kenyon K, Singerman L, et al: Perifoveal vascular leakage and macular edema after intracapsular cataract extraction. *Br J Ophthalmol* 60:765, 1976.

Michels RG, Green WR, Maumenee AE: Cystoid macular edema following cataract extraction: Clinical/histological correlation. *Ophthalmic Surg* 2:217, 1971.

Michels RG, Maumenee AE: Cystoid macular edema associated with topically applied epinephrine in aphakic eyes. *Am J Ophthalmol* 80:379, 1975.

Michels RG, Ryan SJ: Results and complications of 100 consecutive cases of pars plana vitrectomy. *Am J Ophthalmol* 80:24, 1975.

Newsom WA, Hood CI, Horwitz JA, et al: Cystoid macular edema: Histopathologic and angiographic correlations: A clinicopathologic case report. *Trans Am Acad Ophthalmol Otolaryngol* 76: 1005–1009, 1972.

Nicholls JVV: Macular edema in association with cataract extraction. *Am J Ophthalmol* 37:665–672, 1954.

Nicholls JVV: Concurrence of macular edema and cataract extraction. *Arch Ophthalmol* 57:148, 1957.

Norton AL, Brown WJ, Carlson M, et al: Pathogenesis of aphakic macular edema. *Am J Ophthalmol* 80:96–101, 1975.

Notting JG, Pinckers AJLG: Dominant cystoid macular dystrophy. *Am J Ophthalmol* 83:234, 1977.

Pruett RC, Brockhurst RJ, Letts NF: Fluorescein angiography of peripheral uveitis. *Am J Ophthalmol* 77:448, 1974.

Ryan SJ Jr: Cystoid maculopathy in phakic retinal detachment procedures. *Am J Ophthalmol* 76:519, 1973.

Tolentino FI, Schepens CL: Edema of posterior pole after cataract extraction. *Arch Ophthalmol* 74:781, 1965.

West CE, Fitzgerald GR, Sewell JH: Cystoid macular edema following aphakic keratoplasty. *Am J Ophthalmol* 75:77–81, 1973.

Wise GN: Clinical features of idiopathic preretinal macular fibrosis. *Am J Ophthalmol* 79:349, 1975.

Yannuzzi LA, Klein R, Wallyn R, et al: Ineffectiveness of indomethacin treatment in chronic cystoid macular edema. *Am J Ophthalmol* 84:517, 1977.

CHAPTER 10
Miscellaneous

Chapter 10 consists of examples of cases which do not conveniently fall into the previous nine chapters.

Optic Nerve Head Drusen

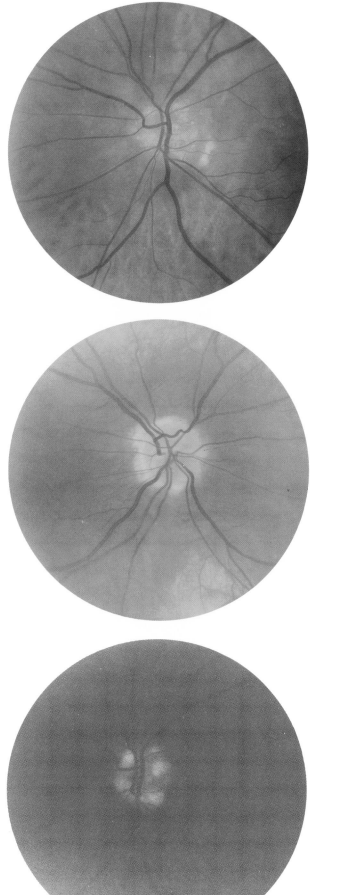

The optic nerve of the left eye demonstrates a fullness with some blurred disc margins which appear scalloped. Small, round, calcific deposits can be seen at the nasal and temporal margins of the nerve. The retinal vasculature appears normal.

The right optic nerve demonstrates some slight blurriness of the disc margin and a scalloped appearance. There also appears to be some very slight peripapillary atrophy. The optic nerve has a yellowish appearance and also appears to be slightly elevated.

Optic nerve head drusen demonstrate autofluorescence, which is obtained prior to injecting the fluorescein dye using the blue excitor filter and the green barrier filter in place.

During the laminar phase of the fluorescein angiogram of the left eye there is some hyperfluorescence surrounding the optic nerve, indicating peripapillary atrophy. There appears to be some slight increase in the hyperfluorescence within the substance of the nerve.

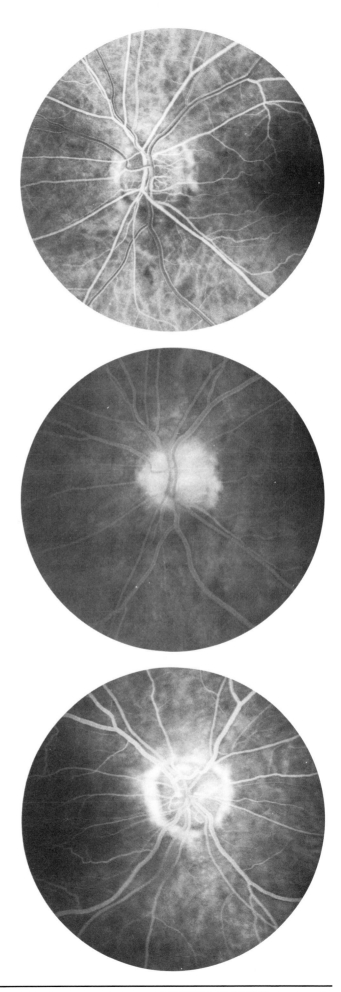

The late angiogram of the left nerve shows an abnormal hyperfluorescence due to the presence of the drusen bodies. The scalloped edge of the nerve is apparent.

The right eye shows small densities of hyperfluorescence within the optic nerve tissue, indicating the presence of the drusen bodies.

AUTHOR'S NOTE

Optic nerve head drusen, as well as astrocytic hamartomas, demonstrate autofluorescence. Optic nerve head drusen must be considered in the differential diagnosis of disc edema. One of the accompanying complications of optic nerve head drusen is the presence of subretinal neovascularization.

Macular Hard Exudate
(secondary to ocular toxoplasmosis)

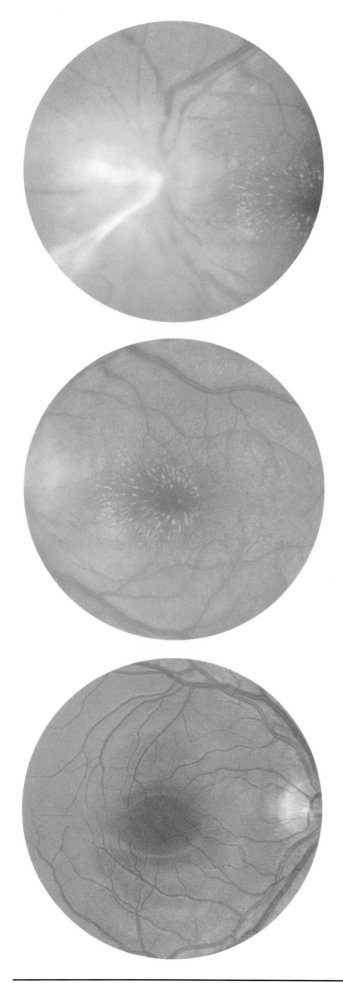

The view of the left optic nerve is somewhat obscured due to the presence of vitreous reaction from intraocular inflammation. Fibrous tissue can be seen in the vicinity of the optic nerve and extending into the vitreous. Nasal to the optic nerve is a whitish, intraretinal inflammatory nodule.

In the macular region of the left eye, there is deposition of intraretinal hard exudate in a ring or star-shaped configuration. Very fine striae at the level of the internal limiting membrane can be seen in the temporal macular region.

The optic nerve, macular region, and retinal vasculature appear normal.

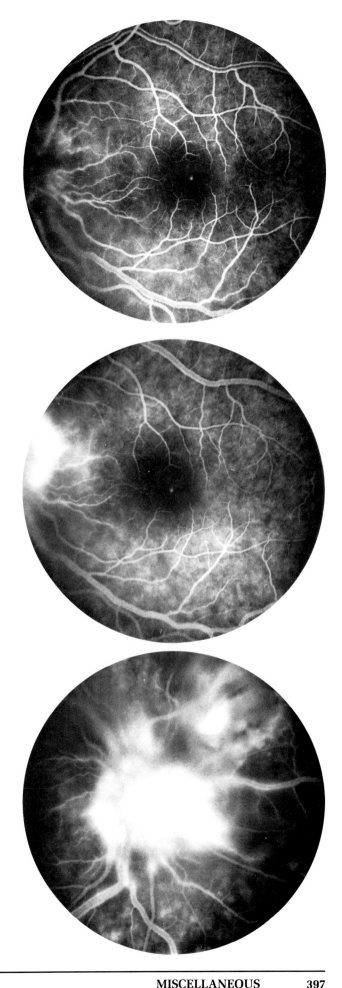

During the laminar phase of the fluorescein angiogram, there is a pinpoint area of hyperfluorescence close to the center of the macula. There appears to be some dilatation of the capillaries with hyperfluorescent change on the temporal aspect of the optic nerve.

Later in the angiogram, there is leakage of fluorescein from the dilated capillaries on the surface of the left optic nerve with staining of the optic nerve tissue. The pinpoint area of hyperfluorescence in the center of the fovea remains essentially the same.

The late angiogram shows diffuse leakage of fluorescein from the dilated capillaries on the surface of the optic nerve. There is also leakage of fluorescein from the inflammatory focus involving the nasal retina. Intraretinal leakage of fluorescein can also be seen inferior nasal to the optic nerve. There is some slight staining of the vein coursing nasal to the optic nerve, indicating a slight breakdown in the blood-retinal barrier from the intraocular inflammation.

AUTHOR'S NOTE

This is an unusual presentation of macular hard exudate associated with ocular toxoplasmosis. This patient has had repeated attacks of ocular toxoplasmosis, which have been diagnosed clinically and also with serologic testing. After implementing the standard quadruple treatment for ocular toxoplasmosis, the intraocular inflammation subsided and the hard exudate in the right eye disappeared.

Macular Neuroretinitis
(unilateral)

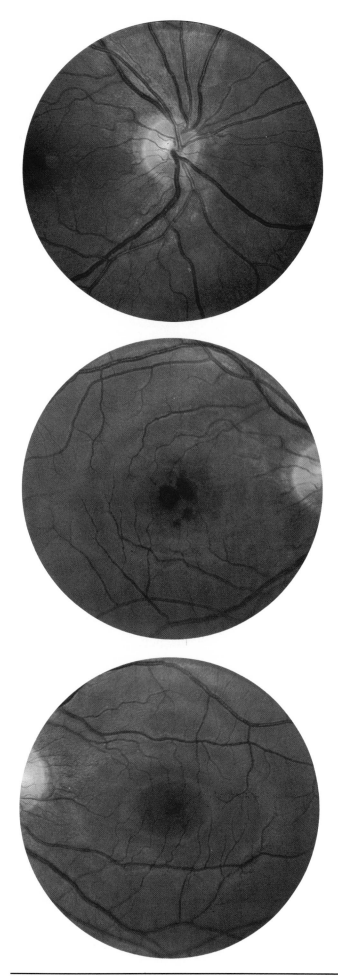

The right optic nerve and retinal vasculature appear normal.

In the macular region of the right eye there are dark brown lesions involving the sensory retina. The lesions are round and wedge-shaped. One of the lesions appears to be directly in the fovea.

The left macular region and retinal vasculature appear normal. The macular ring reflex appears normal.

During the laminar phase of the fluorescein angiogram, there appears to be a normal choroidal filling pattern. There does not appear to be any abnormal hypo- or hyperfluorescent change in the posterior pole.

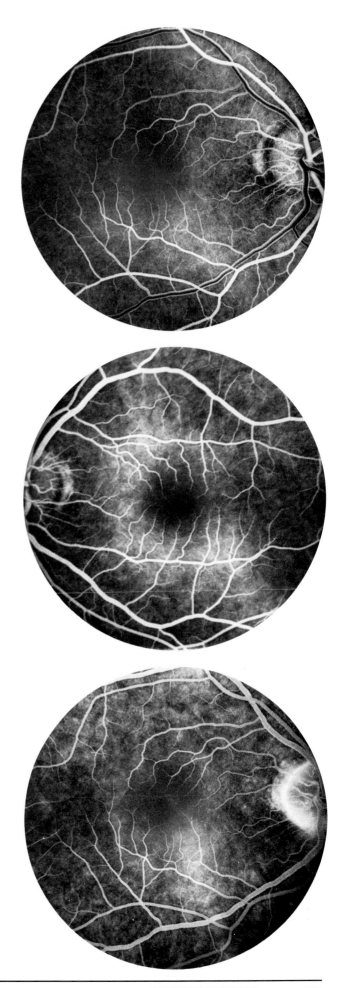

Later in the angiogram, there is no abnormal fluorescent pattern, either at the level of the retinal pigment epithelium or involving the retinal vasculature of the left eye.

The late angiogram shows no abnormal fluorescein pattern. The typical late, mottled fluorescein appearance of the choroid can be seen.

AUTHOR'S NOTE

This 21-year-old white female complained of a dimness of vision in the right eye. A positive history for taking oral contraceptives was obtained. This change can be either unilateral or bilateral.

Macular Neuroretinitis
(bilateral)

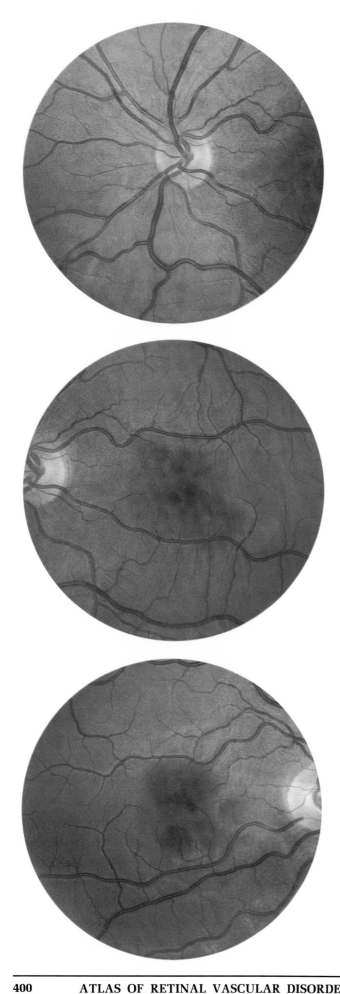

The left optic nerve and major retinal vasculature appear normal.

In the macular region, brownish lesions appear to be present involving the deeper layers of the sensory retina. The retinal vasculature is entirely normal.

In the right macular region, the brownish, round lesions are apparent. No other abnormalities can be seen.

During the laminar phase of the fluorescein angiogram, the choroidal flush in the macular region and filling of the choriocapillaris appear normal. There is no abnormal fluorescent pattern seen.

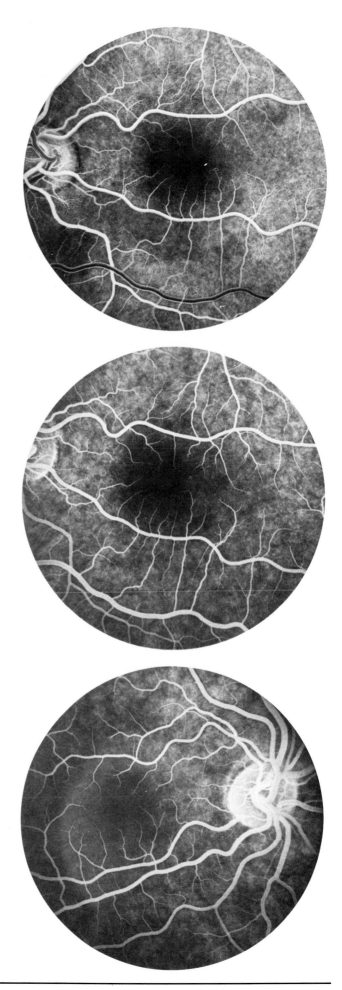

Later in the angiogram, no significant abnormalities can be seen, either at the level of the retinal vasculature or deep to the sensory retina.

The right eye appears entirely normal in the later frames of the fluorescein angiogram.

AUTHOR'S NOTE

This 23-year-old white female has been diagnosed as having macular neuroretinitis. The patient has a history of taking birth control pills. These patients typically show clinical macular changes but normal fluorescein angiography. Therefore, the question arises that perhaps there has been some thinning of the sensory retina in localized areas, making the brown pigment epithelium more apparent. It is also conceivable that there may be some alteration in the xanthophyll pigment, because these changes are well localized to the macular region. To this point in time, there is no histopathology on these cases. The vision is usually reasonably good, but very sensitive visual fields can detect scotomata.

Unilateral Intraretinal Hemorrhages (etiology unknown)

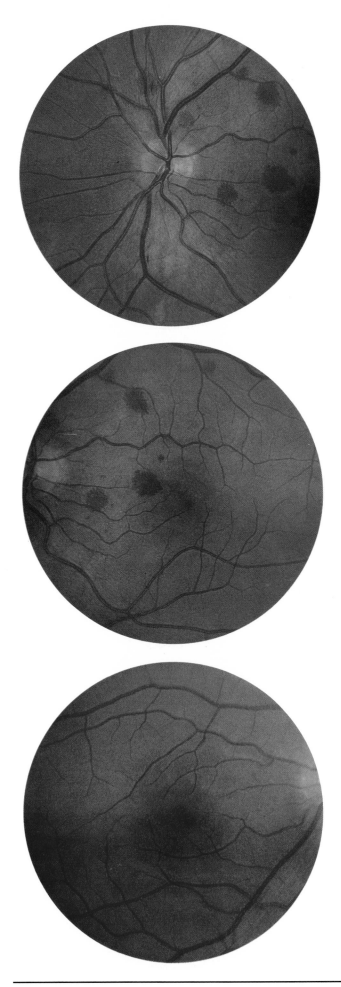

The left optic nerve appears normal. The retinal vasculature shows no significant abnormality. Superior and temporal to the optic nerve are multiple, round, intraretinal blotch hemorrhages. Inferior to the optic nerve is a linear splinter hemorrhage.

The left posterior pole shows the multiple intraretinal blotch and dot hemorrhages. There is some very slight hypopigmentation of the pigment epithelium in the perifoveal region.

The right macula and retinal vasculature appear normal.

During the early laminar phase of the angiogram, there is blockage of the background choroidal fluorescence by the intraretinal hemorrhages. There appear to be a few pinpoint areas of hyperfluorescence in the vicinity of the macula involving the more temporal retina.

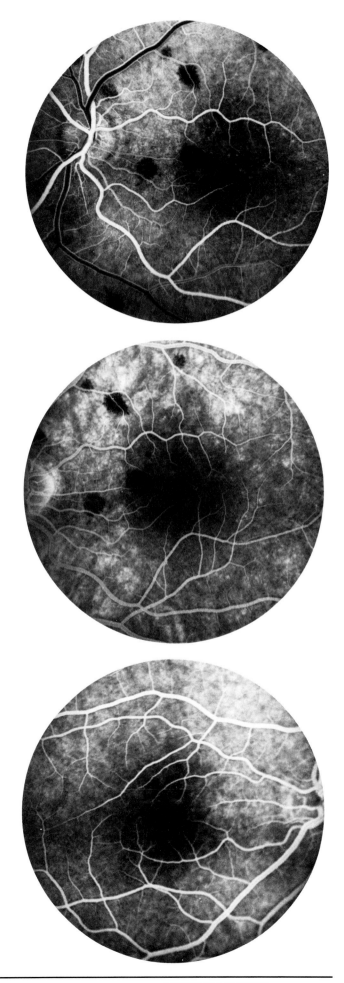

Later in the angiogram, there is continued blockage of the background choroidal fluorescence by the intraretinal hemorrhages. The retinal vasculature appears normal.

The fluorescein pattern of the right eye at the level of the pigment epithelium, choroid, and retinal vasculature appears normal.

AUTHOR'S NOTE

This is a case of an 18-year-old white female who was found to have these intraretinal hemorrhages on a routine examination for glasses. Medical work-up, looking particularly for a hematologic or collagen vascular disorder, was negative. The only possible significant history was the fact that the patient takes birth control pills and also exercises strenuously.

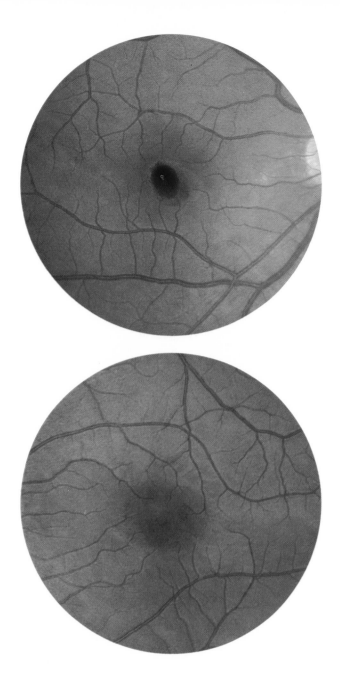

Spontaneous Macular Hemorrhage (etiology unknown)

In the posterior pole of the right eye there is a round, intraretinal hemorrhage which involves the center of the macula. The retinal vasculature appears to be entirely normal.

The macular region and retinal vasculature of the left eye appear normal.

During the laminar phase of the fluorescein angiogram, there is a normal choroidal filling pattern. There is increased blockage of the background choroidal fluorescence by the hemorrhage in the macula.

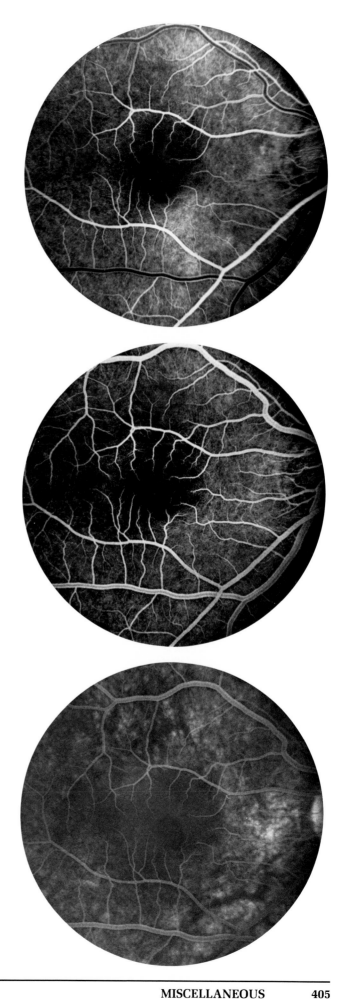

Later in the angiogram, the blockage of the background fluorescence persists in the macula from the intraretinal hemorrhage. No definite vascular abnormality can be seen.

The late angiogram of the right eye shows the typical mottled appearance of the fluorescein within the choroidal vasculature and extravascular space. The hemorrhage continues to block the background choroidal fluorescence. There is no abnormal fluorescence surrounding the hemorrhage or deep to the hemorrhage.

AUTHOR'S NOTE

This is a case of a 26-year-old white male who noticed a sudden drop of vision in his right eye. No cause for the spontaneous macular hemorrhage could be found.

Reader's Notes

General Bibliography

Balantyne AJ, Michaelson IC: *Textbook of the Fundus of the Eye,* ed 2. Baltimore, Williams & Wilkins, 1970.

Duke-Elder S: *System of Ophthalmology,* vol X: *Diseases of the Retina.* St Louis, CV Mosby, 1967.

Fine BS, Yanoff M: *Ocular Histology; A Text and Atlas.* New York, Harper & Row, 1972.

Fine SL, Patz A: *Sights and Sounds in Ophthalmology: Diabetic Retinopathy.* St Louis, CV Mosby, 1980.

Fine SL, Patz A, Orth DH: *Sights and Sounds in Ophthalmology: Retinal Vascular Disorders.* St Louis, CV Mosby, 1976.

Gass JDM: *Stereoscopic Atlas of Macular Diseases.* St Louis, CV Mosby, 1970.

Goldberg MF, Fine SL: *Symposium on the Treatment of Diabetic Retinopathy.* Washington DC, United States Public Health Service, Publication No 1890, 1969.

Hogan MJ, Alvarado JA, Weddell JE: *Histology of the Human Eye; An Atlas and Textbook.* Philadelphia, WB Saunders, 1971.

Hogan JM, Zimmerman LE: *Ophthalmic Pathology,* ed 2. Philadelphia, WB Saunders, 1962.

Krill A: *Hereditary Retinal and Choroidal Diseases,* vol I: *Evaluation.* New York, Harper & Row, 1972.

Krill A: *Hereditary Retinal and Choroidal Diseases,* vol II: *Clinical Characteristics.* Hagerstown, MD, Harper & Row, 1977.

Larsen HW: *The Ocular Fundus.* Philadelphia, WB Saunders, 1976.

L'Esperance FA Jr: *Current Diagnosis and Management of Chorioretinal Diseases.* St Louis, CV Mosby, 1977.

Meyer-Schwickerath G: *Light Coagulation.* St Louis, CV Mosby, 1960.

Nover A: *The Ocular Fundus.* Philadelphia, Lea and Febiger, 1966.

Patz A, Fine SL: *International Ophthalmology Clinic—Interpretation of the Fundus Fluorescein Angiogram.* Boston, Little, Brown, 1977.

Patz A, Fine SL, Orth DH: *Sights and Sounds in Ophthalmology: Diseases of the Macula.* St Louis, CV Mosby, 1976.

Polyak SL: *The Retina.* Chicago, University of Chicago Press,1941.

Polyak SL: *The Vertebrate Visual System.* Chicago, University of Chicago Press, 1957.

Rosen ES: *Fluorescein Photography of the Eye.* London, Appleton-Century-Crofts, 1969.

Schatz H, Burton C, Yannuzzi LA, et al: *Interpretation of Fundus Fluorescein Angiography.* St Louis, CV Mosby, 1978.

Shikano S, Shimizu K: *Atlas of Fluorescein Fundus Angiography.* Tokyo, Ijaku Shoin, 1968.

Wessing A: *Fluorescein Angiography of the Retina.* St Louis, CV Mosby, 1969.

Wise GN, Dollery CT, Henkind P: *The Retinal Circulation.*New York, Harper & Row, 1971.

Yannuzzi LA, Gitter KA, Schatz H: *The Macula—A Comprehensive Text and Atlas.* Baltimore, Williams & Wilkins, 1979.

Index

Page numbers in *italics* denote figures; those followed by "t" or "f" denote tables or footnotes, respectively.